Third Edition

HEALTH PROMOTION *in* NURSING PRACTICE

Third Edition

HEALTH PROMOTION *in* NURSING PRACTICE

Nola J. Pender, RN, PhD, FAAN
Professor and Associate Dean for Academic Affairs and Research
The University of Michigan
School of Nursing
Ann Arbor, Michigan

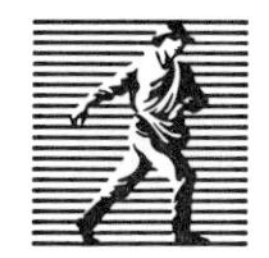

Appleton & Lange
Stamford, Connecticut

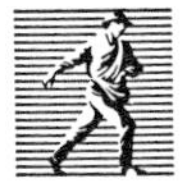

97 98 99 00 / 10 9 8 7 6 5 4 3

Prentice Hall International (UK) Limited, *London*
Prentice Hall of Australia Pty. Limited, *Sydney*
Prentice Hall Canada, Inc., *Toronto*
Prentice Hall Hispanoamericana, S.A., *Mexico*
Prentice Hall of India Private Limited, *New Delhi*
Prentice Hall of Japan, Inc., *Tokyo*
Simon and Schuster Asia Pte., Ltd., *Singapore*
Editora Prentice Hall do Brasil Ltda., *Rio de Janeiro*
Prentice Hall, *Upper Saddle River, New Jersey*

ISBN 0-8385-3659-X

Editor-in-Chief: Sally J. Barhydt
Production Editor: Sondra Greenfield
Production Service: Spectrum Publisher Services, Inc.
Designer: Mary Skudlarek

PRINTED IN THE UNITED STATES OF AMERICA

To Al, my husband and companion in the quest for health, whose support and love are always there for me.

To Brent, my son, and to Andrea and Patrick, my daughter and son-in-law, for whom I wish a happy and healthy life.

To Eileen, my mother and lifelong supporter, and to my father, Frank, who has departed but always believed I could accomplish anything.

Contents

Preface

The scholarly work that I began in the mid-1970s was the start of a knowledge-seeking adventure in a virtually unexplored field—health-promoting behavior. My work predated national and global attention to setting health promotion objectives for the nation that occurred in the mid-1980s and 1990s. It has been exciting to see disease prevention and health promotion move to the forefront of health care policy in the United States during the last quarter of the twentieth century. However, much remains to be accomplished, including the integration of health promotion and disease prevention services into the public and private health care payment systems of the United States. Health care is changing, but it must be further redesigned to provide widespread access to health promotion programs and services for individuals, families, and communities in an increasingly diverse population.

I remember with a smile the nursing leader who told me that health promotion was only a fad and that I was wasting my time conducting research on it. Of course, that leader has been proven completely wrong. Health promotion is here to stay. As an area of inquiry, health promotion is attracting the interests and research efforts of multiple scholars in many fields, all of whom will contribute to a greater understanding among health professionals and consumers of what optimum health is and how it can be attained. Nursing scientists have a myriad of unique and rich opportunities to continue to build the scientific basis for the delivery of quality health promotion care.

The health promotion discoveries of today will be used in a very different health care system of the future—a system in which health care providers and consumers will truly be partners in health care. Instead of consumers coming to health care, health care will come to consumers. Health care will continue to shift to the community and will be increasingly offered in schools, corporations, community health centers, and private homes. Nursing as a profession needs to "spread its wings" and model new systems for primary health care delivery that are focused on promoting health and preventing disease. Now is the time to partner with consumer groups in the community and be innovative and responsive in redesigning health care to meet their needs.

In light of the rapidly changing milieu in health care and the emergence of new opportunities for nurses to collaborate with physicians and other health professionals to provide quality prevention and health promotion services, the purpose of the third edition of this book is fourfold: (1) to provide an overview of major health behavior models and theories developed to date that can guide health promotion interventions; (2) to describe specific strategies and tools that can be used by nursing students and nurses in practice settings for providing health promotive care; (3) to spark the creative energies of nurses everywhere to develop new patient-focused health care systems that meet the health promotion and disease prevention needs of our citizens, particularly the most vulnerable; and (4) to foster critical thinking about what the directions for health promotion research and theory development should be. If I accomplish these objectives in some measure, all the hours of thinking, reading, and writing that went into the preparation of this book will be worthwhile.

The content of the book is organized into five sections. In Part I, various definitions of health are discussed, a number of models from public health, psychology, and nursing relevant to health behavior are presented, and in Chapter 3 the revised health promotion model and related research is described. In Part II, the diversity of health care settings for health promotion are examined. In addition, I discuss strategies for supporting client empowerment and promoting competencies in self-care. Part III presents the critical activities to be completed during the decision-making phase and planning phase of health promotion, which includes assessing health, health beliefs, health behaviors, and most important, developing a health protection and health promotion plan for individuals and for families. In Part IV, interventions for promoting healthy behaviors in relation to exercise, nutrition, stress management, and building social support are described. Finally, in Part V, approaches for promoting a healthier society are critically analyzed.

Throughout this book, as a stimulus for readers to think about the critical nursing research that needs to be conducted to further develop the fields of health promotion and protection, directions for future research are identified at the ends of the chapters.

The term *client* rather than *patient* is used in this third edition to denote individuals, families, groups, and communities who are the recipients of health promotion and prevention services. Health and wellness are used as interchangeable terms.

Appreciation is extended to Sally J. Barhydt, Editor-in-Chief, Nursing, for her prompting me to begin the third edition and her assistance throughout preparation of the book. I am deeply indebted to JoAnn Opstad, who, after the publication of my second edition, spent many hours entering the text of all chapters onto computer files. Her work made preparation of the third edition optimally efficient. The superb work of Becky Ward, BSN, RN, my assistant at the University of Michigan, must be acknowledged. Becky worked with lightning speed to ensure that I had what I needed almost immediately after it was requested. Appreciation is extended to Betty Gadberry and Connie Mason, who keep my life organized so I can write. I also want to thank my nursing colleagues who worked with me at Northern Illinois University in the Health Promotion Research Program and my colleagues at the University of Michigan who make health promotion research at worksites and schools come alive through their exciting research and practice initiatives. Special thanks go to my husband, Al, for being the best coach and supporter I could ever have. He fully supported my writing efforts even when it meant time spent apart from him. He cheered me on and encouraged me. For this, I will always be grateful. My heartfelt appreciation to my son, Brent, and daughter and son-in-law, Andrea and Patrick, who frequently inquired about how the book was coming. I express my deepest appreciation to the above individuals who made the third edition of this book possible.

Nola J. Pender

Third Edition

HEALTH PROMOTION *in* NURSING PRACTICE

Introduction

Health Promotion and Disease Prevention: The Challenge of the 21st Century

A new era in health care is before us in the United States and in the world community, an era in which the promotion of health and prevention of disease will be "front and center" on the health care agenda. This evolution in health care is already in progress and will continue to unfold in the 21st century. No longer will a reactive stance focused exclusively on the treatment of disease dominate the health care system. The challenge of the 21st century will be to provide access to knowledge and services that promote health and prevent disease for all segments of an increasingly diverse world population. This must be accomplished in an environment of economic constraints requiring that the resources spent on health care be balanced with other resource demands.

According to the World Health Organization (WHO), health promotion includes encouraging healthy lifestyles, creating supportive environments for health, strengthening community action, reorienting health services, and building healthy public policy. Health promotion must be geared not only to individuals, but to families and the communities in which they live. Healthy public policy must facilitate and support changes in health behavior norms on a national and international scale.[1]

As opportunities for improving the quality of care and achieving cost savings through primary health care unfold in North America, public support is growing for coverage of health-promotion and illness-prevention services by third-party payors. Increasingly, studies are being undertaken to determine how provision of preventive services affects health care costs within a rapidly evolving managed care environment. To address concerns of policy makers that preventive care may actually increase health care costs, Burton and colleagues[2] examined 2 years of Medicare claims in which preventive visits were included as benefits for over 4000 Medicare recipients. The provision of prevention benefits did not have any negative cost impact. Further, positive health outcomes were demonstrated. The federal government and private insurers should continue to evaluate the impact of providing an array of prevention and health promotion services to individuals and families including the millions of citizens in the United States who are currently uninsured or underinsured.[3]

Public demand is escalating for a health care system that will not only augment longevity but will provide all citizens with the health information needed to extend their productive years and enhance the quality of their lives. In the midst of the information revolution that Toffler and Toffler so aptly describe in their book, *Creating a New Civilization: The Politics of the Third Wave,*[4] electronic media offer unprecedented opportunities to provide health-related information to the public. Innovative use of interactive computer technology and interactive television through worldwide networks is enabling health professionals and consumers to collaborate as never before in the pursuit of health care tailored to the special needs of diverse populations. Health systems can literally "reach around the world." Communication networks provide open access to the latest health knowledge and will increasingly become a national and international resource for informed health care decision making by both providers and consumers.

TOWARD A GLOBAL HEALTH AGENDA

In 1978, at Alma-Ata, Kazakhstan, the nations of the world jointly expressed the urgent need for access to primary health care that would protect and promote the health of the people of the world to enable them to lead socially and economically productive lives. In 1988 at Riga, Latvia, reflections on the progress made since Alma-Ata revealed persistence of gaps in health care, with particular threats to the health of infants, children, and women of childbearing age. Strategies suggested to achieve health for all by the year 2000 included: (1) empowering people by providing information and decision-making opportunities; (2) strengthening local systems of primary health care; (3) improving education and training programs in health promotion and prevention for health professionals; (4) applying science and technology to critical health problems; (5) using new approaches to health problems that have resisted solution; (6) providing special assistance to the least developed countries; and (7) establishing a process for examination of the long-term challenges that must be addressed beyond the year 2000 in achieving health for all.[5]

In the next century, the health-promoting and health-damaging features of social policies, organizations, and environments will receive increased attention. As early as the mid-1980s, when WHO articulated its global commitment to health promotion as a process enabling people to make healthy personal choices within a context of social responsibility for health, the organization emphasized the necessity of going beyond the education of individuals to include organizational changes, community development, and legislation.[6] This broader approach to health promotion is well illustrated by the Healthy Cities Project initiated in 1984 by WHO in Europe. The project stresses a municipal approach to health promotion through extensive community participation, intersectoral cooperation, and the implementation of comprehensive city plans for health promotion. The target end points to be evaluated are not only morbidity and mortality but prevalence of health-promoting behaviors, quality of the physical and social environment, and extent of community empowerment and action.[7] At least 85 cities throughout the world have joined the Healthy Cities Project. These projects focus on health as a central concern to be addressed in political, economic, and social decisions.

A progressive step toward international collaboration among nurses to enhance health promotion and illness prevention services for the world population was the establishment in 1987 of WHO Collaborating Centers for Nursing Development in Primary Health Care. Nurses from centers throughout the world meet regularly to: share information about innovative models of primary health care delivery, plan for computer systems to track global nursing needs, engage in strategic planning for global health care, and design curricula to prepare nurses for delivery of primary health care, including health-promotion and disease-prevention services to the world population. Nurses can play a pivotal role throughout the world in mobilizing forces for change in individual, family, and organizational health behaviors. Thus, the development of nurses for leadership in health promotion is an international priority.[8]

NATIONAL PROGRESS TOWARD HEALTH

In the United States, it is estimated that unhealthy lifestyles are responsible for 54% of the years of life lost prior to age 65, environment for 22%, and heredity for 16%.[9] This is a powerful message that unless the health care system is significantly changed to influence lifestyles and environments, the nation's health profile will continue to deteriorate. What have we done as a nation to meet this challenge? A reflection on our past may be informative at this point.

In 1979, the report *Healthy People: The Surgeon General's Report on Health Promotion and Disease Prevention* introduced a set of broad national goals for improving the health of Americans by 1990.[10] In 1980, a companion document, *Health Promotion—Disease Prevention: Objectives for the Nation,* was published and identified 226 specific health goals in three major areas: health promotion, health protection, and preventive health services.[11] In 1986, a midcourse review of progress toward the objectives indicated that 48% of the health objectives had been or would be achieved by 1990, 26% were unlikely to be achieved, and inadequate data existed to measure the achievement of 26%.[12] The greatest gains were made in the areas of control of high blood pressure, injury prevention, smoking reduction, immunization, and dental health. Death rates for both heart attacks and strokes decreased. Less progress was made in the areas of physical fitness, adolescent pregnancy, and sexually transmitted diseases. Further, few dollars flowed into national prevention and promotion efforts, while costs for illness care continued to escalate.

Because the 1990 objectives were perceived as effective in drawing the nation's attention to the potential of disease prevention and health promotion not only to increase longevity but to improve the quality of lives, in 1987 the effort was begun to develop objectives for the year 2000. In 1990, *Healthy People 2000: National Health Promotion and Disease Prevention Objectives* was published. It identified three broad goals: increase the span of healthy life for Americans, reduce health disparities among Americans, and achieve access to preventive services for all Americans. The plan organizes the 22 priorities for action into the categories of health promotion, health protection, preventive services, and surveillance and data systems.[13] A definition of each category as well as the category-specific priorities are as follows:

Health promotion comprises strategies related to individual lifestyle and personal choices made in a social context that have a powerful influence over one's own health prospects:

1. Physical activity and fitness
2. Nutrition
3. Tobacco
4. Alcohol and other drugs
5. Family planning
6. Mental health and mental disorders
7. Violent and abusive behavior
8. Educational and community-based programs

Health protection includes strategies related to environmental or regulatory measures that confer protection on large population groups:

9. Unintentional injuries
10. Occupational safety and health
11. Environmental health
12. Food and drug safety
13. Oral health

Preventive services consist of strategies that include counseling, screening, immunization, or chemoprophylactic interventions for individuals in clinical settings

14. Maternal and infant health
15. Heart disease and stroke
16. Cancer
17. Diabetes and chronic disabling conditions
18. HIV infection
19. Sexually transmitted diseases
20. Immunization and infectious diseases
21. Clinical preventive services

Surveillance and data systems

22. Surveillance and data systems

The objectives were also organized by developmental stage to indicate those most appropriate for children, adolescents and young adults, middle-aged adults, and older adults. In addition, specific attention was given to the needs of special populations, particularly those who are disadvantaged as a result of low socioeconomic status or disabilities.

The Centers for Disease Control and Prevention have continued since 1990 to work with state and local governments to stimulate use of the national objectives as their framework for prevention and health promotion activities. Special attention is also being devoted to working with private-sector and voluntary organizations to enlist their assistance in realization of the objectives by 2000. Additional comprehensive information tracking systems have been put in place to enable the federal government to track progress toward most of the objectives. Thus, a better data base will exist to track progress and provide a baseline for the national health objectives for the year 2010.

National, state, and local initiatives in prevention and health promotion within both the public and private sectors are increasing rapidly. As the year 2000 approaches, informed individuals and families, activated communities, and concerned health professionals working together can markedly change our nation's and the world's health profiles by improving health throughout the life cycle, extending disability-free years, and enhancing the expression of human potential in all age groups.

• HEALTH PROMOTION AND HEALTH PROTECTION: IS THERE A DIFFERENCE?

The most important difference between health promotion and health protection or illness prevention is in the underlying motivation for the behavior on the part of individuals and aggregates. Health promotion is motivated by the desire to increase well-being and actualize human health potential. Health protection is motivated by a desire to actively avoid illness, detect it early, or maintain functioning within the constraints of illness. Parse describes prevention or health protection as taking action to thwart disease processes—a problem-oriented approach in which emphasis is placed on finding ways to modify the environment, behavior, and bodily defenses so that disease processes are eliminated, slowed, or changed. In contrast, health promotion means to take action to enhance the quality of the flow of life in the human–environment interactive process.[14]

The *stabilizing tendency* underlying health protection is evident in the functioning of homeokinetic mechanisms and is directed toward maintaining balance and equilibrium. The stabilizing tendency is responsible for protective maneuvers, primarily maintaining the internal and external environments within a range compatible with continuing existence. The central question is, What are the conditions that lead to avoidance of disease and injury? The *actualizing tendency* underlying health promotion increases states of positive tension in order to promote change and growth. This increase in tension is often experienced as challenge and facilitates behaviors expressive of human potential. The important question is, What are the conditions that lead to optimal health?

Probably the purest form of motivation for health promotion exists in childhood through young adulthood when energy, vitality, and vigor are important to self-esteem and peer acceptance but the threat of chronic illness seems remote. Youth may engage in health behaviors for the pure pleasure of doing so or for the improvement of physical appearance and attractiveness to others. In the adult years, when human vulnerabilities become more apparent, the two motivations for health behavior usually coexist. For example, an older adult may be motivated to jog in order to improve stamina and energy (health promotion) but also to avoid cardiovascular disease (health protection). Regulatory measures for clean air may be passed to prevent exposure to asbestos as a cancer risk factor (health protection) but also to improve the overall quality of the environment (health promotion). Lester Breslow has described the distinction between health promotion and illness prevention in the following way: "In some important respects, health promotion and disease prevention are two sides of the same coin. Many of the same actions—for example, obtaining adequate exercise and appropriate nutrition—that are aimed at accomplishing one also achieve the other. To the extent that such measures are directed against a particular disease, such as cessation of smoking to minimize the risk of lung cancer, they may be regarded as disease prevention. To the extent that the same measures are aimed at advancing health generally, for example, preserving optimum respiratory and cardiovascular systems, they may be regarded as health promotion."[15]

The reader should note three important theoretical differences between health promotion and health protection. First, health promotion is not illness- or injury-specific; health protection is. Second, health promotion is "approach" motivated, whereas health protection is "avoidance" motivated. Third, health promotion seeks to expand positive potential for health, while health protection seeks to thwart the occurrence of insults to health and well-being. Brubaker[16] has argued that even the dictionary definitions support the differentiation between health promotion and illness prevention. To "prevent" is to keep from occurring, whereas to "promote" is to help or encourage to exist or flourish.

When interventions are being tailored to particular clients, a distinction between the *motivational dynamics* of health promotion and health protection is likely to be helpful. In reality, health promotion and health protection are complementary processes. Both are critical to the quality of life at all developmental stages. More attention will be given to these two concepts throughout the rest of the book.

THE MULTIDIMENSIONAL NATURE OF HEALTH PROMOTION

The health of individuals and families is affected markedly by the community, environment, and society in which they live. The context for living can either sustain and expand health potential or inhibit the emergence of health and well-being. It is important that nurses appreciate and consider the complexity of health promotion endeavors. Dunn has provided the following schema for health promotion efforts[17]:

- Individual wellness
- Family wellness
- Community wellness
- Environmental wellness
- Societal wellness

Individual Wellness

Individuals play a critical role in the determination of their own health status, since self-care represents the dominant mode of health care in our society. Many decisions are made by individuals daily that shape their lifestyle and social and physical environments. Health promotion at the individual level improves personal decision making and health practices. Throughout this book, the frame of reference for individual prevention and health-promotion activities will be the total life span from childhood to the older adult years. Every developmental stage must be considered in formulating national health policy and programs if the quality of life for people of all ages is to be significantly enhanced through health promotion efforts.

Family Wellness

Although the family plays a critical role in the development of health beliefs and health behaviors, there is very little research on the health-promoting role of the family. Almost all individuals can identify with a family group in which members influence one another's ideas and actions. Each family has a characteristic value, role, and power structure as well as unique communication patterns. In addition, families fulfill affective, socialization, health care, and coping functions in varying ways.[18] Parenting styles and family environments can encourage healthy or unhealthy behaviors that may persist throughout the life span. Much more attention should be given to the development of strategies for promoting family wellness.

Community Wellness

According to Dunn, community wellness is achieved by a multiplicity of actions that improve the conditions of family and community life.[17] A number of benefits of community-based health promotion programs can be identified:

1. Enhanced opportunities for information exchange and social support among members of the target population
2. Reduced unit cost of programming because large groups, rather than individuals, receive health promotion services
3. Availability of interorganizational networks that can facilitate and coordinate health promotion efforts
4. Potential for widespread change in social norms regarding health and health behavior
5. Coordinated rather than piecemeal approach to the promotion of health in large populations
6. Access to a broad array of media for dissemination of health information
7. Availability of aggregate indices to be used for tracking the health status of the population
8. Use of the talents and resources of community residents resulting in a sense of commitment to health promotion programming

Community programming for prevention and health promotion can result in rapid dissemination of health information and in marked changes in cultural norms relevant to health and health behavior. The United States is faced with the challenge of moving from heavy reliance on institution-centered health services to greater use of community-based health services. It is time to restructure the health care system from a predominant focus on illness and cure to an orientation toward wellness and care, with services delivered in familiar and convenient community sites such as schools, workplaces, and homes.[19]

Environmental Wellness

The level of environmental wellness affects the extent to which individuals, families, and communities can achieve their optimum potential. "Environment" is a comprehensive term meaning the physical, interpersonal, and economic circumstances in which we live. The quality of the environment is dependent on the absence of toxic substances, the availability of aesthetic or restorative experiences, and the accessibility of human and economic resources needed for healthful and productive living. Socioeconomic conditions such as unemployment, poverty, crime, prejudice, and isolation can have adverse effects on health. Environmental wellness is manifest in harmony and balance between human beings and their surroundings.

Societal Wellness

The wellness of a society depends largely on the passage of laws and the establishment through social action of policies that protect the health and welfare of all age groups. A well society is one in which all members have a standard of living and way of life that allows them to meet basic human needs and engage in activities that express their human potential. Essential to a well society is the collective citizenry's willingness to accept responsibility for health and to foster a level of education commensurate with informed decision making. A well society recognizes the dignity of all human beings, adopts policies to maintain that dignity, and avoids policies and programs that are demeaning or belittling to its members. A well society empowers its members to use their talents throughout the life span without premature retirement or relegation to a status of less value with age. Societal wellness requires involvement of a number of sectors, including those of education, food production, housing, and employment as well as the health sector, in joint efforts to improve the nation's health profile. Prerequisites for a well society include:

1. A belief that disease and illness are not inevitable consequences of human existence
2. A vision for the population beyond that of immediate survival
3. Awareness of the close relationship between individual, family, and community health assets and the well-being and productivity of a society
4. Acceptance of high-level wellness as the goal of the society

Societal wellness provides the framework in which individual, family, community, and environmental wellness can exist. Decisions made at all levels of bureaucracy in the public and private sectors affect the range of health-promoting options available.

Coordinated interventions at all five levels are likely to be the most cost-efficient and effective approach to health promotion. Such interventions are complex but synergistic, optimizing ultimate chances of success.

• THE CONTRIBUTION OF NURSES TO THE PREVENTION AND HEALTH-PROMOTION TEAM

Nurses, because of their biopsychosocial expertise and frequent, continuing contact with clients, have the unique opportunity of providing global leadership to health professionals in the promotion of better health for the world community. Nurses should serve as role models of health-promoting lifestyles and as leaders to activate communities for health promotion. Nurses, as the largest single group of health care providers, will continue to play a vital role in making health promotion and illness prevention reimburseable services and in opening access to such services for all population groups, including those most underserved and vulnerable to illness. Nurses must continue to work to redistribute health care resources so that quality health-promotion and illness-prevention services are available to all. Therein lies the excitement and challenge of being a nurse today as the 20th century draws to a close and the 21st century begins.

REFERENCES

1. Turner J. World Health Organization-charter for health promotion. *Lancet.* 1986;2:1407.
2. Burton LC, Steinwachs DM, German PS, et al. Preventive services for the elderly: would coverage affect utilization and costs under Medicare? *Am J Public Health.* 1995;85:387–391.
3. National Center for Health Services Research and Health Care Technology Assessment. *National Medical Expenditure Survey-A Profile of Uninsured Americans.* Washington, DC: Public Health Service; 1989. US Dept of Health and Human Services 89–3443.
4. Toffler A, Toffler H. *Creating a New Civilization: The Politics of the Third Wave.* Atlanta, Ga: Turner Publishing, Inc; 1995.
5. World Health Organization. *From Alma-Ata to the Year 2000: Reflections at Midpoint.* Geneva, Switzerland: WHO; 1988.
6. *Report of the Working Group on Concepts and Principles of Health Promotion.* Copenhagen, Denmark: WHO; 1984.
7. Ashton J, Grey P, Barnard K. Healthy cities: WHO's new public health initiative. *Health Prom.* 1986;1:319–324.
8. International Council of Nurses. *Nursing in Primary Health Care: Ten Years after Alma-Ata and Perspectives for the Future.* Geneva, Switzerland: ICN & WHO; 1989.
9. Powell KE, Spain KG, Christenson GM, et al. The status of the 1990 objectives for physical fitness and exercise. *Public Health Rep.* 1986;101:19.
10. *Healthy People: The Surgeon General's Report on Health Promotion and Disease Prevention.* Washington, DC: US Public Health Service; 1979. US Dept of Health, Education, and Welfare publication PHS 79-55071.
11. *Promoting Health/Preventing Disease: Objectives for the Nation.* Washington, DC: US Public Health Service; 1980.
12. *The 1990 Health Objectives for the Nation: A Midcourse Review.* Washington, DC: US Public Health Service; 1986.
13. *Healthy People 2000: National Health Promotion and Disease Prevention Objectives.* Washington, DC: US Public Health Service; 1990.
14. Parse R. Promotion and prevention: two distinct cosmologies. *Nurs Sci Q.* 1990;3(3):101.
15. Breslow L. A health promotion primer for the 1990s. *Health Aff (Millwood).* 1990;9(2):6–21.
16. Brubaker BH. Health promotion: a linguistic analysis. *Adv Nurs Sci.* 1983;5(3):1–14.
17. Dunn HL. *High-level wellness.* Arlington, Va: RW Beatty Co., 1973.
18. Friedman MM. *Family nursing: theory and assessment.* New York, NY: Appleton-Century-Crofts; 1981.
19. American Nurses' Association. *Nursing's Agenda for Health Care Reform.* Kansas City, Mo: ANA Publications; 1991.

I

PART ONE

The Human Quest for Health

1

Toward a Definition of Health

Health, person, environment, and nursing constitute the commonly accepted metaparadigm of the discipline of nursing.[1] Although it is the frequently articulated goal of nursing, health still remains a concept that is elusive and operationally ill-defined. This elusiveness may result from the increasingly diverse social values and norms that shape conceptualizations of health in pluralistic societies. What many health professionals once assumed was a universally accepted definition of health, the absence of diagnosable disease, is actually only one of many views of health held among world populations. All people free of disease are not equally healthy. Furthermore, health can exist without illness, but illness never exists without health as its context.[2]

The emergence of health promotion as the central global strategy for improving health has "pushed the envelope" beyond defining health in traditional medical terms (intrapersonal, biologic process). Instead, health is increasingly being investigated as an expansive and much more interesting phenomenon with biopsychosocial, spiritual, environmental, and cultural dimensions. In the context of a multidimensional model of health,

health benefits can potentially be achieved from positive changes in any of the health dimensions.[3] Such a perspective on health is empowering, as it opens up multiple options for improving health status.

During the course of human development, an expansive definition of health appears to emerge over time. As children mature and move into adolescence, their definition of health becomes more inclusive and more abstract.[4] Millstein and Irwin reported that health definitions of adolescents showed a trend toward greater thematic diversity (physical, mental, social, and emotional health) and less emphasis on the absence of illness with increasing age.[5] Conceptions of health need to be studied qualitatively and quantitatively over the life span to understand developmental variations across genders, races, and cultures.

In a positive model of health, emphasis is placed on strengths, resiliencies, resources, potentials, and capabilities rather than on existing pathology. Despite efforts to make a philosophic and conceptual shift in thinking about health, the nature of health as a positive life process is poorly understood empirically. It is almost impossible to find measures of health that do not focus primarily on mortality or on morbidity-related indices such as dysfunction, disability, or impairment. Thus, what are erroneously called "measures of health" are really "measures of illness." Defining health simply in terms of morbidity (prevalence of illness) or mortality (deaths) is inadequate for the 21st century, when for many people "conditions of life" rather than "pathologic states" compromise health. Life conditions positively or negatively impact health long before morbid states are evident.

In a critical review of health measures used in nursing literature, Reynolds found little support for the holistic and expansive views of health to which nurses claim to subscribe. Instead, nurses, just like other professionals, tended to choose empirical indicators for health that were derived from an illness model.[6] New theoretical formulations and measures of health are critically needed. They should (1) characterize health by the conditions defining its presence rather than its absence, (2) identify a spectrum of health states, and (3) reflect a life-span developmental perspective.

The fundamental mechanisms underlying human health processes have only recently received attention from nurse scientists. Many questions remain to be addressed. How is human health expressed biologically and behaviorally? What are the gender-specific, culture-specific, race-specific expressions of health? Are expressions of health qualitatively different at varying points of development? What is maximum human health potential? What are the interactive conditions between the person and the environment that enhance or deplete health? What are the dimensions critical to assessing the health of families? What dimensions are key to evaluating the health of communities? Generating knowledge relevant to these questions is essential to advance nursing science and provide an empirical base for effective health-promoting and health-protecting interventions.

• HEALTH AS AN EVOLVING CONCEPT

A brief review of the historical development of the concept of health will provide the context for examining definitions of health found in professional literature. The word *health* as it is commonly used did not appear in writing until approximately AD 1000. It is derived from the Old English word *hoelth,* meaning being safe or sound and whole of body.[7(p3)] Historically, physical wholeness was of major importance for acceptance in social groups. Persons suffering from disfiguring diseases, like leprosy, or from congenital malformations were ostracized from society. Not only was there fear of contagion of physically obvious disease, there was also repulsion at the grotesque appearance. Being healthy was construed as natural or in harmony with nature, while being unhealthy was thought of as unnatural or contrary to nature.[8]

The concept of mental health as we know it did not exist until the latter part of the 19th century. Individuals who exhibited unpredictable or hostile behavior were labeled "lunatics" and ostracized in much the same way as were those with disfiguring physical ailments. Being put away with little if any human care was considered their "just due," because mental illness was often ascribed to evil spirits or satanic powers. The visibility of the ill only served as a reminder of personal vulnerability and mortality, aspects of human existence that society wished to ignore.

With the advent of the scientific era and the resultant increase in the rate of medical discoveries, illness came to be regarded with less disgust, and society became concerned about assisting individuals to escape its catastrophic effects. *Health* in this context was defined as "freedom from disease." Because disease could be traced to a specific cause, often microbial, it could be diagnosed. The notion that health was a disease-free state was extremely popular into the first half of the 20th century and was recognized by many as *the* definition of health.[9] Health and illness were viewed as extremes on a continuum; the absence of one indicated the presence of the other. This gave rise to "ruling out disease" to assess health, an approach still prevalent in the medical community today. The underlying erroneous assumption is that a disease-free population is a healthy population.

For several decades, the importance of mental health became obscured in the rapid barrage of medical discoveries for treatment of physical disorders. However, the psychologic trauma resulting from the high-stress situations of combat during World War II enlarged the scope of health as a concept to include consideration of the mental status of the individual. Mental health was manifest in the ability of an individual to withstand the stresses imposed by the environment. When individuals succumbed to the rigors of life around them and could no longer carry out the functions of daily living, they were declared to be mentally ill. Despite efforts to develop a more holistic definition of health, the dichotomy between individuals suffering from physical illness and those suffering from mental illness persisted.

In 1974, the World Health Organization (WHO) proposed a definition of health that emphasized "wholeness" and the positive qualities of health: "Health is a state of complete physical, mental, and social well-being and not merely the absence of disease and infirmity."[10] While this definition enlarged the number of factors that needed to be taken into consideration in assessing health, it was difficult to deduce from it the criteria for recognizing health as a positive human experience. The definition was revolutionary in that it did (1) reflect concern for the individual as a total person rather than the sum of parts; (2) place health in the context of the environment; and (3) equate health with productive and creative living.

The WHO definition called attention to the multidimensionality of health. Based on this definition, Ware[11] has proposed five distinct dimensions as a minimum standard for health measures that claim to be comprehensive: physical health, mental health (emotional and intellectual functioning), social functioning, role functioning, and general perceptions of well-being. Parse[12] has questioned the adequacy of this additive approach in accurately reflecting health as the holistic phenomenon that nurses in practice attempt to influence.

Health is increasingly recognized as a concept that is not only multidimensional but applicable to both individuals and aggregates. In the following sections, definitions of health focusing on the individual, family, and community will be discussed. Defining health for individuals has received more attention in nursing and other health disciplines than defining health for families and communities. This is rapidly changing as scholars recognize the critical place that family and community health play in fostering health for large populations across the globe.

• DEFINITIONS OF HEALTH THAT FOCUS ON INDIVIDUALS

Health as Stability

For individuals, stability-based definitions of health derive primarily from the physiologic concepts of homeostasis and adaptation. Dubos, an early advocate of the stability position, defined health as a state or condition that enables the individual to adapt to the environment. The degree of health experienced is dependent on one's ability to adjust to the various internal and external tensions that one faces. Dubos considered optimum health to be a mirage because man in the real world must face the physical and social forces that are forever changing, frequently unpredictable, and often dangerous. According to Dubos, the nearest approach to high-level health is a physical and mental state free of discomfort and pain that permits one to function effectively within the environment.[13]

Definitions of health based on normality can be described as stability-oriented. Statistical norms for a variety of human functions are already well defined. A major problem with normative definitions of health is that they predict "what could be" based on "what is," leaving little room for incorporating growth, maturation, and evolutionary emergence into a definition of health. A norm represents average or middle-range effectiveness rather than excellence or exceptional effectiveness in human functioning.

Parsons defined health in terms of social norms rather than physiologic norms almost three decades ago. He described health as "the effective performance of valued roles and tasks for which an individual has been socialized."[14] According to Parsons, health status can be determined by application of normative standards of adequacy for present and future role and task performance.

Similar to Parsons' sociologic model of health, Patrick, Bush, and Chen have defined health in terms of functional norms. They define health as: ". . . evidence of socially valued function levels in the performance of activities usual for a person's age and social roles with a minimum probability of change to less valued function levels."[15] The desirability of the immediate function level, as well as the probability that the current condition or state will change to a higher or lower preference function level, must be considered in assessing present health status.

A number of nurse-theorists have proposed definitions of health emphasizing stability. Levine defined health as a state in which there is balance between input and output of energy and in which structural, personal, and social integrity exist.[16]

Johnson, in her behavioral system model, does not explicitly define health. A conception of health that focuses on stability can, however, be inferred from her writings. Health or wellness is balance and stability among the following behavioral systems: attachment or affiliative, dependency, ingestive, eliminative, sexual, aggressive, and achievement. Behavioral system balance and stability is demonstrated by efficient and effective behavior that is purposeful, goal-directed, orderly, and predictable.[17] Neuman has defined health or wellness as a condition in which all subsystems—physiologic, psychologic, and sociocultural—are in balance and in harmony with the whole of man. It is also a state of saturation, of inertness, free of disruptive needs. Disrupting forces or noxious stressors with which individuals cannot cope create disharmony, reducing the level of wellness. In a wellness state, total needs are met and more energy is generated and stored than expended. A strong, flexible line of defense is maintained, providing the individual with considerable resistance to disequilibrium.[18]

Roy also subscribes to a stability definition of health. The central concept in Roy's model is adaptation. Health is a state and process of successful adaptation that promotes being and becoming an integrated whole person. The four adaptive modes through which coping energies are expressed are: physiologic, self-concept, role performance, and interdependence modes. Adaptation promotes integrity. Integrity implies soundness or an unimpaired condition that can lead to completeness and unity. The person in an adapted state is freed from ineffective coping attempts that deplete energy. Available energy can be used to enhance health.[19]

Tripp-Reimer proposed a model for health that is stability-oriented. The health state is conceptualized as two-dimensional: an *etic* dimension (disease-nondisease), which reflects the objective interpretation of health state by a scientifically trained practitioner; and the *emic* dimension (wellness-illness), which represents the subjective perception and experiences of an individual and social group as to health state. The various quadrants of the resultant grid—disease-wellness, disease-illness, nondisease-wellness, and nondisease-illness—indicate either congruence or incongruence between the perspectives of client and practitioner. This definition focuses on normality or homeostasis as medically defined. The model is proposed as particularly useful cross-culturally when perceptions of scientifically trained personnel and clients of differing ethnic background may disagree regarding the concept of health or health status.[20]

Health as Actualization

When health is defined more expansively as actualization of human potential, some scholars have proposed that a different term, *wellness,* be used. The argument has been made that a new term must be employed because the definition of health has been so narrowly constrained historically that attempts to expand it will be futile. Despite this legitimate concern, *health* and *wellness* tend to be used interchangeably throughout current scientific writings and will be used interchangeably in this text also.

Halbert Dunn was one of the early advocates for definitions of health emphasizing actualization. Dunn coined the term *high-level wellness,* which he described as integrated human functioning that is oriented toward maximizing the potential of which the individual is capable. This requires that the individual maintain balance and purposeful direction within the environment where he is functioning.[21] While the definition advanced by Dunn identifies balance as a dimension of health, major emphasis is on the realization of human potential through purposeful activity.

Dunn stated that high-level wellness, or optimum health, involves three components: (1) progress in a forward and upward direction toward a higher potential of functioning, (2) an open-ended and ever-expanding challenge to live at a fuller potential, and (3) progressive integration or maturation of the individual at increasingly higher levels throughout the life cycle.[22] Dunn conceptualized wellness as a direction of progress as well as levels to be reached. Well individuals function at a high level amid a dynamic and constantly changing environment. Individuals need freedom to realize personal uniqueness through creative expression and thereby achieve a high level of wellness. Dunn proposes that high-level wellness can only emerge in a favorable environment. Health, according to Dunn, is not simply a "passive state of freedom from illness in which the individual is at peace with his environment,"[23(p4)] it is an emergent process characteristic of the entire life span.

Bermosk and Porter focus on holism and human evolution in their definition of health: Holistic health involves the ongoing integration of mind, body, and spirit. A person evolves from one level of wholeness to another level of wholeness.[24] They view holistic health as integrated energies of mind, body, spirit, and environment. Integration within the human system is synonymous with healing.

Orem, in developing the self-care theory of nursing, used health and well-being to refer to two different but related human states. She defined health as a state characterized by soundness or wholeness of human structures and bodily and mental functions. Well-being was defined as a state characterized by experiences of contentment, pleasure, and happiness; by spiritual experiences; by movement toward fulfillment of one's self-ideal; and by continuing personalization. According to Orem, personalization is movement toward maturation and achievement of human potential. Engaging in responsible self-care and continuing development of self-care competency are facets of the process of personalization. Individuals can experience well-being even under conditions of adversity, including disorders of human structure and function.[25]

Newman, building on the work of Martha Rogers, defined health as the totality of the life process, which is evolving toward expanded consciousness.[26] This definition emphasizes the actualizing properties of individuals throughout the life span. Four dimensions of health as a concept are identified:

1. Health is a fusion of disease and nondisease.
2. Health is the manifestation of an individual's unique pattern.
3. Health is expansion of consciousness. Time is a measure of consciousness, and movement is a reflection of consciousness.
4. Health encompasses the entire life process, which evolves toward higher and greater frequency of energy exchange.

Key life process phenomena include: consciousness, movement, space, and time. Newman's model of health addresses holistic characteristics of human beings. However, empirical referents for many of the terms used within the model need to be identified to facilitate the testing of hypotheses that can be derived from the model.

Parse, in describing her man-living-health theory of nursing, presents five assumptions about health that essentially define the term from her perspective[27]:

1. Health is an open process of becoming, experienced by mankind.
2. Health is a rhythmically coconstituting process of the man–environment relationship.
3. Health is man's patterns of relating value priorities.
4. Health is an intersubjective process of transcending with the possibles.
5. Health is unitary man's negentropic (toward increasing order, complexity, and heterogeneity) unfolding.

The theory proposed by Parse builds on Martha Rogers' theory of unitary man, as did Newman's model of health. Both represent early attempts to define health in terms of the holistic human as opposed to defining health in terms of humankind's component parts. The emergent nature or actualization potential of the healthy individual and the capacity for open energy exchange with the environment are characteristics of both Newman's and Parse's definitions of health.

Health as Actualization and Stability

The definitions of health presented in this section represent mixed models, that is, the definitions incorporate the themes of stability and actualization.

Wu has described health as a feeling of well-being, a capacity to perform to the best of one's ability, and the flexibility to adapt and adjust to varying situations created by the subsystems of humans or the suprasystems in which they exist.[28] Wu proposed that wellness and illness represent distinct entities, with a repertory of behaviors for each. Within this frame of reference, both wellness and illness can exist simultaneously. Evaluation of both are critical to comprehensive health assessment.

King proposed a definition of health that emphasized both stabilizing and actualizing tendencies. She defined health as: a dynamic state in the life cycle of a person that implies adjustment to stressors in the internal and external environment through optimum use of resources to achieve maximum potential for daily living.[29]

Health that encompasses the whole person relates to the way an individual deals with stressors while functioning within the culture to which he or she was born and to which he or she attempts to conform.[30] King indicates that the idea of polarity between health and illness is outmoded. Instead, health should be viewed as a functional state in the life cycle, with illness defined as interference in the cycle.

Smith[31] offered an exposition and analysis of four distinctive ideas (models) of health, three focused on stability and one on actualization. Each of the models of health is defined below by the extremes on the health-illness continuum that it identifies.

- *Clinical model.* Health extreme: absence of signs or symptoms of disease or disability as identified by medical science; illness extreme: conspicuous presence of these signs or symptoms
- *Role-performance model.* Health extreme: performance of social roles with maximum expected output; illness extreme: failure in performance of roles

- *Adaptive model.* Health extreme: the organism maintains flexible adaptation to the environment, interacts with environment with maximum advantage; illness extreme: alienation of the organism from environment, failure of self-corrective responses
- *Eudaimonistic model.* Health extreme: exuberant well-being; illness extreme: enervation, languishing debility

Smith proposes that each model requires distinct approaches to the client. The nature of practice and the modes of intervention are different, depending on which model is being used as the framework for care.

The following definition of health incorporating both actualizing and stabilizing tendencies has been proposed by the author of this book:

> Health is the actualization of inherent and acquired human potential through goal-directed behavior, competent self-care, and satisfying relationships with others while adjustments are made as needed to maintain structural integrity and harmony with relevant environments.

Based on this definition, a system for classifying human expressions of health is proposed (Table 1–1). The major dimensions of health expression include: affect, attitudes, activity, aspirations, and accomplishments. This system is based on the assumptions that health is a manifestation of person and environment interactional patterns that become increasingly complex throughout the life span.

Health is a holistic experience and only becomes fragmented in the minds of health professionals. An expansive view of health and its dimensions is needed that is positive, holistic, and humanistic. This view of health must be developed by nurse scholars.[2] The proposed classification system for expressions of health can be a building block for empirical investigations. The interrelationships between affective, behavioral, and biological expressions of health offer a fascinating area of research.

• THE NEED FOR AN INTEGRATED VIEW OF HEALTH

The importance of nursing's avoiding a fragmented view of health and espousing an integrated biopsychosocial view of human health phenomena has been described by Shaver.[32] Her rationale for an integrated view is summarized in the following four points.

1. The scope of clinical indicators on which diagnostic decisions can be based will be greater. Indicators could include interpersonal behaviors, social support, socioeconomic status, mood state, cognitive efficiency, symptom complaints, hormone levels, neurotransmitter breakdown products, neurochemical substrates, immunoglobulin status, or any combination of these.
2. Study of human response patterns could determine what combination of indicators is predictive of healthy and unhealthy outcomes.
3. An integrated view enlarges the scope of therapeutic options for treating health problems or responses to health problems.

TABLE 1–1. CLASSIFICATION SYSTEM FOR AFFECTIVE AND BEHAVIORAL EXPRESSIONS OF HEALTH

AFFECT

Serenity	Harmony	Vitality	Sensitivity
Calm	Close to God	Energetic	Aware
Relaxed	Contemplative	Vigorous	Connected
Peaceful	At one with the universe	Zestful	Intimate
Content		Alert	Loving
Comfortable		Fit	Warm
Glowing		Buoyant	
Happy		Exhilarated	
Joyous		Powerful	
Pleasant		Courageous	
Satisfied			

ATTITUDES

Optimism	Relevancy	Competency
Hopeful	Useful	Purposive
Enthusiastic	Contributing	Initiating
Open	Valued	Self-motivating
Reverent	Caring	Self-affirming
Trustful	Committed	Innovative
Resilient	Involved	Masterful
		Challenged

ACTIVITY

Positive Life Patterns	Meaningful Work	Invigorating Play
Eating a healthy diet	Setting realistic goals	Having meaningful hobbies
Exercising regularly	Varying activities	Engaging in satisfying leisure activities
Managing stress	Undertaking challenging tasks	Planning energizing diversions
Obtaining adequate rest	Assuming responsibility for self	
Avoiding harmful substances	Collaborating with coworkers	
Building positive relationships	Receiving intrinsic or extrinsic rewards	
Seeking and using health information		
Monitoring health		
Coping constructively		
Maintaining a health-strengthening environment		

ASPIRATIONS

Self-Actualization	Social Contribution
Growth or emergence	Enhancement of global harmony and interdependence
Personal mastery	Preservation of the environment
Organismic efficiency	

ACCOMPLISHMENTS

Enjoyment	Creativity	Transcendence
Pleasure from daily living	Maximum use of capacities	Freedom
Sense of achievement	Innovative contribution	Expansion of consciousness
		Optimized harmony between individual and environment

4. An integrated approach offers greater potential for targeting therapy and individualizing prescriptions for intervention.

An integrated approach represents a step in the direction of a holistic and positive approach to the definition of health.

A conscious effort on the part of nurse scholars to make expansive definitions of health an empirical reality by developing new measurement tools is critical to the advancement of knowledge about human health potential.[33] Further, measures of health must be appropriate to culturally diverse populations, integrating a number of disciplinary perspectives.[34]

HEALTH AND ILLNESS: DISTINCT ENTITIES OR OPPOSITE ENDS OF A CONTINUUM?

The issue of whether health and illness are separate entities or opposite ends of a continuum has fascinated scientists for some time. Are health and illness quantitatively or qualitatively different?

Theorists presenting health and illness as a continuum usually identify possible reference points such as (1) optimum health, (2) suboptimal health or incipient illness, (3) overt illness and disability, (4) very serious illness or approaching death.[7(p5)] This scale has only one point representing health, whereas three points on the scale represent varying states of illness. Dunn proposed construction of continuua that allow the differentiation of varying levels of health as well as varying levels of illness.[23(p5)]

When health and illness are assumed to represent a single continuum, it is difficult to discuss healthy aspects of the ill individual. The presence of illness ascribes the "sick role," and the individual is expected to direct all energies toward finding the cause of the illness and engaging in behaviors that will result in a return to health as soon as possible.

Manifestations of health in the presence of illness have lead some theorists to propose separate but parallel continuua for health and illness. Sorochan commented that everyone free from disease is not equally healthy. He proposed gradations of health separate from gradations of illness, which would allow individuals to be at any stage of health regardless of their position on the illness continuum.[7(p4)] Oelbaum stressed the interrelationship of health and illness, even though she considers the concepts to be separate entities rather than opposite ends of a continuum. She stated that apathy toward the work of wellness is the precursor of disease. The particular health behaviors or functions that are poorly performed will influence the type of disease, disorder, or damage that will follow.[35]

It is the belief of the present author that health and illness are qualitatively different but interrelated concepts. In Figure 1–1, differing levels of health are depicted in interaction with the experience of illness. Illness is diagrammed as representing discrete events throughout the life process, of short or long duration. These illness experiences can thwart or facilitate one's continuing quest for health. Thus, optimum health or poor health can exist with or without overt illness.

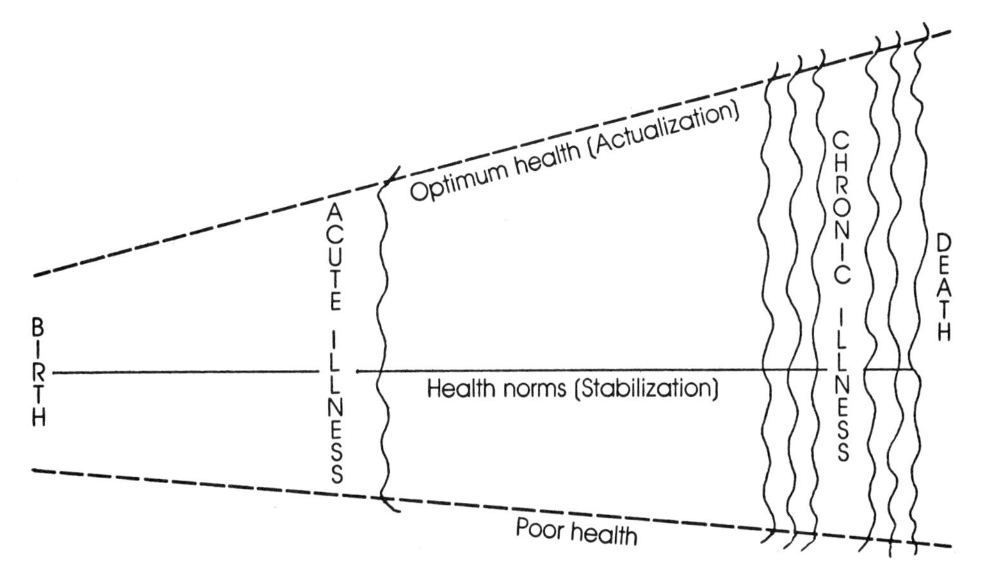

Figure 1–1. The health continuum throughout the life span.

• DEFINITIONS OF HEALTH THAT FOCUS ON THE FAMILY

Much more attention has been given to defining health and wellness as a state or process characteristic of individual human beings than as a state or process descriptive of family systems. Almost all family theorists would agree that health of families is more than a composite of the individual health assessments of family members. Feetham[36] has commented in her review of family research that by focusing on the individual family member, often a member with pathology, family researchers have generated little knowledge about the normal, well-functioning family. Few conceptual frameworks of health proposed for nursing have given attention to the family. The individual system rather than the family system has been the basic unit of analysis. Loveland-Cherry has observed that family health is a concept often referred to as a goal of nursing but seldom defined. Adapting Smith's[31] models of health to families, she has proposed the following four models of **family health**[37]:

- Clinical model: lack of evidence of physical, mental, or social disease, deterioration, or dysfunction of family system
- Role-performance model: ability of family system to carry on family functions effectively and to achieve family developmental tasks
- Adaptive model: family patterns of interaction with the environment characterized by flexible, effective adaptation or ability to change and grow
- Eudaimonistic model: ongoing provision of resources, guidance, and support for realization of family's maximum well-being and potential throughout the life span

This is an excellent start toward specifying the critical dimensions of family health conceptually and putting them into operation.

Other definitions of family health that appear in the literature will be presented here. As a context, a definition of family is essential. A family has been defined as "a small social system made up of individuals related to each other by reason of strong reciprocal affections and loyalties and comprising a permanent household (or cluster of households) that persists over years or decades."[38]

Families as systems are characterized by structure, function, and developmental stages. Families occur in variant forms. It is critical that variation in family structure be taken into consideration in defining and measuring family health.

In discussing the assessment of families, Roberts and Feetham[39] identified three major areas that should be considered in defining family health:

- The relationship between the family and broader social units, such as family and community and family and economy
- The relationships between the family and subsystems, such as parental dyad or sibling subsystem
- The relationships between the family and each individual, focusing on reciprocity

While not specifically defining family health, Wright and Leahey imply that healthy families are characterized by stability and integrity of structure, adaptive rather than maladaptive functioning, and mastery of developmental tasks leading to progressive differentiation and transformation to meet the changing requisites for survival of the system.[40] This definition focuses on stability as the primary criterion for family health.

Petze, in discussing health promotion for the well family, does not provide an explicit definition of family health. However, the following definition of family health focusing on stability can be inferred from the discussion of competent and effectively functioning families:[41]

> An indicator of family health is the continuing viability of the family unit as a functional and productive network. The healthy family has a sense of togetherness that promotes the capacity for change, a balance between mutual and independent action on the part of family members, and adaptation to life events.

Curran, in analyzing opinions of a large number of health professionals regarding defining characteristics for family health, identified 15 traits of healthy families. Examples of these traits include: affirm and support one another, exhibit a sense of shared responsibility, share leisure time, share religious core, and have a strong sense of family with rituals and traditions.[42] These traits seem to address stability of family functioning and balance in interaction among family members.

Smilkstein offered an actualizing definition of family health that can be paraphrased as follows: Family health is a state of cohesiveness in which nurturance and resources necessary for personal growth and sustenance in the face of life's challenges are available to family members.[43]

Another actualizing definition has been offered by Johnson, who defined family health as a process that includes the promotion and maintenance of physical, mental, spiritual, and social health for the family unit and for individual family members. Johnson comments that to achieve wellness, the family must be an integrated unit striving to develop its fullest potential. Family wellness contributes to both individual wellness of family members and the level of wellness within the community.[44]

Many factors influence how family health is defined. Cultural and religious factors play a central role in determining how families view their health. Families' strengths, resources, and competencies are an integral part of a positive conceptualization of health. Defining family health and its aggregate parameters is an ongoing challenge to family researchers in a number of disciplines. It is evident from a review of the literature that family health processes must be given increased attention by nurse researchers along with scientists in other disciplines. The development of models for describing family health will assist health professionals in identifying predictors of family well-being and in promoting the health of families.

• DEFINITIONS OF HEALTH THAT FOCUS ON THE COMMUNITY

The community has been defined as a locality-based entity, composed of systems of formal organizations reflecting societal institutions, informal groups, and aggregates that are interdependent and whose function or expressed intent is to meet a wide variety of collective needs.[45] This definition focuses on the spatial, personal, and functional dimensions of a community.

Community health, a term used increasingly in current literature, is complex and difficult to define. Dever observed that holistic models of health have resulted in new belief systems about what constitutes health for aggregates.[46] Dimensions of community health in a social ecology model have been described in the WHO Ottawa Charter for Health Promotion. Fundamental to community health are peace, shelter, education, food, income, a stable ecosystem, sustainable resources, social justice, and equity. Flynn notes that the responsibility for health is widely shared in the community with collaborative decision making about health issues. Informed political action and healthy public policies are essential to a healthy community.[47]

Goeppinger described community health as having three dimensions that are currently assessed by multiple measures[45]:

1. Status dimension: morbidity, mortality, life expectancy, risk factors, consumer satisfaction, mental health, crime rates, functional levels, worker absenteeism, infant mortality
2. Structural dimension: community health resources measured by utilization patterns, treatment data, and provider : population ratios; social indicators measured by dependency ratios, socioeconomic and racial distributions, and median education level
3. Process dimension: effective community functioning or problem solving that results in community competence as evidenced by: commitment, self–other awareness and clarity of situational definitions, articulateness, effective communication, conflict containment and accommodation, participation, and management of relations with larger society

Incorporating all these dimensions, community health is defined as "the meeting of collective needs through problem identifying and managing interactions within the community and between the community and the larger society."

Archer, Kelly, and Bisch,[48] by describing a community as an open system, imply that community health is characterized by openness to energy exchange, interdependence among community groups, hierarchical organization, self-regulation, dynamic activity, goal-directedness, and the synthesizing processes of wholeness. Community health is more than the sum of the health states of its individual members; it encompasses the characteristics of the community as a whole.

West identified three factors to be used in the assessment of community health[49]:

- Factor One: interaction: exchanging, communicating, and relating patterns within the community
- Factor Two: action: valuing, choosing, and moving
- Factor Three: awareness: walking, feeling, and knowing

West developed a community assessment tool to analyze these dimensions of man–environment interaction or patterns of energy within the community.

In describing a group or community intervention model for the promotion of health, Hogue suggests some group health indicators that might be selected as indices of the health of the community. The indices and examples of measures are presented here.[50]

1. Level of social functioning: work attendance, school attendance, dependency ratio
2. Symptoms and complaints: reasons for absence from school or work, accident rates
3. Disabilities and impairments: proportion of children with learning disabilities or physical, visual, or auditory impairment
4. Biologic correlates of disease or risk factors: blood pressure, cholesterol, triglycerides
5. Disease categories: cases of acute and chronic diseases
6. Mortality: by specific causes
7. Measurements of population growth and pressure: birth, fertility, death rate, divorce rate, proportion living at poverty level, rate of unemployment
8. Measurements of growth and nutritional status: heights and weights of adults and children, iron-deficiency anemia
9. Measures of health care utilization: prenatal care, immunization of infants and children, hospital admissions

According to Hogue, any or all of these indicators could be used to describe the health of a community. The author of this book recommends further expansion of the indices to include dimensions of positive community health.

Individual, family, and community health are intimately related. Changing the environment in which people live changes what they do. Healthy environments support healthy living. Positive community health is expressed in activities such as: on-going analysis of community characteristics, consensus building on strengths and health problems, development and empowerment of community leadership, organized social action, and community influence on public decisions.[51] An expansive definition of community health goes well beyond the health sector of the community to include multiple sectors that impact health and well-being on a daily basis.[52]

It is evident from the various definitions and dimensions of community health described that a multiplicity of approaches are proposed for evaluating the health of a community. Definitions of community health range from those that are highly disease-oriented to those that focus on the actualizing potential of the community. With increasing emphasis on health as more than the absence of disease, community health personnel who rely heavily on disease-oriented indices of community health need to rethink their approach to community assessment. Effective health-promotion interventions must be based on the assessment of a community's competence and actualizing potential. During the next decade, systematic attempts to define community health more holistically and to measure community health as a positive process in all its richness and complexity will be critically needed.

• DIRECTIONS FOR RESEARCH ON THE MEANING OF HEALTH

Cultural models of health need to be clearly defined in order to examine the diversity of health conceptions. Furthermore, longitudinal studies should be conducted to determine the developmental variations in health definitions across the life span. Multidisciplinary research teams are suggested to enrich the exploration of health as a positive construct. Attention should be given to developing more rigorous definitions of family health and community health. The work of scholars cited in this chapter provide a base for further research.

• SUMMARY

Varying definitions of individual, family, and community health have been presented that provide the foundation on which health-promotion efforts for persons and aggregates can be based. To address the promotion of health, one must know what the desired outcome—health—is and how its achievement will be measured at individual, family, and community levels. The survey of existing definitions of health presented in this chapter represents a beginning step toward the specification of health as a dynamic process inherent in the life experience of individuals, families, and communities.

The movement toward positive conceptualization of health and wellness espouses a "competence model" rather than an "illness model." Supporters of this growing movement come from a variety of disciplines and advocate a proactive approach to health that includes building strengths, enhancing resources, and fostering resilience to enhance prospects for effective living.[53]

REFERENCES

1. Fawcett J. *Analysis and Evaluation of Conceptual Models of Nursing.* Philadelphia, Pa: FA Davis Co; 1984.
2. Pender NJ. Expressing health through lifestyle patterns. *Nurs Sci Q.* 1990;3(3):115–122.

3. Benson H, Stuart EM. *The Wellness Book: The Comprehensive Guide to Maintaining Health and Treating Stress-related Illness.* New York, NY: Birch Lane; 1992;8.
4. Millstein SG. A view of health from the adolescent's perspective. In: Millstein SG, Petersen AC, Nightingale EO, eds. *Promoting the Health of Adolescents: New Directions for the Twenty-First Century.* New York, NY: Oxford University Press Inc; 1994;97–118.
5. Millstein SG, Irwin CE. Concepts of health and illness: different constructs or variation in a theme. *Health Psychol.* 1987;6:515–524.
6. Reynolds CL. The measurement of health in nursing research. *Adv Nurs Sci.* 1988;10(4): 23–31.
7. Sorochan W. Health concepts as a basis for orthobiosis. In: Hart E, Sechrist W, eds. *The Dynamics of Wellness.* Belmont, Calif: Wadsworth Inc. 1970.
8. Dolfman ML. The concept of health: an historic and analytic examination. *J Sch Health.* 1973;43:493.
9. Wylie CM. The definition and measurement of health and disease. *Public Health Rep.* February 1970;85:100–104.
10. Tempkin O. What is health? Looking back and ahead. In: Gladston I, ed. *Epidemiology of Health.* New York, NY: Academy of Medicine, Health Education Council; 1953:21.
11. Ware JE. Standards for validating health measures: definition and content. *J Chronic Dis.* 1987;40:473–480.
12. Parse RR. *Nursing Science: Major Paradigms, Theories, and Critiques.* Philadelphia, Pa: WB Saunders Co; 1987.
13. Dubos R. *Man Adapting.* New Haven, Conn: Yale University Press; 1965:349.
14. Parsons T. Definitions of health and illness in the light of American values and social structure. In: Jaco EG, ed. *Patients, Physicians and Illness.* New York, NY: Free Press; 1958:176.
15. Patrick DL, Bush JW, Chen MM. Toward an operational definition of health. *J Health Soc Behav.* 1973;14:6.
16. Levine ME. *Introduction to Clinical Nursing.* 2nd ed. Philadelphia Pa: FA Davis Co; 1973.
17. Loveland-Cherry C, Wilkerson SA. Dorothy Johnson's behavioral system model. In: Fitzpatrick J, Whall A, eds. *Conceptual Models of Nursing: Analysis and Application.* 2nd ed. Norwalk, Conn: Appleton & Lange; 1989.
18. Neuman B. *The Neuman Systems Model: Applications to Nursing Education and Practice.* 2nd ed. Norwalk, Conn: Appleton & Lange; 1995.
19. Roy C. *Introduction to Nursing: An Adaptation Model.* 2nd ed. Norwalk, Conn: Appleton & Lange; 1991.
20. Tripp-Reimer T. Reconceptualizing the concept of health: integrating emic and etic perspectives. *Res Nurs Health.* 1984;7:101–109.
21. Dunn HL. What high-level wellness means. *Can J Public Health.* November 1959;50(11):447–457.
22. Dunn HL. Points of attack for raising the level of wellness. *J Nat Med Assoc.* 1975;49:223–235.
23. Dunn HL. *High-Level Wellness.* Thorofare, NJ: Charles B Slack Inc; 1980.
24. Bermosk LS, Porter SE. *Women's Health and Human Wholeness.* New York, NY: Appleton-Century-Crofts; 1979:11.
25. Orem DE. *Nursing: Concepts of Practice.* 5th ed. New York, NY: McGraw-Hill Inc; 1995.
26. Newman MA. Health conceptualization. In: Fitzpatrick J, Taunton RL, Jacox AK, eds. *Annual Review of Research.* New York, NY: Springer Publishing Co; 1991;9:221–243.
27. Parse RR. *Man-Living-Health: A Theory of Nursing.* New York, NY: John Wiley & Sons; 1981:25–36.
28. Wu R. *Behavior and illness.* Englewood Cliffs, NJ: Prentice-Hall Inc; 1973:112.

29. King IM. *A Theory for Nursing: Systems, Concepts, Processes.* New York, NY: Teachers College Press; 1983;31.
30. King IM. Health as the goal for nursing. *Nurs Sci Q.* 1990;3(3):123–128.
31. Smith J. *The Idea of Health: Implications for the Nursing Profession.* New York, NY: Teachers College Press; 1983:31.
32. Shaver JF. A biopsychosocial view of human health. *Nurs Outlook.* 1985;33(4):186–191.
33. Kulbok PA, Baldwin JH. From preventive health behavior to health promotion: advancing a positive construct. *Adv Nurs Sci.* 1992;14(4):50–64.
34. Landrine H, Klonoff EA. Culture and health-related schemas: a review and proposal for interdisciplinary integration. *Health Psychol.* 1992;11:267–276.
35. Oelbaum CH. Hallmarks of adult wellness. *Am J Nurs.* 1974;74:1623.
36. Feetham SL. Family research: issues and directions for nursing. In: Werley HH, Fitzpatrick JJ, eds. *Annual Review of Nursing Research.* New York: Springer; 1984;3–25.
37. Loveland-Cherry CJ. Family health promotion and protection. In: Bomar PJ, ed. *Nurses and Family Health Promotion: Concepts, Assessment and Interventions.* Baltimore, Md: Williams & Wilkins; 1989:13–25.
38. Terkelson K. Toward a theory of the family lifecycle. In: Carter E, McGoldrick M, eds. *The Family Lifecycle: A Framework for Family Therapy.* New York, NY: Gardner Press Inc; 1980;21–52.
39. Roberts CS, Feetham SL. Assessing family functioning across three areas of relationships. *Nurs Res.* 1982;31:231–235.
40. Wright LM, Leahey M. *Nurses and Families: A Guide to Family Assessment and Intervention.* Philadelphia, Pa: FA Davis Co; 1984.
41. Petze CF. Health promotion for the well family. *Nurs Clin North Am.* 1984;19:229–237.
42. Curran D. *Traits of a Healthy Family.* Minneapolis, Minn: Winston Press Inc; 1983.
43. Smilkstein G. The cycle of family function: a conceptual model for family medicine. *Fam Practitioner.* 1980;11:223.
44. Johnson R. Promoting the health of families in the community. In: Stanhope M, Lancaster J, eds. *Community Health Nursing: Process and Practice for Promoting Health.* 3rd ed. St. Louis, Mo: Mosby Year Book; 1992:330–360.
45. Goeppinger J. Community as client: using the nursing process to promote health. In: Stanhope M, Lancaster J, eds. Community Health Nursing: Process and Practice for Promoting Health. 3rd ed. St. Louis, Mo: Mosby Year Book; 1992:253–276.
46. Dever GEA. *Community Health Analysis: A Holistic Approach.* Germantown, Md: Aspen;1980:12–15.
47. World Health Organization. Ottawa Charter for Health Promotion. *Health Prom.* 1986;1(4):ii–v.
48. Archer SE, Kelly CD, Bisch SA. *Implementing Change in Communities: A Collaborative Process.* St Louis, Mo: CV Mosby Co; 1984:5–6.
49. West M. Community health assessment: the man–environment interaction. *J Community Health Nurs.* 1984;1(2):89–97.
50. Hogue CC. An epidemiological approach to nursing practice. In: Hall JE, Weaver BR. *Distributive Nursing Practice: A Systems Approach to Community Health.* 2nd ed. Philadelphia, Pa: JB Lippincott Co; 1985:293–294.
51. Flynn BC. Healthy cities: the future of public health. *Health Trends Transitions.* 1993;4(3):12–18,80.
52. Flynn BC, Ray DW, Rider MS. Empowering communities: action research through healthy communities. *Health Edu Q.* 1994;21(3):395–405.
53. Seeman J. Toward a model of positive health. *Am Psychol.* 1989;44:1099–1109.

2

Motivation for Health Behavior

- Theories for Understanding Health Protection
  - A. The Health Belief Model
  - B. Protection Motivation Theory
- Theories for Understanding Health Promotion and Health Protection
  - A. Theory of Reasoned Action and Theory of Planned Behavior
  - B. Social Cognitive Theory (Self-Efficacy)
  - C. The Theory of Interpersonal Behavior
  - D. Cognitive Evaluation Theory
  - E. The Interaction Model of Client Health Behavior
  - F. Relapse Prevention
- Factors Influencing Health Behavior Change
- Directions for Research in Health Behavior
- Summary

Scientific knowledge about the determinants of health behavior expanded rapidly during the last two decades of the 20th century. Various behavioral theories and models were applied to a wide range of health behaviors (eg, physical activity, nutritional practices, smoking cessation, and condom use) to determine if their occurrence could be predicted and the underlying motivational mechanisms explained. The intense scientific and clinical interest in health behaviors was spurred by the realization that improving the quality of lives is as important as saving lives. Thus, services provided by health professionals in the United States became increasingly directed toward the goal of assisting individuals, families, and populations to achieve their full health potential. Progress toward this goal requires an understanding of the motivational dynamics underlying actions that damage health and actions that enhance health. This chapter and the subsequent chapter, which focuses on the Health Promotion Model, describe models and theories potentially useful in explaining and predicting health behaviors—those actions motivated by the desire to protect or promote health. It should be noted, however, that some of the general behavioral models presented here are also applicable to health-damaging behaviors. For additional information on problem behaviors, risk-taking behaviors, and health-damaging behaviors, the reader should consult other sources.[1–3]

In the previous edition of this book,[4] a distinction was made between two types of positive health behavior.

Health protection is directed toward decreasing the probability of experiencing health problems by active protection against pathologic stressors or detection of health problems in the asymptomatic stage. Health protection focuses on efforts to move away from or avoid the negatively valanced states of illness and injury.

Health promotion is directed toward increasing the level of well-being and self-actualization of a given individual or group. Health promotion focuses on efforts to approach or move toward a positively valenced state of high-level health and well-being.

In reality, for many health behaviors, both "approaching a positive state" and "avoiding a negative state" serve as sources of motivation for behavior. A **mixed** motivation model (approach and avoidance) may be the rule rather than the exception for most health behaviors of adults who are middle-age or older. In contrast, healthy children provide relatively pure examples of "approach" motivation because negative illness events in the distant future lack the immediacy needed to motivate behavior.

The Health Belief Model and Protection Motivation Theory, discussed in this chapter, are targeted for application to health protection because of their dominant emphasis on **avoidance of negative events.** Other models presented here are not primarily "threat oriented" and thus are applicable to behaviors motivated by either health protection or health promotion or a combination of both when "threat" is not proposed as a salient source of motivation. Since illness frequently thwarts the attainment of high-level well-being, maintaining an illness-free state through health protection is highly desirable. Freedom from illness and the resultant stresses and strains allows individuals and families to direct more energy toward the promotion of health. The terms *health protecting behavior* and *preventive behavior* are used interchangeably in this book.

Three types of health-protection (prevention) have been described in the literature.[5] **Primary prevention** provides specific protection against a disease to prevent its occurrence. Examples include mass immunization (polio, pertussis, diphtheria) to prevent acute infectious diseases; reducing risk factors (inactivity, high dietary cholesterol, high blood pressure), and control of air (passive smoke, asbestos), water (chemical pollutants), and noise (excessive loudness of machinery) pollution to prevent chronic diseases. **Secondary prevention** consists of organized, direct screening efforts or education of the public to promote early case finding of individuals with disease so that prompt intervention can be instituted to halt pathologic processes and limit disability. Public education to promote breast self-examination and testicular self-examination or use of home kits for detection of occult blood in stool specimens are examples of secondary prevention. When primary prevention is not available, secondary prevention (early diagnosis and treatment) represents the first line of defense against disease. In other situations, primary preventive measures may be available but not used, resulting in the need for secondary-level intervention. **Tertiary prevention** is directed toward minimizing residual disability from disease and helping the client learn to live productively with limitations. Cardiac rehabilitation programs following myocardial infarction or cardiovascular surgery are excellent examples of tertiary prevention services.

• THEORIES FOR UNDERSTANDING HEALTH PROTECTION

Understanding the determinants of health-protecting behavior is critical for the development of effective interventions that health professionals can use to assist clients in altering behaviors that increase risk for specific diseases. The Health Belief Model and Protection Motivation Theory are presented here as examples of theoretical explanations for health protection that have been proposed and empirically tested.

The Health Belief Model

The Health Belief Model was proposed in the 1960s as a framework for exploring why some people who are illness-free take actions to avoid illness, while others fail to take protective actions.[6] At the time, a major public health concern was the widespread reluctance of individuals to accept screening for tuberculosis, Pap smear for detection of cervical cancer, immunizations, and other preventive measures that were often free or provided at nominal charge. The model was viewed as potentially useful to predict those individuals who would or would not use preventive measures and to suggest interventions that might increase predisposition of resistant individuals to engage in health-protecting behaviors.

The model is derived from social-psychologic theory, primarily the work of Lewin, who conceptualized that the life space in which an individual exists is composed of regions, some having negative valence, some having positive valence, and others being relatively neutral.[7] Illnesses are conceived to be regions of negative valence that can be expected to exert a force moving the person away from the region. Health-protecting behaviors are strategies for avoiding the negatively valenced regions of illness and disease.[8]

The model as modified by Becker is presented in Figure 2–1. Variables proposed as **directly** affecting predisposition to take action are perceiving a threat to personal health and the conviction that the benefits of taking action to protect health outweigh the barriers that will be encountered. Beliefs about personal susceptibility and the seriousness of a specific disease combine to produce the degree of threat or negative valence of a particular disease. Perceived susceptibility reflects individuals' feelings of personal vulnerability to a specific health problem. Perceived seriousness or severity of a given health problem can be judged either by the degree of emotional arousal created by the thought of having the disease or by the medical and clinical or social difficulties (eg, family and work life) that individuals believe a given health condition would create for them. Perceived benefits are beliefs about the effectiveness of recommended actions in preventing the health threat. Perceived barriers are perceptions concerning the potential negative aspects of taking action such as expense, danger, unpleasantness, inconvenience, and time required.

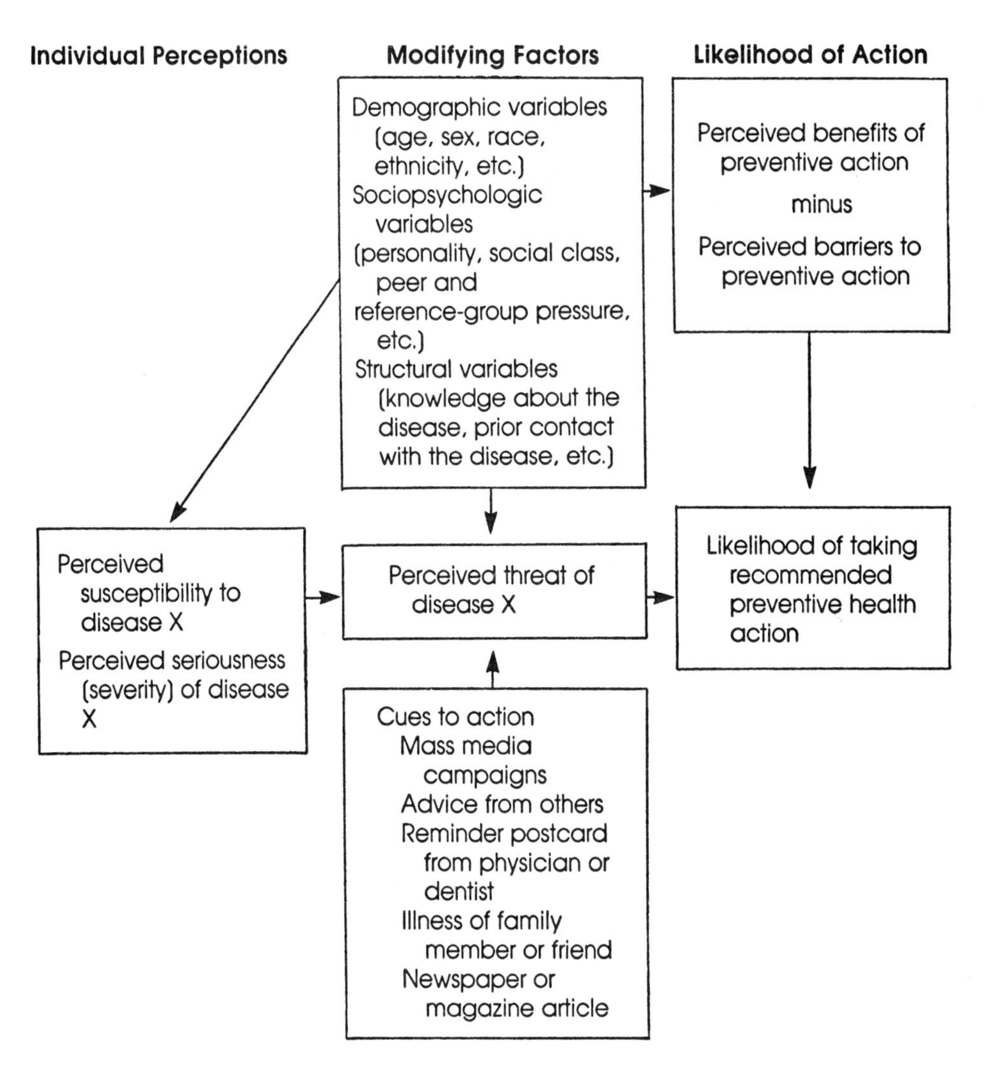

Figure 2–1. The Health Belief Model. (From Becker MH, Haefner DP, Kasl SV, et al. Selected psychosocial models and correlates of individual health-related behaviors. *Med Care.* 1977;15:27–46, with permission.)

Modifying factors such as demographic, sociopsychologic, and structural variables, as well as cues to action, only **indirectly** affect action tendencies through their relationship with perception of threat. The Health Belief Model (HBM) is appropriate as a paradigm for health-protecting or disease-preventing behavior but is clearly inappropriate as a paradigm for health-promoting behavior.[9]

In reviewing 10 years of studies related to the model, Janz and Becker concluded that results of numerous studies, both retrospective and prospective, show **perceived barriers** to be the most powerful of the HBM dimensions in explaining or predicting various health behaviors. **Perceived susceptibility** was also important in understanding preventive behaviors. Both perceived benefits of taking action and perceived seriousness of disease lacked power to explain or predict health-protecting behavior.[9(p2)] Thus, two component variables in the model rather than the whole model appear relevant to designing health-protective interventions. In 1988, Rosenstock et al proposed that self-efficacy be added to the HBM as an explanatory variable and suggested that it be incorporated in interventions based on the model.[10] Burns has suggested further additions to the model such as the variables of emotional response, behavioral norms, and intention.[11] Further research will reveal whether the suggested additions to the model will increase its overall usefulness in developing effective health-protective interventions.

Protection Motivation Theory

Protection Motivation Theory (PMT) offers a social psychologic perspective, similar to the HBM, as an approach to motivating health protective behavior. The theory focuses primarily on health threats or fear appeals to change behavior by emphasizing the harmful personal consequences of health-damaging behaviors. Originally, the theory incorporated three focal cognitive appraisal processes: perceived vulnerability to a health threat, perceived seriousness of the health threat, and perceived effectiveness of responses directed toward preventing the threat (response efficacy).[12]

Subsequently, the theory was revised to incorporate a fourth factor, perceived self-efficacy (beliefs about personal competence) from Bandura's social cognitive theory.[13] In one study applying the theory to persuasive appeals for increasing exercise, 160 undergraduate women read persuasive appeals about exercise and disease that varied on the four dimensions of severity, vulnerability, response efficacy, and self-efficacy. The expectation was that messages high on all four dimensions would be the most effective. The findings indicated that only appeals that emphasized vulnerability to illnesses as a result of sedentary living and self-efficacy enhanced intentions to exercise.[14]

In applying PMT to adolescents, 615 high school students were presented with essay information about cardiovascular disease risk. In the study, the following variables were manipulated in the information given: response efficacy (effectiveness of exercise in preventing cardiovascular disease), response cost (costs associated with taking up a regular exercise program), and self-efficacy (belief in ability to carry out a program of exercise) with two levels (high and low) for each variable. The study purpose was to determine the effects of information on the selection of cognitive coping strategies for cardiovascular disease that were adaptive (intentions to exercise, rational problem solving) or maladaptive (fatalism, avoidance, wishful thinking, and hopelessness). The study revealed that participants in the high self-efficacy condition indicated stronger intentions to exercise, an adaptive coping response. Youth in the low response-efficacy condition were more prone to maladaptive responses such as hopelessness and fatalism. Exercise status, not a component of the model, also exerted a significant effect, with active adolescents more likely to endorse adaptive coping strategies (setting intentions to exercise and rational problem solving) and less likely to endorse the maladaptive coping strategy of fatalism than inactive adolescents. Findings suggest that strategies to promote and maintain high self-efficacy for exercise and high response efficacy for exercise in relation to cardiovascular disease could be effective in increasing exercise among youth.[15]

Studies to date indicate that some of the variables in PMT such as response efficacy and self-efficacy are relevant to health-protecting behaviors. The importance of vulnerability in motivating preventive behavior may depend on the age of the target group. Just as in the HBM, the role of perceived severity or seriousness in facilitating health-protective behaviors can be seriously questioned. Furthermore, it appears that other variables may well need to be considered in a more complex model in order to adequately explain health-protecting behaviors.

Fear and threat are used frequently in health education programs and campaigns, yet they may be of limited effectiveness in achieving desired health behavior outcomes. Job suggests that use of fear to promote health behaviors may do more harm than good unless the following conditions are met: (1) fear onset occurs before a desired coping behavior is offered, (2) the event upon which the fear is based appears to be likely in the not too distant future, (3) a specific desired behavior to alleviate the fear is offered as an integral part of the program or campaign, (4) the level of fear induced should only be such that the suggested behaviors can substantially reduce it, and (5) a noticeable decrease in fear is experienced, reinforcing the behavior and confirming its effectiveness. Job concludes that given the difficulties involved in fear- or threat-based health programs such as regulating the "dose" of fear or threat administered and the potential harm that could occur, the focus on removing unhealthy behaviors should be resisted in favor of promoting healthy alternative behaviors.[16] It is toward this direction that the present discussion of health behavior models now turns.

• THEORIES FOR UNDERSTANDING HEALTH PROMOTION AND HEALTH PROTECTION

The models and theories discussed in this section can be used to understand both health promoting and health protecting behaviors. Thus, they can be applied clinically across a wide range of health behaviors.

Theory of Reasoned Action and Theory of Planned Behavior

In 1975, Ajzen and Fishbein proposed the Theory of Reasoned Action (TRA) to explain the role of beliefs and attitudes in determining behavior.[17] Beliefs constitute the fundamental building blocks in this conceptual structure, with behavioral intention the immediate determinant of behavior. The model for predicting intentions and, in turn, behavior is as follows:

$$B \approx I = [A_{act}]w_1 + [SN]w_2$$

in which

B = target behavior
$\approx$ = is a function of
I = intention to perform the behavior
A_{act} = attitude toward the behavior
SN = subjective norm in relation to the behavior
w_1, w_2 = empirical weights determined by regression analysis

Intentions are directly influenced by attitudes and subjective norms. Attitude toward a behavior is a multiplicative function of its component parts: beliefs concerning the consequences of performing the behavior (b) and evaluation of these consequences, either positive or negative (e).

$$A_{act} = \Sigma b \times e$$

The second determinant of intention is subjective norms, a multiplicative function of what significant others expect a person to do (nb) and the motivation of the individual to comply with their expectations (m).

$$SN = \Sigma nb \times m$$

This theory assumes that behavior is under volitional control, that is, that there are no barriers to performance of the intended behavior. This may or may not be true for different health behaviors at varying points in time. Ajzen, in a critique of the TRA, commented that the theory assumes that behavior is completely under the control of the individual. This may not always be the case. Thus, Ajzen added a third variable of perceived behavioral control to the original Fishbein and Ajzen concepts of attitude and subjective norms, resulting in three proposed predictors of behavioral intentions. He labeled the extended theory, the Theory of Planned Behavior (TPB).[18,19]

In a field study that examined factors associated with testicular self-examination (TSE) among 232 college students, instructors provided information on testicular cancer and assigned reading materials on testicular cancer and TSE. A questionnaire measuring components of TRA and TPB was administered. Both attitude and normative beliefs contributed significantly to the prediction of TSE, with attitudes being the strongest predictor. Ajzen's extension of the TRA to the TPB was also tested in this study by adding a measure of perceived behavioral control. When TSE knowledge and perceived behavioral control were added to the regression equation, there was a substantial increase in the power to predict TSE. Thus, both TRA and its extension, TPB, were partially supported in this study.[20]

A great deal of research has tested the applicability of the TRA to various health behaviors. An overview of related research findings indicates that intentions are, for the most part, moderately to highly correlated with behavior, attitudes are moderately correlated with behavior, and subjective norms are uncorrelated to moderately correlated with behavior. Relationships vary by type of health behavior studied and study methods. Intervention studies in which variables in the TRA have been manipulated have had some reported successes in bringing about behavior change. The TPB has received considerably less testing to date. Needed are further prospective studies that test the usefulness of these theories in explaining the occurrence of various health behaviors. Study findings should be incorporated into research that tests interventions for behavior change based on the TRA and the TPB singly and in combination.

Social Cognitive Theory (Self-Efficacy)

Social cognitive theory is a broad theoretical approach to explaining human behavior. Within this perspective, individuals are neither driven by inner forces nor automatically controlled by external stimuli. Human behavior is explained in terms of triadic reciprocal determinism, in which behavior, cognition and other personal factors, and environmental events all operate as interacting determinants of each other. Basic human capabilities undergirding regulation of behavior include symbolization, forethought, vicarious learning, self-regulation, and self-reflection. Self-efficacy, a form of self-knowledge, is a central concept in the theory.[21] This concept will be the focus of the presentation here.

Perceived self-efficacy is a judgment of one's ability to accomplish a certain level of performance in executing a specific behavior. Efficacy expectations (judgments of personal efficacy) are distinct from outcome expectations (judgments concerning behavioral consequences). Efficacy expectations are proposed by Bandura as a primary determinant of behavior. Sources of efficacy expectations include performance attainments (mastery experiences), vicarious experiences (observing the behavior of others), verbal persuasion (being convinced by others of capabilities), and physiologic states (aversive arousal: stress and anxiety, fatigue, or pain). Individuals derive their sense of self-efficacy for a given behavior by weighing and integrating efficacy information from these diverse sources. According to social cognitive theory, the cumulative perception of efficacy determines predisposition to undertake a given behavior.[21(pp390–453)] For further discussion of self-efficacy, the reader is referred to Schwarzer and colleagues, who offer a comprehensive examination of the concept.[22]

A growing number of studies support the importance of self-efficacy in the explanation and prediction of behavior. For example, among sedentary women, self-efficacy has been identified as a significant predictor of exercise levels.[23] Further, in another study of adults participating in an organized exercise program, self-efficacy directly predicted exercise and mediated the effects of social support on exercise. The measurement of self-efficacy in the latter study included the component of exercise efficacy (perceived capability of achieving progressively more difficult levels of exercise) and barriers to efficacy (perceived capabilities of overcoming time, cost, and inconvenience barriers to exercise).[24] Other health behaviors reported to be predicted by self-efficacy include breast self-examination,[25] safe sex,[26] and smoking cessation.[27]

Self-efficacy should be considered an important concept for manipulation in health protection and health promotion interventions. The interaction of self-efficacy with other predictors of health behaviors needs to be explored further to understand the intricate nature of the motivational dynamics underlying health behavior. The effects of high versus low levels of efficacy on immune processes has been explored recently. Initial studies of efficacy-enhancing interventions in stressful situations have shown positive effects on immunocompetency.[28] This potential biobehavioral connection merits further study and may offer new perspectives on mind-body relationships.

The Theory of Interpersonal Behavior

Triandis offers a model of behavior that incorporates affective and physiologic dimensions as well as habit strength into the explanation of behavior.[29] These are factors given less attention in other models of behavior. Facione has recently reviewed this model and cites two equations that depict the model variables[30]:

$$B = w(I) + w(H) + w(F) + w(P)$$

in which

B = target behavior
I = intention to perform target behavior
H = previous habit of performing behavior
F = facilitating factors in the environment that assist or constrain the behavior
P = arousal to perform the behavior
w = corresponding regression coefficients

Intentions are predicted by the following equation:

$$I = w(C) + w(A) + w(S)$$

in which

I = intention to perform target behavior
C = beliefs about the consequences of performing the behavior
A = affect toward the behavior
S = social influences on the behavior such as normative beliefs and role expectations
w = corresponding regression coefficients

Since some behaviors can be performed with little conscious awareness, the number of times that a behavior has been performed determines its habit strength. With repeated performance of a behavior, Triandis proposes that habit may replace intention.[31] Further explication of the role of affect toward a behavior as a determinant of health behavior performance would augment knowledge gained from models that focus primarily on cognitive influences on behavior. A unique feature of Triandis's work is his emphasis on explicating the model variables within the culture to be studied, or "cultural fitting" of the model. This important consideration is not explicitly addressed by other theorists whose work is presented in this chapter.

Cognitive Evaluation Theory

According to this theory proposed by Deci and Ryan,[32] human motivation is based on a set of innate or acquired psychologic needs: for self-determination, competence, and interpersonal relatedness. Self-determination and intrinsic motivation (IM) are central concepts in the theory. Intrinsic motivation is energized by the need to be self-determining and competent in relation to personally valued behaviors. Interests, personal challenge, and desire for mastery provide direction to internal motivation and determine behavioral choices. Deci and Ryan contrast internal motivation processes for behavior with external motivational and amotivational processes:

- Internal motivational processes—doing an activity for its own sake, for its inherent interest and the spontaneous cognitions and affects that accompany it—reflects self-determined causality
- External motivational processes—doing an activity to attain extrinsic rewards or to comply with external demands—reflects control causality.
- Amotivational processes result when a person is not in control and perceives no way of being in control of a given behavior; the environment allows neither self-determination nor behavioral competence.

Deci and Ryan propose that extrinsic rewards, when unassociated with positive feedback about competence, may decrease IM; whereas, positive feedback about competence increases IM. Ego involvement in a task (perception that success or failure is particularly critical to self-esteem) and disposition to public self-consciousness (marked internalization of the standards of others) has been shown to decrease IM. Behavioral challenges undertaken, including health behavior change, should be in the optimal range: neither too easy, which causes boredom and decreases IM, or too hard, which causes distress and decreases IM.

Efforts to make this theory operate in relation to health behavior are best illustrated in the model development and nursing research activities of Cox, who suggests that intrinsic motivation should be the primary motivational construct used to explain health behavior. Thus, at this point, attention is turned to the Interaction Model of Client Health Behavior.[33]

The Interaction Model of Client Health Behavior

The Interaction Model of Client Health Behavior (IMCHB) focuses on both characteristics of the client and factors external to the client to provide a comprehensive explanation of actions directed toward risk reduction and health promotion. Client background variables included in the model are demographic characteristics, social influence, previous health care experience, and environmental resources. These background variables and the intrinsic motivation, cognitive appraisal, and affective response of the client in regard to a particular behavior interface with elements of client-professional interaction (affective support, health information, decisional control, and professional technical competencies) to affect health outcomes. Critical elements of health outcomes are use of health care services, clinical health status indicators, severity of health care problems, adherence to the recommended care regimen, and satisfaction with care. The model is depicted in Figure 2–2.

A Health Self-Determinism Index (HSDI) has been derived from the cognitive evaluation framework proposed by Deci and Ryan as an approach to measuring intrinsic motivation. The four subscales constituting the instrument are: self-determined health judgments, self-determined health behavior, perceived competency in health matters, and internal and external cue responsiveness. A Health Self-Determinism Index for Children (HSDI-C) has also been developed to measure their intrinsic motivation in health behavior. The psychometric characteristics of both instruments are reported elsewhere.[34,35] In examining alcohol and tranquilizer use and current smoking behavior of 379 older adults ranging in age from 50 to 101 years, Cox et al found that the more self-determined the older people's behavior, the less likely they were to smoke or take tranquilizers. Alcohol use was unrelated to HSDI scores.[36]

A number of tests of the model have been published. For example, the model has been applied to explain the decision of at-risk women to request an amniocentesis. Findings revealed that 22 of the 35 hypothesized causal paths were significant and over half of the variance in the women's decisions was explained.[37,38] Troumbley and Lenz applied the IMCHB to explaining relationships between client singularity variables (demographic characteristics, intrinsic motivation, cognitive appraisal of designating self as overweight or normal weight, and affective response of psychologic distress to weight concerns) and health outcomes (health risk and health status) among enlisted US Army

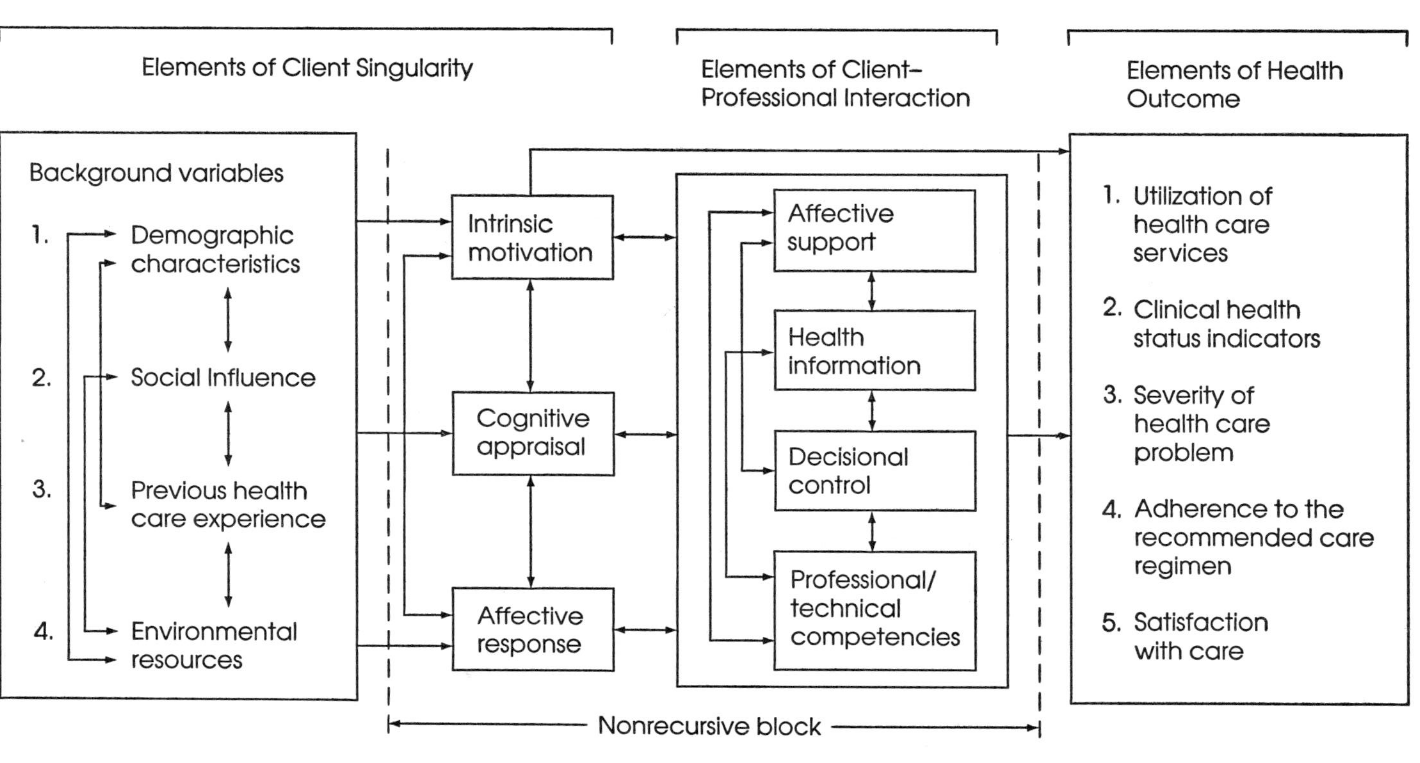

Figure 2–2. Interaction model of client health behavior. (From Cox[33][p47], with permission from Aspen Publishers.)

soldiers. Client singularity variables were explanatory of both health status and health risk.[39] The IMCHB was tested among a sample of 260 fourth-grade children and their mothers to determine its explanatory potential for a composite of 36 health behaviors. Because of redundancy among independent and dependent measures, an attempt was made to reduce redundancy prior to model testing. Health perception exerted the only direct effect on health behaviors, among girls as well as among boys. Relationship patterns among the model variables received differential support across genders.[40]

Initial tests indicate that the IMCHB offers a framework that merits further exploration in prospective studies to determine its explanatory potential for health behaviors. The model may yield critical variables that should be incorporated in health-protective and health-promotive nursing interventions.

Relapse Prevention

The final theoretical model to be examined in this chapter is Relapse Prevention proposed by Marlatt and Gordon.[41] Prevention of relapse is a daunting challenge, particularly for addictive behaviors such as alcoholism, smoking, obesity, and drug dependency. Because of the addictive nature of these behaviors and the high rates of recidivism, researchers have focused on understanding various factors that predispose to relapse after cessation of health-damaging behaviors and on designing interventions to prevent relapse. Theory-based strategies for relapse prevention are critically important to the effectiveness of health professionals in working with addicted clients.

In understanding the natural history of relapse, it is important to differentiate between lapse and relapse. A lapse is a "slip" that results in a single repeat of the addictive behavior. In relapse, the clients not only return to the behavior they are trying to abandon, but continue to engage in the behavior with increasing frequency. Marlatt and Gordon have indicated that by allowing room for mistakes to occur but providing clients with preparatory training (coping responses) to deal with these lapses, relapses can be prevented.[41(pp32–33)] For example, the client in a smoking cessation program who has been abstinent and suddenly finds him- or herself smoking a cigarette, if taught appropriate coping responses, may smoke no additional cigarettes and feel efficacious or competent in being able to stop after one smoke. According to the theory, this should result in a decreased probability of experiencing relapse. In contrast, the client who lapses and has no coping responses to draw upon is likely to experience decreased self-efficacy for quitting, positive effects from return to substance use, and the abstinence violation effect (AVE) of feeling guilty and "out of control." Such feelings are likely to lead to continuing performance of the behavior the client is trying to eliminate, despite the voluntary choice of the client to try to change. The cognitive-behavioral model of the relapse process appears in Figure 2–3.

Marlatt and Gordon propose that individuals experience enhanced self-efficacy and personal control from maintaining abstinence. Perceived control will continue to strengthen but can be threatened by a high-risk situation. A high-risk situation is defined as any one that threatens self-control and can potentially trigger relapse. Three categories of events that are associated with high rates of relapse are: negative emotional states (anger, frustration, depression, boredom), social situations (negative situations such as interpersonal conflict with significant other, friend, family member, or employee; or positive situations, such as partying or relaxing with friends, where social pressure is exerted

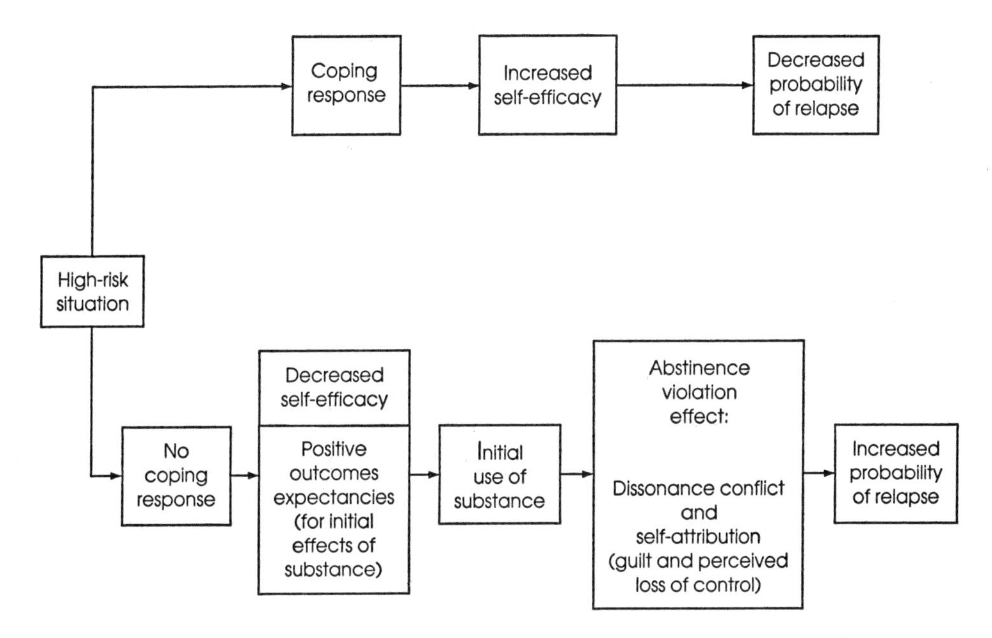

Figure 2–3. A cognitive behavioral model of the relapse process. (From Marlatt & Gordon[41[p38]], with permission).

by others to engage in the health-damaging behavior), and physical craving (withdrawal symptoms and physical response to cues). In these situations, use of coping responses that have been learned and rehearsed as part of relapse-prevention training can prevent a lapse from becoming a relapse. Specific relapse-prevention strategies that are suggested include: self-monitoring, relaxation training, relapse rehearsal, contracts, reminder cards, and cognitive restructuring. Although in-depth discussion of these techniques is beyond the scope of this book, the reader is referred to Chapter 8 and to other sources for further information about the relapse-prevention process and associated strategies.[42]

The Relapse-Prevention Model may also be applicable to behaviors that are motivated by the desire to promote health as well as protect health. Few attempts have been made to apply relapse prevention in health promotion programs. For example, does use of relapse prevention techniques foster continuation of exercise among children and young adults or healthy nutritional practices among individuals at or near recommended weight? With development of this model in the context of addictive behaviors, rigorous testing with differing populations is essential to determine if it can be used by health professionals and clients in maintaining positive health actions and lifestyles as well as in the cessation of health-damaging behaviors. Intervention studies that focus on relapse prevention are beginning to appear in the literature. Investigative work needs to continue in this important area.

• FACTORS INFLUENCING HEALTH BEHAVIOR CHANGE

Increasing healthy behaviors and decreasing risky or health-damaging behaviors is the major challenge facing health professionals and populations globally during the next several decades. Thus, a critical question is what major theories or constructs identified through research to date seem to explain or influence health behavior and health behavior change? In a theorist's workshop held in 1991, Martin Fishbein, Albert Bandura, Harry Triandis, Frederick Kanfer, and Marshall Becker analyzed their own theoretical work to identify variables in their theories or models that they viewed as primary determinants of behavior and behavior change. The following eight variables and client conditions or states required for change were identified[43]:

1. Intention: The person has made a commitment to perform the behavior.
2. Environmental constraints: No external conditions or circumstances exist that make it impossible for the behavior to occur.
3. Ability: The person has the skills necessary to perform the behavior.
4. Anticipated outcomes: The person believes that the advantages (benefits) of performing the behavior outweigh the disadvantages (costs); the person has a positive attitude toward performing the behavior.
5. Norms: The person perceives more social pressure to perform the behavior than not perform the behavior.
6. Self-standards: The person perceives performance of the behavior as more consistent than inconsistent with his or her self-image.
7. Emotion: The person's emotional reaction to performing the behavior is more positive than negative.
8. Self-efficacy: The person perceives that he or she has the capabilities for performing the behavior under a number of different circumstances.

Although this list of variables can be instructive for structuring interventions using concepts from various theories as building blocks, new models or theories are needed that combine potentially powerful variables from diverse theories into integrated and coherent frameworks on which interventions to change behavior can be based. For example, relapse prevention, self-efficacy, and the transtheoretical model (stages of change) have been combined by some investigators focusing on smoking cessation.[44] Further, the "net" should be cast much wider than it has been to date to identify theories and concepts relevant to health behavior. The preponderance of theories have come from psychology and public health. Other theoretical perspectives such as that of nursing, social work, sociology, anthropology, political science, and the biologic sciences should be examined and tested to determine their potential usefulness. Moving to the next step in generation of knowledge about factors influencing health behavior change will require creative interdisciplinary research and theory building.

• DIRECTIONS FOR RESEARCH IN HEALTH BEHAVIOR

Attention has increasingly focused on the redundancies and similarities across existing theories. Weinstein has proposed that a number of concepts in existing models have the same underlying meaning and are measured by questions that are indistinguishable from one theory to another.[45] Questions that need to be addressed include:

1. What are the differences and similarities between perceptions of self-efficacy (social cognitive theory) and behavioral control (TPB)?
2. How does response efficacy (health-protection theory) differ from perceived benefits (HBM)?
3. Are perceived benefits and barriers to preventive action (HBM) conceptually similar to attitudes (TRA)?
4. What are the conceptual differences, if any, between intention in the theory of interpersonal behavior and in the TPB?
5. Are social influences (theory of interpersonal behavior) the same as normative beliefs (TPB)?

Have theories progressively expanded our understanding of human health behavior to date through introducing new concepts or integrating existing concepts in new ways or has redundancy in concepts across theories retarded progress? Needed is research that looks at the intercorrelations among measures of similar concepts from several theories to address the redundancy issue. Furthermore, there is a need for studies that move beyond testing one theory to examining the predictive validity and intervention utility of combining several theories.[45(pp329–332)]

Another important issue that must be addressed is whether extant theories have relevance across genders and across cultures that vary in race, ethnicity, and other dimensions. It is likely that across cultures there will be equivalency for some theories and concepts and lack of equivalency for others. Determination of cultural relevancy and equivalency is important when concepts and instruments that have been developed and normed primarily on a homogeneous population are used, rather than those developed with diverse populations of study. Further, in developing new instruments, a culturally grounded approach is recommended to see where there are conceptual points of cultural convergence and divergence. Cultural sensitivity and cultural competence must characterize health-promotion and health-protection research if it is to make a difference in the health experiences of individuals, families, and communities from diverse settings and life circumstances. Collaboration among "communities of interest" and health professionals is essential to shape emerging science with the cultural relevance needed for developing meaningful and effective health-protection and health-promotion interventions.

• SUMMARY

This chapter has presented an overview of a number of models and theories relevant to health behavior and health behavior change. An attempt has been made where adequate data exist to indicate the strength of predictive variables from the various theories and models. Models relevant primarily to health protection and models and theories relevant to both health protection and health promotion have been presented. With advances in information technology, the future effectiveness of interventions may not depend on adopting one entire model rather than another but on identifying the constellation of critical determinants across models for a given individual for a particular health behavior and tailoring the intervention to target those specific variables. Continuing attempts should be made to develop integrated theories that incorporate a wider range of powerful explanatory and predictive variables as a basis for highly effective health promotion and risk-reduction interventions.

REFERENCES

1. Jessor R, Jessor SL. *Problem Behavior and Psychosocial Development: A Longitudinal Study of Youth.* New York, NY: Academic Press Inc; 1977.
2. Lipsitt LP, Mitnick LL, eds. *Self-regulatory Behavior and Risk-Taking: Causes and Consequences.* Norwood, NJ: Ablex Publishing Corp; 1991.
3. Yates JF, ed. *Risk-Taking Behavior.* New York, NY: John Wiley & Sons; 1992.
4. Pender NJ. *Health Promotion in Nursing Practice.* 2nd ed. Norwalk, Conn: Appleton & Lange; 1987.
5. Shamansky SL, Clausen CL. Levels of prevention: examination of the concept. *Nurs Outlook.* 1980;28:104–108.
6. Rosenstock IM. Why people use health services. *Milbank Mem Fund Q.* 1966;44:94–127.
7. Lewin K, Dembo T, Festinger L, et al. Level of aspiration. In: Hunt J, ed. *Personality and the Behavioral Disorders: A Handbook Based on Experimental and Clinical Research.* New York, NY: Ronald Press; 1944:333–378.
8. Davidhizar R. Critique of the health belief model. *J Adv Nurs.* 1983;8:467–472.
9. Janz NK, Becker MH. The health belief model: a decade later. *Health Educ Q.* 1984;11(1):1–47.
10. Rosenstock IM, Strecher VJ, Becker MH. Social learning theory and the Health Belief Model. *Health Educ Q.* 1988;15(2):175–183.
11. Burns AC. The expanded health belief model as a basis for enlightened preventive health care practice and research. *J Health Care Market.* 1992;12(3):32–45.
12. Rogers RW. A protection motivation theory of fear appeals and attitude change. *J Psychol.* 1975;91:93–114.
13. Maddux JE, Rogers RW. Protection motivation and self-efficacy: a revised theory of fear appeals and attitude change. *J Exp Soc Psychol.* 1983;19:469–479.
14. Wurtele SK, Maddux JE. Relative contributions of protection motivation theory components in predicting exercise intentions and behavior. *Health Psychol.* 1987;6:453–466.
15. Fruin DJ, Pratt C, Owen N. Protection motivation theory and adolescents' perceptions of exercise. *J Appl Soc Psychol.* 1991;22:55–69.
16. Job RFS. Effective and ineffective use of fear in health promotion campaigns. *Am J Public Health.* 1988;78:163–167.
17. Fishbein M, Ajzen I. *Belief, Attitude, Intention and Behavior: An Introduction to Theory and Research.* Reading, Mass: Addison-Wesley Publishing Co Inc; 1975.
18. Ajzen I. From intentions to actions: a theory of planned behavior. In: Kuhl J, Beckmann J, eds. *Action - control: From cognition to behavior.* Heidelberg, Germany: Springer Verlag; 1985:11–39.
19. Ajzen I. *Attitudes, Personality, and Behavior.* Chicago, Ill: Dorsey Press; 1988.
20. Brubaker RG, Wickerman D. Encouraging the practice of testicular self-examination: a field application of the theory of reasoned action. *Health Psychol.* 1990;9(2):154–163.
21. Bandura A. *Social Foundations of Thought and Action: A Social Cognitive Theory.* Englewood Cliffs, NJ: Prentice-Hall Inc; 1986.
22. Schwarzer R, ed. *Self-efficacy: Thought Control of Action.* Washington, DC: Hemisphere Publishing Corp.; 1992.

23. McAuley E, Jacobson L. Self-efficacy and exercise participation in sedentary adult females. *Am J Health Prom.* 5(3), 1991, 185–191.
24. Duncan TE, McAuley E. Social support and efficacy cognitions in exercise adherence: a latent growth curve analysis. *J Behav Med* 1993;16(2):199–218.
25. Seydel E, Taal E, Wiegman O. Risk-appraisal, outcome and self-efficacy expectancies: cognitive factors in preventive behavior related to cancer. *Psychol Health.* 1990;4:99–109.
26. McKusick L, Coates TJ, Morin SF, et al. Longitudinal predictors of reductions in unprotected anal intercourse among gay men in San Francisco: the AIDS behavioral research project. *Am J Public Health.* 1990;80:978–983.
27. Kok G, DeVries H, Mudde AN, et al. Planned health education and the role of self-efficacy: Dutch research. *Health Educ Res.* 6(2):1991;231–238.
28. Wiedenfeld SA, O'Leary A, Bandura A, et al. Impact of perceived self-efficacy in coping with stressors on components of the immune system. *J Pers Soc Psychol.* 1990;59:1082–1094.
29. Triandis HC. *Interpersonal Behavior Theory.* Monterey, Calif: Brooks/Cole Publishing Co; 1977.
30. Facione NC. The Triandis model for the study of health and illness behavior: a social behavior theory with sensitivity to diversity. *Adv Nurs Sci.* 1993;15(3):49–58.
31. Godin G. Social-cognitive theories. In: Dishman RK, ed. *Advances in Exercise Adherence.* Champaign, Ill: Human Kinetics; 1994:123.
32. Deci EL, Ryan RM. *Intrinsic Motivation and Self-Determination in Human Behavior.* New York, NY: Plenum Press, 1985.
33. Cox C. An interaction model of client health behavior: theoretical prescription for nursing. *Adv Nurs Sci.* 1982;5:41–56.
34. Cox C. The health self-determinism index. *Nurs Res.* 1985;34(3):177–183.
35. Cox CL, Cowell JM, Marion LN, et al. The health self-determinism index for children. *Res Nurs Health.* 1990;13(4):237–246.
36. Cox CL, Miller EH, Mull CS. Motivation in health behavior: measurement, antecedents and correlates. *Adv Nurs Sci.* 1987;9(4):1–15.
37. Cox CL, Sullivan JA, Roghmann KL. A conceptual explanation of risk-reduction behavior and intervention development. *Nurs Res.* 1984;33(3):168–173.
38. Cox CL, Roghmann KJ. Empirical test of the interaction model of client health behavior. *Res Nurs Health.* 1984;7(4):275–285.
39. Troumbley PF, Lenz ER. Application of Cox's interaction model of client health behavior in a weight control program for military personnel: a preintervention baseline. *Adv Nurs Sci.* 1992;14(4):65–78.
40. Farrand LL, Cox CL. Determinants of positive health behavior in middle childhood. *Nurs Res.* 1993;42(4):208–213.
41. Marlatt GA, Gordon JR. *Relapse Prevention: Maintenance Strategies in the Treatment of Addictive Behaviors.* New York, NY: Guilford Press; 1985.
42. Brownell KD, Marlatt GA, Lichtenstein E, et al. Understanding and preventing relapse. *Am Psychol.* 1986;41:765–782.
43. Fishbein M, Bandura A, Triandis HC, et al. Factors influencing behavior and behavior change: final report of theorist's workshop on AIDS-related behaviors. Washington, DC: October 3-5, 1991. National Institute of Mental Health, National Institutes of Health.
44. Velicer WF, DiClemente CD, Rossi JS, et al. Relapse situations and self-efficacy: an integrative model. *Addict Behav.* 1990;15:271–283.
45. Weinstein ND. Testing four competing theories of health-protective behavior. *Health Psychol.* 1993;12:324–333.

3

The Health Promotion Model

- The Theoretical Basis for the Health Promotion Model
  - A. Expectancy-Value Theory
  - B. Social Cognitive Theory
- Assumptions of the Health Promotion Model
- Tests of the Health Promotion Model
  - A. Explaining and Predicting Health-Promoting Lifestyles
  - B. Explaining and Predicting Exercise Behavior
  - C. Predicting Use of Hearing Protection
- Implications of Research Findings
- The Revised Health-Promotion Model
  - A. Individual Characteristics and Experiences
  - B. Behavior-Specific Cognitions and Affect
  - C. Behavioral Outcome
- Directions for Research
- Summary

In the early 1980s, the Health Promotion Model (HPM) first appeared in nursing literature. It was proposed as a framework for integrating nursing and behavioral science perspectives on factors influencing health behaviors. The framework was offered as a guide for exploration of the complex biopsychosocial processes that motivate individuals to engage in behaviors directed toward the enhancement of health.[1] The term "health behavior" was being used with increasing frequency in health literature and there was renewed interest in earlier work by Dunn[2,3] on high-level wellness and related behavior that was motivated by a desire to promote personal health and well-being in the absence of illness.

In the late 1980s, public attention to health promotion continued to escalate and people were intrigued by the idea of health as a positive state. Still, little was understood about what motivated people to seek to express their health potential. In 1987, the HPM, with minor revisions, appeared in the second edition of this book.[4] That version of the model is shown in Figure 3–1. It stimulated a number of studies to determine the power of its component constructs to explain and predict health behaviors. The studies reported here test this version of the model.

The HPM is a competence- or approach-oriented model. Unlike the Health Belief Model and Protection Motivation Theory described in the previous chapter, the HPM does not include "fear" or "threat" as sources of motivation for health behavior. Although immediate threats to health have been shown to motivate action, threats in the distant future lack the same motivational strength. Thus, avoidance-oriented models of health be-

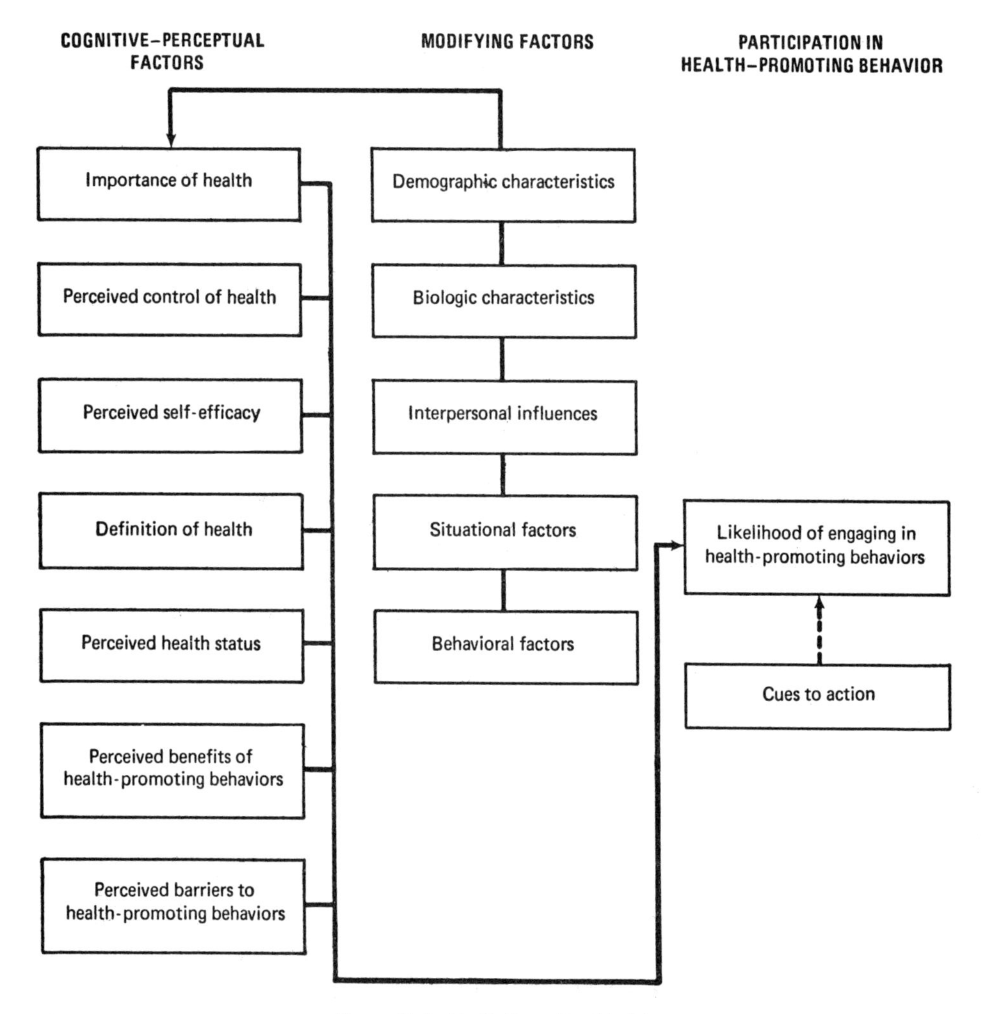

Figure 3–1. Health Promotion Model.

havior are of limited usefulness in motivating overall healthy lifestyles in people in youth and early adulthood as well as in other individuals who for varying reasons perceive themselves to be invulnerable to illness. Because the HPM does not rely on "personal threat" as a primary source of health motivation, it is a model with potential applicability across the life span. In reality, the sources of health behavior motivation for any given individual have unique combinational properties, from predominantly health-promotion or approach-oriented motives, through mixed motives of both approach *and* avoidance, to predominantly avoidance-oriented or protective motives. The HPM is applicable to any health behavior in which "threat" is not proposed as a major source of motivation for the behavior.

• THE THEORETICAL BASIS FOR THE HEALTH PROMOTION MODEL

The HPM is an attempt to depict the multidimensional nature of persons interacting with their environment as they pursue health. The model integrates a number of constructs from expectancy-value theory and social learning theory (now renamed social cognitive theory), within a nursing perspective of holistic human functioning. Expectancy-value theory and social cognitive theory will be briefly described here.

Expectancy-Value Theory

Many conceptions of goal-directed behavior, including social cognitive theory, are based on the expectancy-value model of human motivation described by Feather.[5] According to the expectancy-value model, behavior is rational and economical. Specifically, a person will engage in a given action and will persist in it to the extent that (a) the outcome of taking action is of positive personal value, and (b) based on available information, taking this course of action is likely to bring about the desired outcome. Thus, individuals will not invest their effort and personal resources in working toward goals that are of little or no value to them. Furthermore, most individuals will not invest their efforts in goals that, despite their attractiveness, are perceived as impossible to achieve. Personal change can best be understood within this theoretical framework by considering the subjective value of the change and the subjective expectancy of achieving it.[6] The motivational significance of the **subjective value of change** is based on the supposition that the more a person is dissatisfied with his or her present situation in a particular domain, the greater will be the rewards or benefits associated with favorable change. This subjective value of change can be viewed as comparable to the perceived benefits of engaging in a given health behavior. The motivational significance of the **subjective expectancy of successfully obtaining the change** or outcome is based on prior knowledge of personal successes or the successes of others in attaining the outcome and the personal confidence that one's success will be the same or even superior to others.[6] This concept is similar to the concept of self-efficacy in social cognitive theory.

Social Cognitive Theory

Social cognitive theory presents an interactional model of causation in which environmental events, personal factors, and behavior act as reciprocal determinants of each other.

The theory places major emphasis on self-direction, self-regulation, and perceptions of self-efficacy. Social cognitive theory, proposes that human beings possess the following basic capabilities[7]:

1. Symbolization: processing and transforming transient experiences into internal models that serve as guides for future action
2. Forethought: anticipating likely consequences of prospective actions and planning future courses of action to achieve valued goals
3. Vicarious learning: acquiring rules for the generation and regulation of behavior through observation without the need to engage in extensive trial and error
4. Self-regulation: using internal standards and self-evaluative reactions as a means to motivate and regulate behavior; arranging the external environment to create incentives for action
5. Self-reflection: thinking about one's own thought processes and actively modifying them

Given these basic capabilities, behavior is neither solely driven by inner forces nor automatically shaped by external stimuli. Instead, cognitions and other personal factors, behavior, and environmental events are interactive. Behavior can modify cognitions and other personal factors as well as change the environment. On the other hand, the environment can augment or constrain behavior. This dynamic interactional causality provides a rich array of human possibilities.[8]

According to social cognitive theory, self beliefs formed through self-observation and self-reflective thought powerfully influence human functioning. These self beliefs include: self-attribution, self-evaluation, and self-efficacy. Beliefs concerning self-efficacy are particularly important. Perceived self-efficacy is a judgment of one's ability to carry out a particular course of action. Perceptions of self-efficacy develop through mastery experiences, vicarious learning, verbal persuasion, and somatic responses to particular situations. Marked overestimation of competencies can result in failure and marked underestimation can result in lack of challenge and resultant growth. Efficacy judgments that appear to be most functional are those that slightly exceed present capabilities. Such judgments facilitate undertaking realistically demanding tasks that build competencies and confidence. The greater the perceived efficacy, the more vigorous and persistent individuals will be to engage in a behavior, even in the face of obstacles and aversive experiences. Self-efficacy is a central construct in the HPM. For a comprehensive description of social cognitive theory, the reader is referred to the book, *Social Foundations of Thought and Action*, by Albert Bandura.[7(pp393–401)]

• ASSUMPTIONS OF THE HEALTH PROMOTION MODEL

The HPM is based on the following assumptions, which reflect both nursing and behavioral science perspectives:

1. Persons seek to create conditions of living through which they can express their unique human health potential.

2. Persons have the capacity for reflective self-awareness, including assessment of their own competencies.
3. Persons value growth in directions viewed as positive and attempt to achieve a personally acceptable balance between change and stability.
4. Individuals seek to actively regulate their own behavior.
5. Individuals in all their biopsychosocial complexity interact with the environment, progressively transforming the environment and being transformed over time.
6. Health professionals constitute a part of the interpersonal environment, which exerts influence on persons throughout their life span.
7. Self-initiated reconfiguration of person-environment interactive patterns is essential to behavior change.

These assumptions emphasize the **active role** of the client in shaping and maintaining health behaviors and in modifying the environmental context for health behaviors.

• TESTS OF THE HEALTH PROMOTION MODEL

The HPM as depicted in Figure 3–1 has been used as a framework for research aimed at predicting overall health-promoting lifestyles as well as specific behaviors, such as exercise and use of hearing protection. In some of the studies, a small set of variables has been selected from the model to test as predictors of a given behavior. Other studies have tested the majority of variables in the model. A number of these studies that have been published as articles or government reports are presented here. It is beyond the scope of this chapter to review the many theses and dissertations that have been based on the HPM.

Explaining and Predicting Health-Promoting Lifestyles

Achieving a healthy lifestyle in major behavioral domains should be the goal of individuals of all ages. In order for nurses to assist clients in accomplishing this, determinants of healthy lifestyles need to be identified.

Health-Promoting Lifestyles of Blue-Collar Workers

Race and ethnicity are viewed as powerful influences on health behaviors. Increasingly in the United States, information is becoming available not only on the morbidity and mortality experiences of racial and ethnic groups but on their risk behaviors and health behaviors. Weitzel[9] in a study of a multicultural population of 179 European-American (51%), Hispanic (27%) and African-American (20%) blue-collar workers examined the prediction of a health-promoting lifestyle using the HPM. Specifically, four of seven cognitive-perceptual variables were tested: importance of health, perceived control of health, perceived self-efficacy, and perceived health status. Modifying factors studied were the demographics of gender, age, education, and income. All variables were assessed by questionnaire.

Both total and subscale scores on the Health-Promoting Lifestyle Profile (HPLP)[10] were regressed on the cognitive-perceptual factors and modifying factors. All of the cognitive-perceptual variables examined were predictive of one or more health-promoting behaviors. Health status, self-efficacy, importance of health, and education were the stongest predictors of total HPLP scores, explaining 20% of the variance. Of the HPLP subscales, the model best predicted nutrition behaviors, with 28% of the variance explained.

Pender and her colleagues conducted a research program funded by the National Center for Nursing Research (now the National Institute of Nursing Research), National Institutes of Health, to evaluate the HPM in four different populations: working adults; older, community-dwelling adults; ambulatory cancer patients; and cardiac rehabilitation patients.[11] The following brief descriptions report the major findings of their work.

Health-Promoting Lifestyle of Worksite Fitness Program Participants

Workplace health-promotion programs have emerged as a prominent component of employer-sponsored health care benefits primarily in response to increasing evidence that lifestyle can positively influence health status. Although many employees initially enroll in workplace health-promotion efforts, the problems of erratic participation and dropouts plague many programs. In this study, researchers evaluated the HPM's explanatory potential for health-promoting lifestyles in a sample of 589 employees enrolled in six employer-sponsored corporate health promotion programs in a large metropolitan area. All cognitive-perceptual factors in the HPM except benefits and barriers were measured in the study. In terms of modifying factors, selected demographic characteristics and the behavioral factor of stage of exercise (acquisition or maintenance) were also measured. Data were collected using questionnaires and the daily exercise records maintained by all the participating fitness programs.

When the data were analyzed using multiple regression analysis, 31% of the variance in current health-promoting lifestyle patterns was explained with personal competence (a proxy for self-efficacy in relation to overall lifestyle), definition of health, health status, control of health, gender, age, and the behavioral factor of stage of exercise being significant explanatory factors.[12]

Causal path modeling using LISREL, a computer program for structural equation analysis, revealed that the majority of indirect and direct paths proposed in the model were significant. However, the demographic characteristics of age and gender had significant direct paths as well as significant indirect paths to health-promoting lifestyles. The direct paths from the modifying factors to health-promoting behavior were not consistent with the HPM suggesting a possible need for modifications in the model.

Health-Promoting Lifestyles Among Community-Dwelling Older Adults

Healthy aging is highly dependent on acceptance of responsibility for initiating and maintaining healthy lifestyles by individuals themselves. Although older adults report a high level of interest in what they can do to promote their own health, only recently have elderly Americans been included in health-promotion programming and research efforts. The purpose of this study was to test the usefulness of selected variables from the HPM (definition of health, importance of health, control of health, perceived health status, and selected demographics) in explaining the frequency of health-promoting lifestyle behaviors among 361 community-dwelling older adults (55 years or above) as well as in predicting health-promoting lifestyles at a later point in time. Quota sampling was used to achieve representation across age ranges. Subjects were recruited from various community settings in a midwestern state. Questionnaire booklets were used for data collection.

Hierarchic multiple regression analysis revealed that the selected cognitive-perceptual and modifying factors from the HPM explained 28% of the variance in lifestyle with definition of health, control of health, gender, and age making statistically significant contributions to the regression equation. Self-motivation, an added exploratory personal characteristic, contributed an additional 6% explained variance for a total explained variance of 34%. This suggests that individual characteristics other than demographics should be considered as potential determinants of health behaviors. The same set of variables predicted 29% of the variance in lifestyle 12 months later. Structural equation modeling using LISREL revealed that only some of the indirect and direct paths proposed in the model were significant. Age had no significant direct paths to any of the cognitive-perceptual variables and gender and socioeconomic status had significant direct paths, as well as the hypothesized indirect paths to health-promoting lifestyle. Perceived health status did not have a significant direct path to health-promoting lifestyle. Thus, some proposed paths were supported, others were not.

Health-Promoting Lifestyles of Cardiac Rehabilitation Program Participants

Cardiac rehabilitation programs began in the 1960s when prescriptions for physical activity and exercise replaced recommendations for long-term rest after myocardial infarction. Many programs now include numerous activities directed toward fostering healthy lifestyles. The purpose of this study was to determine the usefulness of the HPM in explaining the occurrence of health-promoting lifestyles among cardiac rehabilitation participants and predicting lifestyle at a later time. Participants were recruited from individuals enrolled in fifteen Phase II and Phase III cardiac rehabilitation programs in a midwestern state. Each participant identified his or her significant other, who was also invited to participate. Of the volunteer participant–significant-other pairs, 576 pairs, predominantly European-Americans, provided complete data for this study. Participants ranged in age from 30 to 84 years of age. Data were collected using questionnaire booklets.

Hierarchic multiple regression was conducted with four of seven HPM cognitive-perceptual variables (importance of health, control of health, definition of health, and health status), demographic characteristics, interpersonal influences, and behavioral factors entered into the regression. Self-motivation, an individual characteristic not in the HPM, was entered on an experimental basis. Cognitive-perceptual and modifying factors explained 21% of the variance in lifestyle, with self-motivation contributing an additional 6% explained variance. Significant HPM predictors for lifestyle scores were definition of health, control of health, demographics (age, education, gender), interpersonal influences (lifestyle of significant other), and behavioral factors (phase of cardiac rehabilitation). This total set of variables predicted 25% of the variance in health-promoting lifestyle 3 months later. In structural equation modeling using LISREL, only some of the hypothesized direct and indirect paths were supported. The modifying factors of age and socioeconomic status had direct paths to lifestyle as well as the hypothesized indirect paths.

Perceived control of health did not have a direct path to lifestyle. This study raised a question concerning the appropriateness of the model for predicting health-related lifestyles among cardiac rehabilitation populations. Although some cardiac rehabilitation patients report a shift in their motivation from fearing recurrence of a coronary event to desire to optimize their personal health, it is possible that disease avoidance still remains a major motivational dynamic underlying health behaviors for these clients. If so, "avoidance models" or a "mixed model" might provide a better framework for explaining and predicting variance in the lifestyle of this group as well as that of other groups in whom a recent occurrence of catastrophic illness may make avoidance motives predominant.

Health-Promoting Lifestyles Among Ambulatory Cancer Patients

Cancer is now routinely treated in the community as people maintain their lifestyles during therapy. Cancer self-help groups that place emphasis on health promotion and wellness also exist throughout the nation. Thus, health professionals should place primary emphasis on working with cancer patients to foster healthy lifestyles and augment their mental and physical well-being. This study tested the HPM as a model to explain and predict the occurrence of health-promoting lifestyles among 385 ambulatory cancer patients receiving chemotherapy and radiation in outpatient settings. The cancer patients were selected from those undergoing treatment in 13 clinical sites in the midwestern United States. HPM variables tested in the study were importance of health, control of health, health definition, health status, and selected demographics. Data were collected via questionnaire.

Multiple regression revealed that 24% of the variance in health-promoting lifestyle was explained by the HPM cognitive-perceptual variables of perceived control of health, definition of health, and perceived health status, and the modifying factors of education, income, age, and employment. All of these variables made significant but modest contributions to the explained variance. Importance of health was not associated with a health promoting lifestyle.[13] Using structural equation modeling, a number of hypothesized indirect and direct paths were significant. However, age and socioeconomic status both had significant direct paths to health-promoting lifestyle. This was inconsistent with the proposed indirect relationships in the HPM.

Health-Promoting Lifestyles of Participants in the National Survey of Personal Health Practices and Consequences 1979–1980

Johnson et al[14] attempted to evaluate the HPM using secondary analysis on data from 1290 respondents to the National Survey of Personal Health Practices and Consequences 1979–1980, a telephone survey of 3025 individuals between the ages of 20 to 64. Only one to two items from the survey, rather than well-established scales, were used as indicators of each of the HPM variables: control of health, self-efficacy, and perceived health status. Modifying variables of demographics (gender, age, income, marital status, and education) and biologic characteristics (body mass index) were also included in the analysis. Proxy measures of one to three items were selected for five of the six proposed dimensions of a health-promoting lifestyle. These proxy items were not aggregated as a measure of overall health-promoting lifestyle, nor did they capture the multiple dimensions of each lifestyle domain.

Using structural equation analysis (LISREL), all modifying variables were found to have direct paths as well, as the HPM hypothesized indirect paths to the proxy measures of health-promoting behaviors. Three of seven cognitive-perceptual variables and two of five modifying variables were tested. This limited set of variables predicted 5.3% to 12.6% of the variance in the proposed proxy measures of single HPLP subscales. Study findings agree with results of a number of studies that indicate the need to build into the model "direct" effects of the proposed modifying factors on health behavior. The questionable validity and reliability of the cognitive-perceptual and outcome measures used may well have contributed to the extremely low explained variance observed.

Explaining and Predicting Exercise Behavior

Pender and colleagues conducted a series of studies within the same National Institute of Nursing Research (NINR) funded research program to determine if the HPM was useful in explaining or predicting the specific behavior of exercise. These studies are summarized below.

Exercise Among Worksite Fitness Program Participants

The HPM was used as the conceptual framework for exploring the frequency of exercise among 539 predominantly European-American working adults participating in corporate fitness programs in six midwest corporations. All model variables except cues to action were measured in the study. The study participants were divided into two groups by exercise stage, acquisition (N = 208) and maintenance (N = 331). In the first stage of data analysis, hierarchic multiple regression was used, with 3-month exercise frequency regressed on cognitive-perceptual variables entered first and modifying variables entered last. In the acquisition group, 22% of the variance in exercise was explained with exercise efficacy, benefits, and the modifying behavioral factor of prior exercise behavior (measured by a single, self-report item) being significant. In the maintenance group, 21% of the variance in exercise was explained with perceived control of **physical fitness,** exercise efficacy, barriers, control of health, and prior exercise behavior being significant. The acquisition and maintenance groups were combined, and structural equation analysis using LISREL was performed on the data. As predicted, the modifying variables of gender and socioeconomic status had only significant indirect paths to exercise.

Next, actual fitness center exercise records for the previous month (rather than a single, self-report item) were used to measure prior exercise behavior. With refinement in the measure of prior exercise behavior, HPM variables predicted 59% of the variance in exercise frequency. This major increase in variance explained should caution researchers concerning use of single items to measure model variables. Barriers, personal competence (general self-efficacy measure), age, and prior exercise behavior were significant direct predictors, with prior exercise being the most powerful (manuscript submitted for publication). These findings support the existence of a direct **"habit"** effect on exercise rather than the proposed indirect effect of behavioral factors as proposed in the HBM.

Exercise Patterns of Community-Dwelling Older Adults

This study was conducted to determine the extent to which the HPM would explain exercise adherence among older adults in the community. A total of 361 adults aged 55 and over were recruited from urban, suburban, and rural communities in a midwestern state. Study participants had to be ambulatory without assistive devices and able to participate in a program of exercise. Most were of European-American descent. Six cognitive-perceptual factors (importance of health, perceived control of health, definition of health, health status, benefits, and barriers to exercise) were assessed by questionnaire. Self-motivation and preferred level of exertion, not in the HPM, were included as exploratory variables. Modifying factors of demographic and biologic characteristics and behavioral factors were also assessed. Exercise was measured by the exercise subscale of the HPLP. In hierarchic multiple regression analysis, exercise scores were regressed on both cognitive-perceptual variables and modifying variables. The selected HPM variables explained 24% of the variance in exercise. Self-motivation and preferred exertion added an additional 10%. Preferred exertion could be interpreted as an indirect measure of the biologic characteristic of energy reserve for older adults and thus legitimately included as a modifying factor.

Structural equation analysis using LISREL was performed on the data. Benefits and barriers had significant direct paths to exercise but control of health, health status, and definition of health did not.

Exercise Behavior of Cardiac Rehabilitation Program Participants

The purpose of this study was to determine the usefulness of the HPM in explaining the frequency of exercise behaviors among cardiac rehabilitation program participants. Study volunteers were recruited from individuals enrolled in 15 Phase II and Phase III cardiac rehabilitation programs in a midwestern state. The 511 cardiac rehabilitation patients who agreed to participate ranged in age from 31 to 84 years and were predominantly European-American. All variables were measured by questionnaires. All HPM variables were measured except situational factors and cues to action. Exercise frequency was measured over a 12-week period by cardiac rehabilitation program attendance and by the exercise subscale of the HPLP. The significant other's exercise behavior was measured as an indication of interpersonal influence (modeling).

Components of the HPM explained 23% of the variance in exercise behavior measured by the HPLP exercise subscale and 20% when measured by high or low cardiac program attendance. Exercise efficacy, barriers to exercise, importance of health, and phase of exercise had significant beta weights. Structural equation analysis using LISREL revealed that as hypothesized, gender and socioeconomic status has only indirect effects on exercise. However, the direct effects of perceived control of health, perceived health status, and definition of health were not supported.

Exercise Patterns of Ambulatory Cancer Patients

A focus on "wellness" or health promotion rather than on illness has progressively occurred during the last decade among people with cancer. This has been the result of changes in survival, improvement in cancer treatments, and changes in the settings where cancer treatments are delivered. Exercise is one recognized component of healthy lifestyle among cancer patients. Patients who have been sedentary may actually begin exercising during the period of therapy. The purpose of this study was to test the usefulness of the HPM in explaining the occurrence of reported exercise behavior among ambulatory cancer patients receiving chemotherapy and radiation in outpatient settings. Predictor variables were measured by questionnaire administered to 385 predominantly European-American patients undergoing treatment for their disease in 13 clinical sites in the midwestern United States. Two measures of exercise behavior were used, the exercise subscale of the HPLP and the health diary or daily record of health-related events that the individual filled out each day for a month's period of time.

Using hierarchic multiple regression, the exercise subscale of the HPLP was regressed on the cognitive-perceptual factors of importance of health, control of health, definition of health, health status, benefits, and barriers as well as the modifying variables of demographic characteristics (marital status, employment, gender, education, age, and income) and reaction to diagnosis as an additional cancer-specific variable. Cognitive-perceptual variables from the HPM combined to explain 42% of the variance in exercise with modifying factors and reaction to the diagnosis explaining negligible variance. Benefits and barriers alone explained 38% of the variance in exercise. Perceived health status was the only other HPM factor with a significant beta weight in the regression. The direct and indirect paths among the HPM variables were explored using structural equation analysis (LISREL). Both gender and socioeconomic status had the HPM-proposed indirect paths to exercise. However, the HPM-proposed direct paths of perceived control of health and definition of health to exercise were not supported.

Adolescents' Exercise Beliefs and Prediction of Their Exercise Behavior

A team of scientists at the University of Michigan Child/Adolescent Health Behavior Research Center, funded by the NINR, are exploring the determinants of health behaviors and risk behaviors among preadolescents and adolescents. The HPM provides the organizing framework for several of these studies.

Garcia and colleagues[15] examined gender and developmental differences in exercise-related beliefs and exercise behaviors of 286 racially diverse youth: 30% African-Americans, 63% European-Americans, and 7% of other racial heritage. It is well known that physical activity declines almost 50% during adolescence, with females becoming increasingly more sedentary than males. The HPM provided the basis for the model of exercise prediction tested in this study. Those fifth-, sixth-, and eighth-grade students who had parental consent and assented to participate completed the questionnaire designed to assess model variables. The HPM variables assessed were perceived health status, previous exercise, exercise benefits and barriers, exercise self-efficacy, interpersonal influences (exercise models, norms, and social support), and situational influences (sedentary time, and access to facilities and programs). The modifying factors of gender, grade, and race were also assessed. Eight weeks later, students completed an exercise log for 7 consecutive days. They completed the logs at school for the previous day.

Regression analysis revealed that only 19% of the variance in exercise was explained. Although low, this is comparable to the amount of explained variance found in many other adolescent exercise studies. Significant predictors of exercise were gender, the exercise benefits and barriers differential, and access to facilities and programs. Previous exercise came close but failed to reach significance. Surprisingly in an adolescent population, self-efficacy did not directly predict exercise behavior. An exploratory path analysis revealed that the effects of grade, perceived health status, self-efficacy, social support for exercise, and exercise norms indirectly affected exercise through the exercise benefits and barriers differential.

Predicting Use of Hearing Protection

Repetitive exposure to high noise levels can cause psychologic distress and hearing loss. In the United States, 14 million workers are exposed to hazardous noise where they work.[16] Noise-induced hearing loss can be prevented, but once it has occurred it is irreversible. Occupational health nurses can intervene to reduce hearing loss and its associated medical costs and impaired quality of life by motivating employees to regularly use hearing protection devices. However, to optimize the effectiveness of interventions, it is important for nurses to understand those factors that affect hearing protection practices.[17]

Predicting Use of Hearing Protection Among Factory Workers

Lusk et al[18] tested the HPM as a causal model to predict workers' use of hearing protection devices. This behavior may well represent a mix of both health-protecting and health-promoting motivation. Workers could select personal hearing protection from a variety of earplugs and earmuffs provided by the plant. A convenience sample of 561 workers provided data for the study. The cognitive-perceptual variables of perceived control of health, perceived self-efficacy, definition of health, perceived health status, perceived benefits, and perceived barriers were used as predictors along with the modifying variables of demographic characteristics and situational factors. Use of hearing protection was measured by the workers' self-reports of the percent of time (0% to 100%) they used hearing protection during the past week, the past month, and the past 3 months. Data were analyzed by structural equation modeling. The model implied by the HPM accounted for 49% of the variance in use of hearing protection. Value of use (benefits), barriers, self-efficacy, and health competence were found to have significant direct paths to use of hearing protection. Situational factors (accessibility) and demographic characteristics (gender, age, education, and job category) had significant indirect paths. When exploratory causal modeling including all theoretically specified paths and, in addition, all direct paths from modifying factors was used to examine use of hearing protection, 53% of the variance was explained. Significant predictors of use were self-efficacy, value of use (benefits), perceived barriers, health competence, education, age, gender, and situational factors.

Predicting Use of Hearing Protection Among Construction Workers

Lusk and colleagues used the HPM as a conceptual framework for studying the use of hearing protection among 359 construction workers in the Midwest (unpublished data, 1995). All variables in the model except importance of health, behavioral factors, biologic characteristics, and cues to action were assessed using questionnaires. Use of hearing protection was measured by workers' self-report of percent of time (0% to 100%) that they used hearing protection during the past week, the past month, and the past 3 months in high-noise areas. Structural equation modeling revealed that the path model implied by the HPM fit fairly well, accounting for 36% of the variance in use. Value of use, barriers, self-efficacy, and perceived health status had significant direct paths to use. When an exploratory model was employed, with all predictors having direct paths to use, three of the original predictors (value of use, barriers, and self-efficacy) and two additional ones (interpersonal support for behavior [modeling] and situational influences on behavior [noise exposure]) were found to have significant direct paths to use of protection. This exploratory model with additional direct paths explained over 50% of the variance in use of hearing protection.

Predicting Use of Hearing Protection Among Mexican-American Industrial Workers

Kerr, a member of Lusk's research team, tested the cross-cultural applicability of the HPM in a study that aimed to identify components of the HPM that were most strongly related to use of hearing protection among Mexican-American workers.[19] Mexican-Americans are the largest Hispanic subgroup and fastest growing ethnic and racial minority in the United States, comprising 13.5 million people. Thus, occupational health professionals need to understand the factors influencing the use of hearing protection among Mexican-American workers in order to develop more effective programs to increase use. A sample of 119 workers was recruited from a garment industry in the southwestern United States where Mexican Americans constituted a large portion of the work force. Participants needed to be able to read English, but assistance was provided as needed. Questionnaires and focus group sessions were used for collection of data. The HPM variables included in the study were interpersonal influences (support, norms, models), situational factors, control of health, self-efficacy, definition of health, perceived health status, benefits, value of use, and barriers. Use of hearing protection was measured by the workers self-report of the percent of time (0% to 100%) they actually used hearing protection during the past week, the past month, and the past 3 months when they were in their work areas.

Self-efficacy in the use of hearing protection, a clinical conception (definition) of health, benefits of use of hearing protection, and a higher perceived health status were positively related to use and perceived barriers negatively related to use. A path model consistent with the HPM resulted in explanation of 25% of the variance in use of hearing protection. When a second model was tested allowing direct paths from modifying factors to use of hearing protection, 55% of the variance in use of hearing protection was explained by three variables representing four cognitive-perceptual factors in the model: benefits minus barriers, clinical conception of health, and perceived health. The modifying factor of situational influences (hearing protection requirement and plant site) also contributed to the explained variance.

An overview of all the studies reported in this section of the chapter appears in Table 3–1. The table reports for each study, the population, dependent variable, and independent variables studied. Significant predictor variables are identified and the percent of variance explained reported. Across the various studies, multiple regression analysis, path analysis, and structural equation analysis were the statistical methods employed.

• IMPLICATIONS OF RESEARCH FINDINGS

In the studies conducted to date to test the HPM, 5 to 12 variables have been studied at any given time. None of the reported studies have tested the effects of "cues to action." In the studies in which most of the HPM variables were tested, the variance explained ranged from 19% to 59%. It should be noted that the predictive performance of the HPM

TABLE 3–1. SUMMARY OF FINDINGS FROM STUDIES USING THE HEALTH PROMOTION MODEL

AUTHOR	POPULATION	DEPENDENT VARIABLE	VARIABLES STUDIED	VARIANCE EXPLAINED
Health-Specific Outcome Measures				
Weitzel[9]	Blue-collar workers	Health-promoting lifestyle	1,6,7,8,10	20%
Pender et al[12]	White-collar workers	Health-promoting lifestyle	1,5,6,7,8 9,10	31%
Walker[11]	Community-dwelling older adults	Health-promoting lifestyle	1,6,7,9,10	28%
Sechrist[11]	Cardiac rehabilitation participants	Health-promoting lifestyle	1,3,5,6,7, 9,10	21%
Frank-Strnmborg et al[13]	Ambulatory cancer patients	Health-promoting lifestyle	1,6,7,9,10	24%
ohnson et al[14]	National data sample	Health-promoting lifestyle	1,2,7,8,10 (proxy items used)	Not reported for HPLP total score
Behavior-Specific Outcome Measures				
Exercise				
Pender[11]	White-collar workers	Exercise frequency (acquisition stage)	1,2,3,4,5*, 6,7,8,9,10, 11,12,	22%
		Exercise frequency (maintenance stage)	1,2,3,4,5* 6,7,8,9,10. 11,12,	21%
Pender et al (Unpublished data)	White-collar workers	Exercise frequency (total group with stages combined)	1,2,3,4,5†, 6,7,8,9,10 11,12	59%
Walker[11]	Community-dwelling older adults	Exercise frequency	1,2,5,6,7, 9,10,11,12	24%
Sechrist[11]	Cardiac rehabilitation patients	Exercise frequency	1,2,3,5,6, 7,8,9,10, 11,12	23%
Frank-Stromborg[11]	Ambulatory cancer patients	Exercise frequency	1,6,7,9,10, 11,12	42%
Garcia et al[15]	Preadolescents and adolescents	Exercise frequency and intensity	1,3,4,5,8, 10,11,12	19%
Use of Hearing Protection				
Lusk et al[18]	Factory workers (skilled trades)	Use of hearing protection	1,4,7,8,9, 10,11,12	49%
			(Modifying factors allowed to have direct paths to use)	53%

TABLE 3–1. SUMMARY OF FINDINGS FROM STUDIES USING THE HEALTH PROMOTION MODEL (Continued)

AUTHOR	POPULATION	DEPENDENT VARIABLE	VARIABLES STUDIED	VARIANCE EXPLAINED
Lusk (Unpublished data)	Construction workers	Use of hearing protection	1,3,4,7,8,9, 10,11,12	36%
			(Modifying factors allowed to have direct paths to use)	51%
Kerr[19]	Mexican-American industrial workers	Use of hearing protection	3,4,7,8,9, 10,11,12	25%
			(Modifying factors allowed to have direct paths to use)	55%

KEY 1 = Demographic characteristics
2 = Biologic characteristics
3 = Interpersonal influences
4 = Situational factors
5 = Behavioral factors
6 = Importance of health
7 = Perceived control of health
8 = Perceived self-efficacy
9 = Definition of health
10 = Perceived health status
11 = Perceived benefits
12 = Perceived barriers
13 = Cues to action

Underlined number indicates significant predictor of dependent variable
*Prior exercise measured by self-report on a single item
†Prior exercise measured by fitness center exercise records from previous month

in relation to hearing protection was considerably enhanced when modifying factors were allowed to directly affect the target behavior (36% explained variance increased to 51%; 25% explained variance increased to 55%).

An analysis of the studies reported indicate that the behavior-specific variables of **perceived self-efficacy, benefits** and **barriers** were empirically supported as predictors of health behaviors in the majority of studies in which they were included. Self-efficacy and barriers received the strongest support, with benefits receiving moderate support.

On the other hand, the results of the studies indicate that the health-specific variables need to be reevaluated as to their centrality in predicting health-promoting and protecting behaviors. **Importance of health** failed to explain health behavior in 9 of the 11 studies in which it was included. The reason for lack of explanatory power was clear. Participants in all studies ranked "health" so high as a value in relation to other personal values that without variance, this variable was not useful as a predictor. **Perceived control of health** contributed to the explanation of health-promoting lifestyle in a majority of the studies but by and large did not contribute to the explanation of specific health behaviors. When perceived control of health was a significant predictor, the direction of the relationship was sometimes other than that predicted. This inconsistency of performance has been reported in other studies. **Definition of health** was predictive of health-promoting lifestyle in all the studies reported but was explanatory or predictive in only two of nine studies when specific behaviors were being predicted. **Perceived health**

status was a significant predictor of the target behaviors in a number of studies and was predictive both in those studies of health-promoting lifestyle and in studies of specific behaviors such as exercise and use of hearing protection. However, only limited variance was explained. Thus, perceived health status might best be reinterpreted as a psychological personal factor that can either directly or indirectly affect health behavior when current health status is relevant to performance of a given health action. For example, health status may be relevant to vigorous exercising but not relevant to brushing one's teeth.

Given that the HPM evolved from social learning theory, **interpersonal, situational,** and **behavioral influences** on health behaviors are of high theoretical importance. Significant effects of these variables on health behaviors in a number of the studies reported provide empirical evidence that they should be retained but positioned to have direct as well as indirect effects on health-promoting behavior. Repositioning the above three variables does not violate the theoretical integrity of the model and is consistent with social learning theory, in which the environment (situational and interpersonal influences) and prior behavior (behavioral factors) affect subsequent behavior. Development of rigorous measures of these variables relevant to various health behaviors is needed.

Cues to action are transient stimuli that are difficult to identify and measure reliably. Thus, the utility of this variable in the model can be questioned.

In the revised HPM, importance of health, perceived control of health, and cues to action will be deleted from the model. Definition of health, perceived health status, and demographic and biologic characteristics will be repositioned in the model and included in a category of personal factors from which can be selected variables that are considered relevant influences on a particular health behavior in a given target population. The revised HPM is presented in the next section of this chapter.

• THE REVISED HEALTH-PROMOTION MODEL

The revised HPM appears in Figure 3–2. The variables in the revised HPM and their interrelationships are described below. Three new variables have been added to the model: activity-related affect, commitment to a plan of action, and immediate competing demands and preferences. It is beyond the scope of this chapter to describe approaches to measuring each variable, but information regarding measurement of variables that is not already reported in the literature can be obtained from the author.

Individual Characteristics and Experiences

Each person has unique personal characteristics and experiences that affect subsequent actions. The importance of their effect will depend on the target behavior being considered. The aspects of prior behavior or individual characteristics selected for measurement provide flexibility in the HPM to capture variables that may be highly relevant to a particular health behavior but not to all health behaviors or in a particular target population but not in all populations.

Prior Related Behavior

Behavioral factors have been retained in the HPM as "prior related behavior." Empirical studies indicate that often the best predictor of behavior is the frequency of the same or a

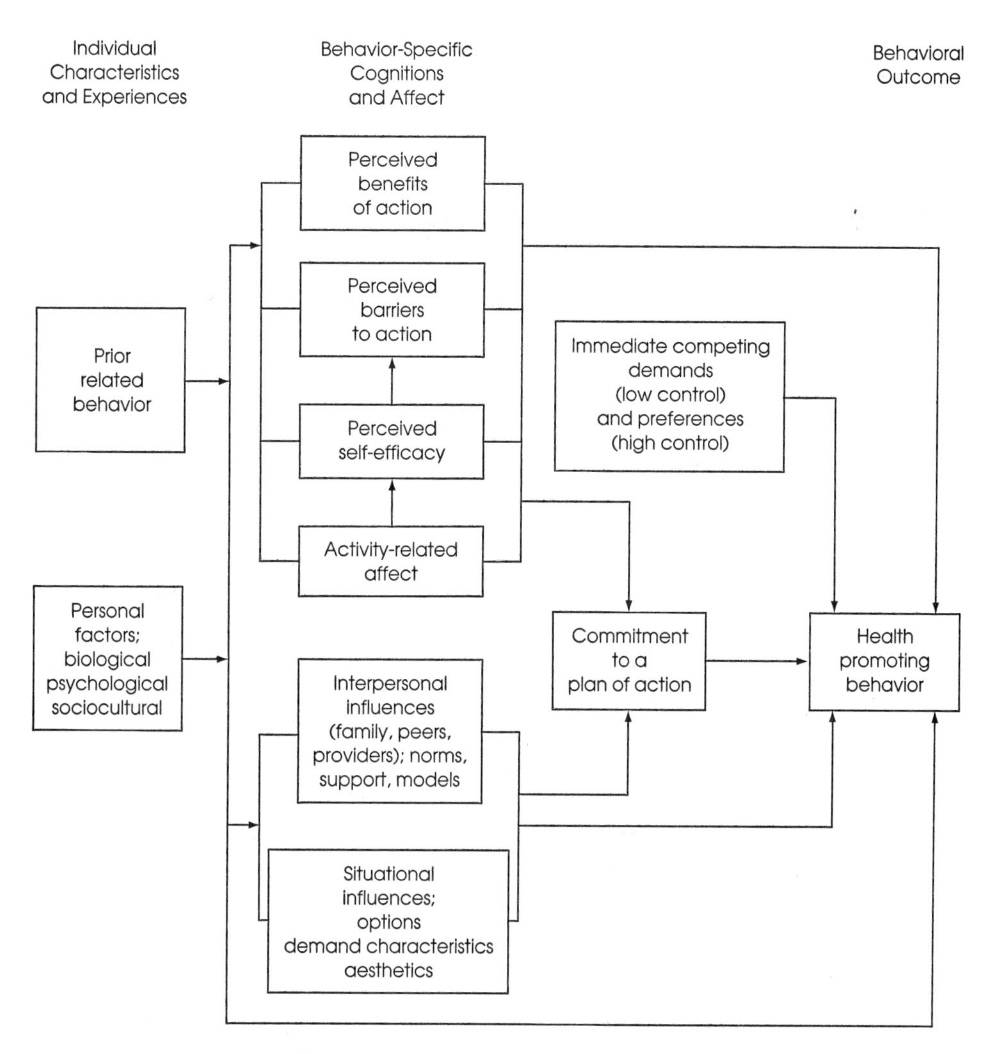

Figure 3–2. Revised Health Promotion Model.

similar behavior in the past. Prior behavior is proposed as having both direct and indirect effects on the likelihood of engaging in health-promoting behaviors. The direct effect of past behavior on current health promoting behavior may be due to habit formation, predisposing one to engage in the behavior automatically, with little attention to the specific details of its execution. Habit strength accrues each time the behavior occurs and is most facilitated by concentrated, repetitive practice of the behavior.

Consistent with social cognitive theory, prior behavior is proposed as also having an indirect influence on health-promoting behavior through perceptions of self-efficacy, benefits, barriers, and activity-related affect. According to Bandura,[7] actual enactment of a behavior and its associated feedback is a major source of efficacy or "skill" information. Anticipated or experienced benefits from engaging in the behavior are referred to by Bandura as outcome expectations. If desired short-term benefits are experienced early in the course of the behavior, the behavior is more likely to be repeated. Barriers to a given behavior are experienced and stored in memory as "hurdles" that need to be overcome to successfully engage in the behavior. Every incident of a behavior is also accompanied by emotions or affect. Positive or negative affect either before, during, or following the behavior is encoded into memory as information that is retrieved when engaging in the behavior is contemplated at a later point in time. Prior behavior is proposed as shaping all of these behavior-specific cognitions and affect. The nurse can help the client shape a positive behavioral history for the future by focusing on the benefits of a behavior, teaching clients how to overcome hurdles to carrying out the behavior, and engendering high levels of efficacy and positive affect through successful experiences of performance and positive feedback.

Personal Factors

The relevant personal factors predictive of a given behavior are shaped by the nature of the target behavior being considered. In the revised HPM, personal factors have been categorized as biologic, psychologic and sociocultural. Personal biologic factors include variables such as age, gender, body mass index, pubertal status, menopausal status, aerobic capacity, strength, agility, or balance. Personal psychologic factors can include variables such as self-esteem, self-motivation, personal competence, perceived health status, and definition of health. Personal sociocultural factors include variables such as race, ethnicity, acculturation, education, and socioeconomic status. Since numerous personal factors exist, those factors to be included in any given study should be limited to the few that are theoretically relevant to explanation or prediction of a given target behavior. The difference in behavioral relevance of these factors is illustrated by the fact that aerobic capacity may directly influence participation in vigorous exercise but is unlikely to directly influence eating a nutritious diet. Personal factors are proposed as directly influencing both behavior-specific cognitions and affect as well as health-promoting behavior. Although personal factors may influence cognitions and affect and predict health behaviors, some personal factors cannot be changed; thus, they are seldom incorporated into health-behavior change interventions.

Behavior-Specific Cognitions and Affect

This category of variables within the HPM is considered to be of major motivational significance. Furthermore, these variables constitute a critical "core" for intervention, as they are subject to modification through nursing actions.

Perceived Benefits of Action

One's plan to engage in a particular behavior often hinges on the anticipated benefits or outcomes that will occur. Anticipated benefits of action are mental representations of the positive or reinforcing consequences of a behavior. According to expectancy-value theory, the motivational importance of anticipated benefits is based on personal or vicarious experience of outcomes from prior direct experience with the behavior or observational learning from others engaging in the behavior. Beliefs in benefits or positive outcome expectations have generally been shown to be a necessary although not sufficient condition for engagement in a specific health behavior. Individuals tend to invest time and resources in activities with a high likelihood of increasing their experience of positive outcomes. The motivational importance of perceived benefits of action has been supported in the majority of HPM studies in which it has been tested.

Benefits from performance of the behavior may be intrinsic or extrinsic. Examples of intrinsic benefits include increased alertness and decreased feelings of fatigue. Extrinsic benefits can include monetary rewards or social interactions possible as a result of engaging in the behavior. Initially, extrinsic benefits of health behaviors may be of high motivational significance, whereas intrinsic benefits may be more powerful in motivating continuation of health behaviors. The expected magnitude of benefits and the temporal relation of benefits to action impact the potency of anticipated benefits as a determinant of health behavior. In the HPM, perceived benefits are proposed as directly motivating behavior as well as indirectly motivating behavior through determining the extent of commitment to a plan of action to engage in the behaviors from which the anticipated benefits will result.

Perceived Barriers to Action

Anticipated barriers have been repeatedly shown in empirical studies to affect intentions to engage in a particular behavior and the actual execution of the behavior. In relation to health-promoting behaviors, barriers may be imagined or real. They consist of perceptions concerning the unavailability, inconvenience, expense, difficulty, or time-consuming nature of a particular action. Barriers are often viewed as the blocks, hurdles, and personal costs of undertaking a given behavior. Loss of satisfaction from giving up health-damaging behaviors such as smoking or eating high-fat foods to adopt a healthier lifestyle can also constitute a barrier. Barriers usually arouse motives of avoidance in relation to a given behavior.

When readiness to act is low and barriers are high, action is unlikely to occur. When readiness to act is high and barriers are low, the probability of action is much greater. Perceived barriers to action as depicted in the revised HPM affect health-promoting behavior directly by serving as blocks to action as well as indirectly through decreasing commitment to a plan of action.

Perceived Self-Efficacy

Self-efficacy, as defined by Bandura,[7] is the judgment of personal capability to organize and execute a particular course of action. It is concerned not with the skill one has but with judgments of what one can do with whatever skills one possesses. Judgments of personal efficacy are distinguished from outcome expectations. Perceived self-efficacy is a judgment of one's abilities to accomplish a certain level of performance, whereas an outcome expectation is a judgment of the likely consequences (eg, benefits, costs) such behavior will produce. Perceptions of skill and competence in a particular domain motivate individuals to engage in those behaviors that they excel in. Feeling efficacious and skilled in one's performance is likely to encourage one to engage in the target behavior more frequently than feeling inept and unskilled.

Personal knowledge about one's self-efficacy is based on four types of information: (1) performance attainments from actually engaging in the behavior and evaluating performance in relation to some self-standard or external feedback given by others, (2) vicarious experiences of observing the performance of others and their related self-evaluation and feedback, (3) verbal persuasion on the part of others that one does possess the ability to carry out a particular course of action, and (4) physiologic states (eg, anxiety, fear, calm, tranquility) from which people judge their competencies.[20] In the HPM, perceived self-efficacy is proposed as being influenced by activity-related affect. The more positive the affect, the greater the perceptions of efficacy. In turn, self-efficacy is proposed as influencing perceived barriers to action, with higher efficacy resulting in lowered perception of barriers to the performance of the target behavior. Self-efficacy motivates health-promoting behavior directly by efficacy expectations and indirectly by affecting perceived barriers and commitment or persistence in pursuing a plan of action.

Activity-Related Affect

Subjective feeling states occur prior to, during, and following a behavior, based on the stimulus properties of the behavior itself. These affective responses may be mild, moderate, or strong and are cognitively labeled, stored in memory, and associated with subsequent thoughts of the behavior. Affective responses to a particular behavior consist of three components: emotional arousal to the act itself (activity-related), the self acting (self-related), or the environment in which the action takes place (context-related). The resultant feeling state is likely to affect whether an individual will repeat the behavior again or maintain the behavior long-term.[21] Behavior-contingent feeling states have been explored as determinants of health behaviors in recent studies.[21–25] The affect associated with the behavior reflects a direct emotional reaction or gut-level response to the thought of the behavior, which can be positive or negative—is it fun, delightful, enjoyable, disgusting, or unpleasant? Behaviors associated with positive affect are likely to be repeated, whereas those associated with negative affect are likely to be avoided. For some behaviors, both positive and negative feelings states will be induced. Thus, the relative balance between positive and negative affect prior to, during, and following the behavior is important to ascertain. Activity-related affect is different from the evaluative dimension of attitude as proposed by Fishbein and Ajzen.[20] The evaluative dimension of attitude reflects affective evaluation of the specific outcomes of a behavior rather than the response to the stimulus properties of the behavior itself.

For any given behavior, the full range of negative and positive feelings states should be elaborated so that both are adequately measured. In many instruments proposed to measure affect, negative feelings are elaborated more extensively than positive feelings. This is not surprising since anxiety, fear, and depression have been studied much more than joy, elation, and calm. Based on social cognitive theory, there is a relationship proposed between self-efficacy and activity-related affect. McAuley and Courneya[22] found that positive affective response during exercise was a significant predictor of postexercise efficacy. This is consistent with Bandura's proposal that emotional responses and their induced physiologic states during a behavior serve as sources of efficacy information.[7] Thus, activity-related affect is proposed as influencing health behavior directly as well as indirectly through self-efficacy and commitment to a plan of action.

Interpersonal Influences

According to the HPM, interpersonal influences are cognitions concerning the behaviors, beliefs or attitudes of others. These cognitions may or may not correspond with reality.

Primary sources of interpersonal influence on health-promoting behaviors are families (parents or siblings), peers, and health care providers. Interpersonal influences include: norms (expectations of significant others),[20] social support (instrumental and emotional encouragement), and modeling (vicarious learning through observing others engaged in a particular behavior).[7] These three interpersonal processes have been shown to affect individuals' predisposition to engage in health-promoting behaviors in a number of health-related studies. Social norms set standards for performance that individuals can adopt or reject. Social support for a behavior taps the sustaining resources offered by others. Modeling portrays the sequential components of a health behavior and is an important strategy for behavior change in social cognitive theory. Interpersonal influences affect health-promoting behavior directly as well as indirectly through social pressures or encouragement to commit to a plan of action.

Individuals vary in the extent to which they are sensitive to the wishes, examples, and praise of others. However, given sufficient motivation to behave in a way consistent with interpersonal influences, individuals are likely to undertake behaviors for which they will be admired and socially reinforced. In order for interpersonal influences to have an effect, individuals must attend to the behaviors, wishes, and inputs of others; comprehend them; and assimilate them into cognitive representations related to given behaviors. Susceptibility to the influence of others may vary developmentally and be particularly evident in adolescence. Some cultures may place more emphasis on interpersonal influences than others. For example, *familismo* among Hispanic populations may encourage individuals to engage in a particular behavior for the good of the family rather than for personal gain.

Situational Influences

Personal perceptions and cognitions of any situation or context can facilitate or impede behavior. Situational influences on health-promoting behavior include perceptions of options available, demand characteristics, and aesthetic features of the environment in which a given behavior is proposed to take place. Kaplan and Kaplan,[26] in their work on restorative natural environments, have heightened awareness of how environments or situational contexts can impact health and health-related behaviors. Individuals are drawn to and perform more competently in situations or environmental contexts in which they feel compatible rather than incompatible, related rather than alienated, safe and reassured rather than unsafe and threatened. Environments that are fascinating and interesting are also desirable contexts for the performance of health behaviors.

In the revised HPM, situational influences have been reconceptualized as direct and as indirect influences on health behavior. Situations may directly affect behaviors by presenting an environment "loaded" with cues that trigger action. For example, a "no smoking" environment creates demand characteristics for nonsmoking behavior. Company regulations for hearing protection to be worn create demand characteristics that regulations be obeyed. Both situations enforce commitment to health actions.

Situational influences have been given little attention in prior studies of the HPM and are worthy of further exploration as potentially important determinants of health behavior. They may hold an important key to developing new and more effective strategies for facilitating the acquisition and maintenance of health behaviors.

Behavioral Outcome

Commitment to a plan of action initiates a behavioral event. This commitment will propel the individual into and through the behavior unless a competing demand that the individual cannot avoid or a competing preference that the individual does not resist intervenes.

Commitment to a Plan of Action

Human beings generally engage in organized rather than disorganized behavior. According to Ajzen and Fishbein, intentionality is a major determinant of volitional behavior.[27] **Commitment to a plan of action** in the revised HPM implies the underlying cognitive processes: (1) commitment to carry out a specific action at a given time and place and with specified persons or alone, irrespective of competing preferences, (2) identification of definitive strategies for eliciting, carrying out, and reinforcing the behavior. The requirement of identification of specific strategies to be used at different points in the behavioral sequence goes beyond intentionality to further the likelihood that the plan of action developed by nurse and client will be successfully implemented. For example, the strategy of contracting consists of a mutually agreed-on set of actions to which one party commits with the understanding that the other party will provide some tangible reward or reinforcement if the commitment is sustained. Strategies can be selected by clients to energize and reinforce health behaviors according to their own preferences and the stage of change that they are at. Commitment alone without associated strategies often results in "good intentions" but failure to perform a valued health behavior.

Immediate Competing Demands and Preferences

Immediate competing demands or preferences refer to alternative behaviors that intrude into consciousness as possible courses of action immediately prior to the intended occurrence of a planned health-promoting behavior. Competing demands are viewed as those alternative behaviors over which individuals have a relatively low level of control because of environmental contingencies such as work or family care responsibilities. Failure to respond to a demand may have untoward effects for the self or for significant others. Competing preferences are viewed as alternative behaviors with powerful reinforcing properties over which individuals exert a relatively high level of control. They can derail a health-promoting behavior in favor of the competing behavior.[28] The extent to which an individual is able to resist competing preferences depends on his or her ability to be self-regulating. Examples of "giving in" to competing preferences are: selecting a food high in fat rather than low in fat because of taste or flavor preferences; driving past the recreation center where one usually exercises to stop at the mall (a preference for browsing or shopping rather than exercising). Both competing demands and preferences can derail a plan of action to which one has committed. Competing demands can be differentiated from barriers in that the individual must carry out an unanticipated behavior based on external demand or untoward results are likely to occur. Competing preferences can be differentiated from barriers such as lack of time, because competing preferences are last-minute urges based on one's preference hierarchy that derail a plan for positive health action.

Individuals vary in their ability to sustain attention and avoid disruption. Some individuals may be predisposed developmentally or biologically to be more easily swayed from a course of action than others. Inhibiting competing preferences requires the exercise of self-regulation and control capabilities. Strong commitment to a plan of action may sustain dedication to complete a behavior in light of competing demands or preferences. In the HPM, immediate competing demands and preferences directly affect the probability of occurrence of health behavior as well as moderate the effects of commitment.

Health-Promoting Behavior

This variable in the model has been addressed extensively throughout the book so needs little further discussion here. Health-promoting behavior is the end point or action outcome in the HPM. However, it should be noted that health-promoting behavior is ultimately directed toward **attaining positive health outcomes** for the client. Health-promoting behaviors, particularly when integrated into a healthy lifestyle that pervades all aspects of living, result in a positive health experience throughout the life span.

• DIRECTIONS FOR RESEARCH

The revised HPM presented in this chapter incorporates the outcome expectancies of expectancy-value theory and self-efficacy expectancies for mastery of social cognitive theory. Further, interpersonal, situational, and behavioral factors, as well as cognitive and other personal factors delineated in social learning theory are integral to the HPM. Thus, it is theoretically consistent with these frameworks. The model has been refined to focus on 10 determinants or categories of determinants of behavior rather than the previous 13 determinants. The revised model needs to be tested empirically. Before testing the model with any specific health behavior, it is suggested that rigorous measures of behavior-specific variables be developed if they do not already exist. This may involve eliciting appropriate content for the instruments prior to their design. Relationships among the variables should be tested in predictive studies. Where there is already evidence supporting the predictive validity of constructs in the HPM, such as perceived barriers to action, perceived benefits of actions, perceived self-efficacy, interpersonal influences, and situational influences, health promotion intervention studies should be designed incorporating these variables. The extent to which the revised HPM is useful in explaining, predicting, and altering health-promoting behaviors will be determined through further empirical studies.

• SUMMARY

The theoretical underpinnings and assumptions of the HPM have been presented in this chapter as well as the results of a number of studies testing the HPM. The revisions of the model to increase its potential utility for prediction and intervention are presented with a rationale for the revisions.

REFERENCES

1. Pender NJ. *Health Promotion in Nursing Practice.* Norwalk, Conn: Appleton-Century-Crofts; 1982.
2. Dunn HL. What high-level wellness means. *Can J Public Health.* 1959;50(11):447–457.
3. Dunn HL. High-level wellness for men and society. *Am J Public Health.* 1959;49(6):786–792.
4. Pender NJ. *Health Promotion in Nursing Practice.* 2nd ed. Norwalk, Conn: Appleton & Lange; 1987.
5. Feather NT, ed. *Expectations and Actions: Expectancy-Value Models in Psychology.* Hillsdale, NJ: Lawrence Erlbaum Associates Inc; 1982.
6. Klar Y, Nader A, Mallor TE. Opting to change: student's informal self-change endeavors. In: Klar Y, Fisher JD, Chinsky JM, et al, eds. *Self-change: Social and Psychological Perspectives.* New York, NY: Springer-Verlag; 1992:63–83.
7. Bandura A. *Social Foundations of Thought and Action: A Social Cognitive Theory.* Englewood Cliffs, NJ: Prentice-Hall Inc; 1986.
8. Bandura A. Self efficacy: toward a unifying theory of behavioral change. *Psychol Rev.* 1977;84:191–215.
9. Weitzel MH. A test of the Health Promotion Model with blue collar workers. *Nurs Res.* 1989;38(2):99–104.
10. Walker SN, Sechrist KR, Pender NJ. The Health-Promoting Lifestyle Profile: development and psychometric characteristics. *Nurs Res.* 1987;36(2):76–81.
11. Pender NJ, Walker SN, Sechrist KR, et al. *The Health Promotion Model: Refinement and Validation.* Final Report to the National Center for Nursing Research, National Institutes of Health (Grant no. NR01121) Dekalb, IL: Northern Illinois University Press; 1990.
12. Pender NJ, Walker SN, Sechrist KR, et al. Predicting health-promoting lifestyles in the workplace. *Nurs Res.* 1990;39(6):326–332.
13. Frank-Stromborg M, Pender NJ, Walker SN. Determinants of health-promoting lifestyles in ambulatory cancer patients. *Soc Sci Med.* 1990;31:1159–1168.
14. Johnson JL, Ratner PA, Bottorff JL, et al. An exploration of Pender's Health Promotion Model using LISREL. *Nurs Res.* 1993;42(3):132–138.
15. Garcia A, Norton-Broda MA, Frenn M, et al. Gender and developmental differences in exercise beliefs among youth and prediction of their exercise behavior. *J School Health.* 1995,65(6):213–219.
16. Occupational Safety and Health Administration. *Noise Control: A Guide for Workers and Employers.* Washington DC: US Department of Labor; 1980.
17. Lusk SL. *Preventing Noise-Induced Hearing Loss.* Final report to the National Institute of Nursing Research, National Institutes of Health, (Grant No. NR02050); 1994.
18. Lusk SL, Ronis D, Kerr MJ, et al. Test of the health promotion model as a causal model of workers' use of hearing protection. *Nurs Res.* 1994;43(3):151–157.
19. Kerr MJ. *Factors Related to Mexican-American Workers' Use of Hearing Protection.* Ann Arbor, Mich: University of Michigan; 1994. *Dissertation Abstracts International,* 1994, University Microfilms No. 9501083.
20. Fishbein M, Ajzen I. *Belief, Attitude, Intention and Behavior: An Introduction to Theory and Research.* Boston, Mass: Addison-Wesley Publishing Co Inc; 1975.
21. Gauvin L, Rejeski WJ. The exercise-induced feeling inventory: development and initial validation. *J Sport Exerc Psychol.* 1993;15:403–423.
22. McAuley E, Courneya KS. Self-efficacy relationships with affective and exertion responses to exercise. *J Appl Soc Psychol.* 1992;22:312–326.

23. Hardy CJ, Rejeski WJ. Not what, but how one feels: the measurement of affect during exercise. *J Sport Exerc Psychol.* 1989;11:304–317.
24. Godin G. Importance of the emotional aspect of attitude to predict intention. *Psychol Rep.* 1987;61:719–723.
25. Rejeski WJ, Gauvin L, Hobson ML, et al. Effects of baseline responses, in-task feelings, and duration of activity on exercise-induced feeling states in women. *Health Psychol.* 1995; 14:350–359.
26. Kaplan R, Kaplan S. *The Experience of Nature: A Psychological Perspective.* Cambridge, England: Cambridge University Press; 1989.
27. Ajzen I, Fishbein M. *Understanding Attitudes and Predicting Social Behavior.* Englewood Cliffs, NJ: Prentice-Hall Inc; 1980.
28. Vara LS, Epstein L. Laboratory assessment of choice between exercise or sedentary behaviors. *Res Q Exerc Sport.* 1995;64:356–360.

II

PART TWO

Health Empowerment in Diverse Settings

4

Settings for Health Promotion

- Health Promotion in Families
- Health Promotion in the School
- Health Promotion at the Worksite
- Health Promotion in Nursing Centers
- The Community at Large as a Setting for Health Promotion
- Directions for Research on Settings for Health Promotion
- Summary

More than ever before, the value of health-promotion services for improving the health of populations is recognized worldwide. Increasingly, third-party payors are including health-promotion benefits in their plans as reimbursable services. The many settings in which health promotion is now delivered offer the possibility for achieving an integration of effort across sites and among health professionals that has never been achieved before. If people of all ages are to benefit from quality health-promotive care, gender- and culture-sensitive services should be delivered at sites where people are, where they spend many of their waking hours. Thus, schools and worksites are logical locations for well-designed health-promotion programs. The purpose of this chapter is to provide an overview of health-promotion settings from families and schools to the community at large.

To provide cost-effective, seamless health-promotive care to clients, information technology that supports the transportability of patient records must be used to facilitate care. For example, the school health record of the child should be readily available to the nurse practitioner in the community nursing center so that care is coordinated between the school and the clinic. Community-wide collaboration in health care delivery will be the key to developing a system of health-promotion services that is user-friendly and well integrated.

• HEALTH PROMOTION IN FAMILIES

Health values, attitudes, and behaviors are learned in the family context. The place of health in the family value structure and the extent to which health-promoting knowledge and skills are transmitted to offspring determine the degree of impact that families have on the health potential of future generations. While the family provides a context for individual health actions, it is a unit of health behavior analysis in its own right. Further, the relationship between family health and individual health is multivariate and complex, an exciting area for investigation by nurse scientists.[1] Just as individuals must assume increased responsibility for their own health status, so families must assume similar responsibilities for the family structure as a whole. Structural and functional features of the family that must be considered when attempting to influence health practices include value structure, role structure, power structure (decision-making patterns), communication patterns, affective function, socialization function, health care function, and coping function. Specific questions that should be explored in relation to family values, beliefs, and lifestyle include:

1. How does the family unit define health?
2. What health-promoting behaviors does the family engage in regularly?
3. What health-promoting behaviors are particularly enjoyable to family members?
4. Do all family members engage in these behaviors or are patterns of participation highly variable throughout the family system?
5. Is there consistency between family health values as stated and their health actions?
6. What are the explicit or implicit goals of the family in the area of health?

Variant family forms are common in today's society. Family units may be: one-parent families (most often mother only), blended families (parts of two preexisting families), extended families (nuclear plus a relative, often older), augmented families (additional members, not blood relations), married adult dyads, and unmarried adult dyads (blood and nonblood relations). Families are as diverse as individuals and need to be actively involved in planning their health promotion activities so that they have a high probability of success with the plan developed. The nurse working with families in the area of health promotion must be sensitive to both the commonalities and differences across varying family forms. Studies of family form and related lifestyles are critical to the formulation of theories helpful in understanding the milieu for the promotion of health in families of varying types.

Rather than focusing only on the high-risk individual, Knutsen and Knutsen[2] used the family as the unit of intervention directed toward reducing coronary risk factors. Through a primary care intervention delivered to families, the goal was to reduce coronary risk by reducing sugar intake, energy intake from dietary fat, and smoking and increasing the amount of exercise. Families were randomly assigned to intervention and control groups. The intervention families were informed that they were at increased risk for coronary heart disease because of a shared family lifestyle. The intervention consisted of home visits and counseling, with special emphasis on diet. Smoking and exercise were also discussed, but in less detail. Based on dietary information from the family, the dietitian gave specific advice, using food models and other audiovisuals to reinforce her message regarding good nutrition. At rescreening approximately 5 years later, significantly lower risk factor levels were found in the men and their spouses in the intervention group compared with the control group. For children in the family, the difference in overall risk factors was minimal and generally nonsignificant. The entire families in the intervention group reported more positive health practices in relation to diet than in the control group. No differences were found between the two groups in smoking and exercise behavior. This study indicated that a family approach to risk reduction and health promotion is well accepted, moderately effective, and feasible in primary care.

Baranowski and colleagues[3] designed and implemented a center-based program for exercise change among African-American families. Ninety-four families were recruited and assigned to an intervention or control group. The intervention was designed to be culture-sensitive to meet the needs of the participants. The intervention consisted of two fitness sessions and one education session with individual counseling each week for 14 weeks, small group education, and an aerobic activity. Free transportation, free babysitting services, and reminders were offered to promote attendance. Participation on the part of the families tapered off rapidly so that by the end of the program only 20% of the original attendees were still participating. As a result of the extremely high dropout rate, no differences in fitness were detected between intervention and control groups. In analyzing postprogram interview data to determine what went wrong, the investigators concluded that they may have underestimated the magnitude of the barriers to participation. Participants had frequent changes in work schedules, precluding attendance in many instances. Furthermore, relatively high body weights at the beginning of the program indicated greater difficulty for heavy people attempting to initiate an exercise program. The investigators concluded that center-based exercise programs may not be appropriate to meet the needs of families in some segments of the population because of frequent work schedule changes. It is highly possible that a church-based or home-based exercise program would have been more effective. Further studies could determine if this is indeed true.

Nurses should heed what has been learned through the studies cited as well as other studies evaluating the success of family health promotion interventions. Planning programs directly with participants and tailoring the programs to their specific needs to the extent possible is likely to result in better participation. When a family can communicate freely, articulate shared goals, plan together to achieve goals, implement plans, evaluate goal attainment, and revise goals as necessary, behavior change is more likely to occur and persist.

Nursing care is frequently delivered to families during transition periods such as transition to parenthood or developmental transitions of children. Nursing care directed at health promotion is no exception. Important steps in transitions in the family unit include: evaluating current lifestyle, planning for behavior change, implementing changes to enhance family health, evaluating family outcomes. Through supportive-educative care, family members can be encouraged to perceive themselves as competent and in control of family health status even during potentially stressful transitions.

The well family demonstrates a spectrum of abilities, insights, and strengths. The challenges for the nurse is to assist the family unit in identifying relevant health goals, planning for developmental and other transitions so that they are minimally disruptive, and planning for positive lifestyle changes that will not only begin but continue as an ongoing family commitment. For further discussion concerning the nurses' role in family health promotion the reader is referred to work by Bomar.[4]

• HEALTH PROMOTION IN THE SCHOOL

With a majority of the nation's children enrolled in elementary and secondary schools, school-based health promotion programs can exert a major influence on the acquisition of health-promoting behaviors among children and adolescents. Children spend thousands of hours throughout childhood and adolescence in school,[5] therefore, schools should be health-promoting environments. They should build resilience as well as teach children how to deal with problems such as substance abuse, postponement of sexual involvement, and avoidance of delinquent behavior. Schools should promote success and bonding rather than failure and alienation.[5(p178)] School competence is highly related to life competence. Teachers and school health personnel should both set the normative expectations for healthy behaviors and serve as role models of health-enhancing lifestyles. Creating healthy environments may include restructuring school routines so that the emphasis is on the learner, not the content to be learned. Healthy schools also have parents who are interested and involved. Fostering parental participation is key to creating healthy lifestyles that carry over into the home environment. Of critical importance is creating positive peer influences that foster health-promoting rather than health-damaging behaviors.

Health promotion programs in school settings are often not integral to the instructional program of the school. As long as this condition is allowed to persist, health education will be thought of as an "add on" rather than as a vital part of instructional programming. Critical functions of comprehensive school health promotion programs include:

1. Promote acquisition of knowledge and skills for competent self-care and informed decision making about health.
2. Reinforce positive health attitudes.
3. Structure environment and social influences to support health-promoting behaviors.
4. Facilitate growth and self-actualization.
5. Sensitize students to aspects of their environment and culture that are detrimental to health and well-being.
6. Foster positive life skills that enhance successful coping.

Health-promoting behaviors are acquired more readily in childhood, when routines and habits are less stabilized. In addition, habits or behaviors developed in childhood and adolescence are more likely to persist as an integral part of lifestyle than changes made in health behaviors later in the adult years.

Perry and Murray[6] stress the importance of considering the developmental stages of children and adolescents in structuring school health-promotion programs. They identify four environmental structures of influence that affect the health behaviors of the school-age population. The most important is the **model structure,** which includes the actual behavior of significant others. Children are greatly influenced by the food selections, exercise habits, coping methods, smoking habits, and alcohol use of parents, teachers, and friends. The **network structure** consists of loosely organized groups that interact regularly with one another, such as peer groups, neighborhoods, and organizations to which children or adolescents may belong. Establishing health promotion programs in existing support networks may lead to more successful development of health behaviors than randomly grouping the school-age population for purposes of behavior change. The **social system structure** of which the child or adolescent is a member plays a critical role in health. For instance, the school as a social system regulates to a considerable degree the options and choices available to the school-age population for a major portion of each day. Schools can have psychologically, socially, and ecologically unhealthy environments that pose threats to students' well-being. The **community message structure** is the fourth influence on health behaviors of school-age children. Television programming, advertisements, community resources, and government regulations shape attitudes toward health behaviors.

With increasing concern about the future of our nation's children, new models of school health services are evolving with a vision for schools as the primary care and health-promotion education and service delivery sites of the future for children and families.[7] Tragically, one in five children in the United States lives in poverty, only half of all poor children receive Medicaid coverage, and many children are uninsured. To make matters even worse, in the inner city dropout rates can reach 80%. Even those who remain in school struggle with math, science, and communication skills. When future prospects for employment are dim, the resources to support personal well-being and that of dependent others is greatly compromised. Adolescents and young adults become prey for criminals and can initiate early a life of crime and welfare dependency. All of this does not bode well for the future of our nation's youth.[8]

Youth health-promotion programs can address many of the pressing problems that today's youth face. Responding to the challenge of promoting the health of adolescents will not be easy. It will require integration of knowledge from various disciplines including a solid research base on adolescent health and development, developmental patterns of healthy and risky behaviors, and effectiveness of theory-based health promotion interventions with diverse populations of adolescents. Millstein and colleagues suggest the following guidelines for successful programs.[9] The programs should be:

1. Highly responsive to the population for whom they are developed, recognizing age-related differences
2. Sensitive to the diverse cultural and social contexts in which youth live
3. Inclusive of many individuals and institutions that affect the lives of youth
4. Responsive to the need for continuing education of parents, teachers, and health professionals to enable them to use "state of the science" strategies and interventions to meet the needs of youth

To address the pressing health problems of youth, Uphold and Graham propose that traditional school health services be restructured as family service centers to help families solve their interrelated educational, social, economic, and health care problems. Although school health centers have greatly increased accessibility of health care to children and adolescents, some of the problems that youths face will not be solved until families and communities get more involved. The authors described the Family Services Center located at a middle-school in Gainesville, Florida. The primary objective of the center is to empower families to make substantial life and health behavior changes and to escape the cycle of poverty. When a family seeks service at the center, a family liaison specialist completes a needs assessment and develops a contract that addresses issues such as parenting skills, literacy, substance abuse, and various aspects of health care. The specialist may conduct home visits as needed and referrals are made to other agencies for services not provided at the center. Adult education and job training are a central focus of the center. An education specialist works with parents to improve their ability to help their child succeed academically. Peer counseling, mental health counseling, social work, and health care services are available. Transportation is provided for families to the center and referral agencies. A school nurse specialist and health room aides develop and implement care plans for families. Nurse practitioners and school nurses are an ideal team to provide leadership to a collaborating group of health professionals and lay workers in developing family service centers that are school-based or school-linked.[8]

Igoe[10] described empowerment programs for health consumers of school age as essential components of health promotion. She identifies the knowledge base for such empowerment programs as an understanding of: (1) the knowledge, beliefs, and attitudes of children and adolescents about health and illness, including their sense of vulnerability for health problems and (2) the health behaviors of youth in varying circumstances. The HealthPACT (Participatory and Assertive Consumer Training) program developed by Igoe and her colleagues is directed toward assisting youth to develop interactive skills that will enable them to communicate with health care providers. The program was developed by school nurse-practitioner faculty at the University of Colorado after a review of children's literature revealed the passive role depicted for children in interaction with health professionals. The program is flexible and can be offered in school settings or adapted to clinics or physician's offices. The emphasis of the program on the assertive consumer who employs health professionals as consultants on personal health matters is philosophically in harmony with current illness-prevention and health-promotion efforts that focus on individual responsibility for health status.

The communication code taught to children for use during appointments is TLADD. The acronym serves as a memory device for *T*alk, *L*isten and learn, *A*sk, *D*ecide, *D*o. It covers the four basic consumer rights to be informed, to choose, to be heard, and to be safe. Social learning theory with its emphasis on efficacy and mastery provides the theoretical underpinnings for the program. Program components include: role modeling, rehearsal, cuing, and other behavioral training and prompting strategies. A 3-year national study of the program revealed that it was successful in achieving behavioral change with statistically significant effect across four of the seven study sites. The program appeared to achieve its greatest success in the fourth grade. Further diffusion of the program to other schools is warranted based on study results.

The final program to be described is Project Model Health (PMH), a middle school health-promotion program.[11] The pilot program consisted of 32 hours of classroom instruction and activities provided in 64 sessions over the course of the semester. Eighth-grade students were taught by teams of college-age instructors of both genders. The units covered nutrition, tobacco, marijuana, alcohol, and sexuality. To promote the development of positive behaviors in each of these areas, the following strategies were used: (1) instructors served as positive, high-status role models, (2) focus was directed toward understanding and interpreting media messages about the targeted behaviors, (3) peer refusal skills were practiced, (4) information on peer norms for the targeted behaviors were discussed, (5) short-term results were emphasized, (6) students' public commitment to change their behavior was used to support adherence, and (7) students were engaged in projects advocating healthy behaviors in their school and in their community. A comparison group was used for purposes of evaluation. Results of follow-up 20 months later revealed that the PMH group significantly reduced their rate of cigarette use and showed significant improvement in food choices. Results were suggestive of a decrease in sexual intercourse among the PMH group and the increase in use of marijuana was less for the PMH group than for the comparison group. The program was marginally successful in reducing alcohol use, with results falling just short of statistical significance. Claims for the success of the program are tempered by methodologic issues related to consistent implementation, selection process for comparison groups, etc. Further study of the intervention is needed, with refinements made as indicated from the pilot study of the program.

In examining comprehensive health and social programs for adolescents at-risk, Dryfoos[12] identified several characteristics of programs that work. The programs that work provide: (1) individual attention to children, (2) are multicomponent, multiagency, community-wide programs, (3) focus on intervention as early as preschool, (4) promote acquisition of basic academic skills, (5) create healthy school climates, (6) promote "real" parental involvement with paid or volunteer positions, (7) promote active peer involvement, (8) connect to the real world of work, (9) provide social and life skills training, and (10) attend to the needs of staff for training and supervision. These characteristics should be built in to school health-promotion programs to optimize their chances of success and meaningful impact on the youth that they serve.

• HEALTH PROMOTION AT THE WORKSITE

With the escalating cost of health insurance benefits, employers are attracted to worksite prevention and health-promotion initiatives as a means of controlling costs and maintaining a healthy and productive workforce. Accumulating evidence suggests that such programs may increase productivity, decrease abstenteeism, decrease use of expensive medical care, and lower disability claims. More than ever before, the global competitiveness of corporations in the United States depends on a healthy, productive workforce.

A definite advantage of health-promotion activities at the worksite is that they create a cultural milieu that supports and rewards health-promoting behaviors. The social and physical environments of corporations can be altered to increase their health-enhancing potential. Offering a variety of health-promotion programs at the worksite, using differing approaches, increases the appeal of the program to employees of varying cultural backgrounds and of differing ages. The following characteristics of effective programs have been identified: strategies and incentives that motivate employees to participate, focus on immediate personal benefits from participation, minimal barriers to participation, and programs tailored to the preferences of individual participants. Advantages that worksite health-promotion programs offer include[13]:

1. Most employees go to the workplace on a regular schedule, facilitating regular participation in the programs.
2. Contact with coworkers can provide reinforcing social support, a primary force in sustaining lifestyle change.
3. The workplace offers many opportunities for environmental supports, such as healthy food in the cafeteria, office policies regarding smoking, and aesthetic work space.
4. Opportunities abound for positive reinforcement for employees participating in the program.
5. Programs in the workplace are generally less expensive for the employee than comparable programs in the community.
6. Programs in the workplace are conveniently located.

The unique features of worksite wellness programs will likely mean that they will continue to be a highly viable component of comprehensive health promotion programming in the United States in the years ahead. Corporations find such facilities to be a useful recruitment tool as well as a resource to improve the mental and physical well-being of employees. Several major corporations have comprehensive health-promotion programs that are regarded as the "standard of excellence" in worksite wellness. Major corporations with large facilities and staffs often broaden their health promotion programming to include activities for family members as well as employees. In addition, insurance companies are beginning to reimburse for health education and health-promotion services. This could cast a new light on the economics of worksite health promotion in the near future.

Worksite health-promotion programs share many common components such as nutrition education, physical fitness facilities, and stress management programs. However, they also have interesting differences. For example, in some companies the primary focus is on the health of the individual employee; in others, the environment is the primary focus; still others combine both emphases into comprehensive programming. An overview of several programs is presented below to inform the reader of the range of approaches that can be used to promote wellness at the worksite.

Sorensen and colleagues[14] described a company-wide nonsmoking policy change program implemented across 600 sites with 27,374 employees. Smoking was banned in all work areas except for designated sections in cafeterias and lounges. A full-time field manager was appointed for 18 months to facilitate implementation and enforcement of the policy. Free on-site smoking-cessation classes were offered. Approximately 20 months later, a study was conducted to examine the effects of this policy on employee smoking behavior. A random sample of approximately 1500 employees was surveyed. Of the respondents, 21% who were smokers when the program was implemented were not smoking at the time of the survey. Nine percent reported that they actually quit smoking because of the policy. The program provided 38% of respondents classified as smokers with cessation assistance. Smokers attending smoking-cessation programs were more likely to quit than those who did not seek help. This overall quit rate of 21% is much higher than the spontaneous quit rate in the population, which is about 2% to 5% per year. This program is interesting in that it leveraged a policy change into environmental modifications that appeared, in turn, to trigger smoking-cessation behavior. Clearly, the findings of this study suggest that a thoughtful and well-supervised worksite nonsmoking policy, accompanied by cessation assistance, can increase smoking cessation among employees.

Another approach to worksite health-promotion programming is depicted by the Healthy Worker Project conducted in a seven-county metropolitan area surrounding Minneapolis-St. Paul, Minnesota.[15] Worksites with between 400 and 900 employees were recruited into the study. The primary objective of this program was to reduce the smoking and mean body weight of employees in intervention sites compared with control sites. The study included 32 worksites. The sites included those in businesses of insurance, financial services, manufacturing, education, government, etc. Sites were randomized to either an intervention or no-treatment group for 2 years. In a baseline survey, health habits, smoking and weight-loss histories, diet and exercise habits, job characteristics, and job satisfaction were assessed. Height and weight were measured. The intervention was based on the results of several successful pilot studies. Classes held on-site and on employee time focused on smoking cessation and healthy weight loss using behavior change principles. An incentive system was organized through payroll deduction. Participants selected an amount of money to be deducted from each paycheck. Employees in the weight loss program received a refund at each session if they had made progress toward their weight loss goals. Expired carbon monoxide was measured to validate smoking status, and employees in the smoking cessation program received a refund at each session their carbon monoxide values were less than 8 ppm (no-smoking level). Women were more likely to participate in the programs than men, professional, clerical, and sales personnel were 1.6 times as likely as blue-collar workers to participate in the weight loss program, and professionals were 2.6 times more likely than clerical and sales or blue-collar workers to participate in the smoking-cessation program. Across the 2-year period, 43% of smokers quit, as indicated by a carbon monoxide of 8 ppm or less at the last session attended. The average per-person weight loss in the weight program was 4.8 pounds. In a critique of the program impact, it appeared that some employees quit smoking as a result of the program, whereas for others, the presence of the program may have served as a cue to quit on their own. The authors make a point that should not be overlooked—program popularity should not be confused with program effectiveness. The weight loss program was by far the more attractive, but the smoking program was more effective in terms of results.

Erfurt and colleagues[16] evaluated a menu approach with follow-up counseling in a 3-year intervention study in four manufacturing facilities with predominantly blue-collar workers. The intent was to test different program models that required differing levels of staffing to determine their relative effectiveness in changing smoking behaviors and weight status of employees. The four sites were randomly assigned to one of the four program models, followed by risk-factor screening and counseling for employees at all four sites. Site 1 (control site) offered an "advice only" model in which people identified as having health risks were counseled about them, with health-education classes offered on-site. No further follow-up was used; employees could seek information or assistance as needed but had to take the initiative. Site 2 (health-education site) used multimedia throughout the time period to encourage employees to participate in health-education classes. Classes were offered twice a year and were widely marketed. A monthly newsletter containing articles about health was instituted. A health fair and other promotional events were held at intervals. Site 3 (risk-reduction site) used a model that was based on the assumption that behavior change requires not only awareness but support, encouragement, and assistance with problem solving. This program was identical to that at site 2 but added wellness counselors who contacted employees and offered to assist them with behavior change. They provided a menu of approaches including guided self-help manuals, minigroups, one-on-one sessions, and large group classes. Site 4 (full-service site) used a health-promotion model that incorporated all the features of the site 3 program but went beyond risk reduction and encouraged employees to build new health behaviors and to support one another in behavior change. The model emphasized learning positive substitutes for risky behaviors. Strategies used included health communication networks, competitions, buddy systems, and other support programs.

The site 3 and 4 models were much more successful than the site 1 and 2 models in engaging employees in health-promotion and risk-reduction efforts. Sites 3 and 4 actually engaged 50% of the overweight and almost 50% of the smokers in risk-reduction activities, whereas the other sites engaged less than 10% in similar activities. The more intensive one-to-one sessions were critical to engaging "reluctant" employees in self-change. Although the more intensive programs were more costly, long-term evaluation may indicate that dollar for dollar, they are more cost-effective.

Including families in worksite health-promotion programs is of interest to many employers because 50% of their outlay for health care costs is for family members. Studies have shown that smokers are more likely to have spouses who smoke and that individuals with physically active spouses are more likely to be active themselves, and their children are likely to be more active. McCauley[17] reports that companies are reaching out to families with health-promotion efforts. The health publications, health events, and health-promotion programs of many companies are geared to families. For example, Kimberly Clark has a special series of health activities on Saturdays called "Kids Care," which include clowns, games, health demonstrations attractive to children, and take-home activities. A number of companies offer prenatal and parenting classes to give the next generation a healthy start. Increasingly, primary care services are offered on-site for all family members. This provides convenient health care and may well represent an emerging model of full-service worksites similar to full-service schools. Some companies have also invited teachers from local schools to participate in their training programs so that health-promotion concepts in schools and worksites are consistent and integrated. This effort, if greatly expanded, could give rise to "seamless" health-promotion programming that would accelerate behavior change efforts in communities.

Worksite health-promotion programs will expand in the future. Exciting possibilities exist for integrating these programs into a coordinated community effort. The effectiveness of worksite programs will continue to be evaluated as more and more companies adopt this approach to promoting the health of employees and containing health-care costs. For an overview of health and cost-effective outcome studies conducted at the worksite, the reader is referred to a review and analysis of these programs by Pelletier.[18]

• HEALTH PROMOTION IN NURSING CENTERS

Nursing centers represent an ideal setting for health-promotion activities. While many nursing centers are relatively new, there are approximately 100 centers throughout the United States. Such centers offer a spectrum of services, from health promotion and primary care to counseling and support for the chronically ill. The goals of most nursing centers incorporate both health-promotion and health-protection services. Nursing centers provide health services to a diverse range of populations. The focus on the "individual and family" rather than on "the presenting illness" has enhanced the appeal of nursing centers for the delivery of care to a broad sector of the population. For example, many women prefer to obtain health care from nurse practitioners in a setting that is user-friendly and respectful of both their unique assets and needs. Women's health clinics are geared to accommodate to the work demands of women (over 60% in the workforce), offer warm and hospitable environments, provide educational self-help materials for women, offer gender-appropriate health education counseling and classes, enhance the self-esteem and self-efficacy of clients, and help women gain a sense of control over their health and their lives. This is a welcome approach, compared to the indifference that women often encounter in the health care system.

Nursing centers provide family-oriented care that is culturally sensitive. With the diversity of populations today and the variation in composition of family units, most families need assistance with healthy parenting and with meeting the health-promotion needs of all family members. The nature of health problems experienced today have their roots in early family habits and lifestyles. From habits of physical activity to approaches for dealing with interpersonal conflicts, families play a critical role in fostering health. Thus, a majority of nursing centers include in their services not only direct care but education classes on highly relevant topics, small group-support sessions, and family and individual counseling. Family-centered activities of nursing centers serve as excellent care-delivery models. They illustrate the directions that health reform should take, if health care is to be cost-effective and relevant to the people that it serves.

The University of Michigan School of Nursing and Medical Center founded a North Campus Nursing Center in 1991 to provide health care to international students living on campus. These students and their families may have a limited command of English, have minimal incomes, and feel alienated in a culture different from their home culture. The center, staffed by nurse practitioners and community health nurses, provides an array of services to international student families. Immunizations and well-baby checkups are available, as is personalized care for other family members. The center is located in an apartment in the campus housing area so it is maximally convenient to students and their families. The reception and examination rooms are welcoming and attractive. A living room and play area has been furnished to encourage informal conversations among clients and health care workers. The center is currently funded by a health maintenance organization (HMO), Medicaid, and various state and federal programs. Fee for service for the uninsured is on a sliding scale based on ability to pay.

Nursing centers can be established in many different environments readily accessible to the people that they are intended to serve. For example, some nursing centers are set up at or near schools so that the pressing health needs of children and adolescents can be met in a confidential and developmentally appropriate manner. Locating nursing centers in malls or storefronts where people congregate or spend time when not at school or work also provides easy accessibility. Ultimately nursing centers should offer new alternatives of care to diverse populations, family-focused care that enhances the health and well-being of all family members, interdisciplinary care that provides a range of health and social services, and integrated care that covers the life span of families and individuals.

With major national emphasis on cost containment in health care, community nursing centers are particularly appealing as integral components of the health care system. They provide quality care to families that is preventive and health promotive in orientation, technologically of low intensity for the most part, highly acceptable, and effective. Thus, health insurers, HMOs, and Medicare and Medicaid are increasingly interested in incorporating nursing centers into the cadre of health care providers. Innovative models of nursing centers are being established throughout the United States and other countries as a positive alternative or complement to existing models of health care. Particularly appealing are the opportunities to link universities and nursing centers together so that "state of the science" care can be implemented and evaluated in terms of client and family outcomes. Computerized tracking systems will be particularly critical to collect the data needed to evaluate the quality and cost-effectiveness of health care delivered in nursing centers.

Nurses need to address the legislative impediments that unduly constrain the establishment of nursing centers and the provision of a range of services to individuals and families. In an increasing number of states, nurse practitioners have prescriptive authority and are identified as primary care providers. As managed care becomes a reality, health professionals at nursing centers are uniquely positioned in the health care system to negotiate with managed care organizations to be primary care providers to a growing segment of the population. Health professionals in nursing centers, the nursing profession, and lay organizations should continue concerted efforts to bring nursing centers into the mainstream of health care delivery.

• THE COMMUNITY AT LARGE AS A SETTING FOR HEALTH PROMOTION

The idea of changing the behavior of communities rather than of individuals or small groups is based on the efficiency gained by using community organizations, media, and information dissemination and support structures to mobilize large groups of individuals, in the effort to improve the health of the environment and of subgroups, families, and individuals. Community-based health promotion programs have many advantages over programs directed toward smaller aggregates or individuals. Weiss[19] has cited a number of benefits of the community-based intervention model:

1. It enhances opportunities for information exchange and social support among members of the target community.
2. It reduces the unit cost of health-promotion programming because large groups rather than individuals are the recipients of services.

3. It allows for observation of the efficacy of health-promotion efforts and related health outcomes that may have policy implications.
4. Societal norms regarding health behavior are amenable to change over time as a result of community-wide programming.
5. Comprehensive rather than piecemeal approaches to promotion of health can be implemented.
6. Powerful interorganizational systems within the community can be used to facilitate health-promotion efforts.

Community-based health promotion and prevention programs encompass a range of activities aimed at creating a health-enhancing environment and healthy behaviors for populations. Activities include community-wide health-education, health-enhancement, and risk-reduction intervention programs, environmental awareness and "care" programs, and activities among the citizens of a community to change laws or regulatory policy to be supportive of health. The community-based approach offers a strategy for achieving substantial health gains through community organization techniques to mobilize community leadership and resources for assessment, intervention, and evaluation activities. Community activation, as a health-promotion strategy, includes organized efforts to increase community awareness and consensus about health problems, coordinate planning of health-promotion and environmental change programs, achieve interorganizational allocation of resources, and promote citizen involvement in these processes. Community activation is most closely associated with a social planning model that places emphasis on organizational change and the development of rational planning strategies to achieve goals.[20] A critical feature of community activation is matching programming to "real" community needs identified by those who reside in the community. Community empowerment, a topic to be addressed in a later chapter, is the essence of community activation. It is critical to keep in mind that a community is a "living" organism with interactive webs among organizations, neighborhoods, families, and friends. The health of the community as an organism is directly related to the health of its members. The health of all is enhanced through effective social change.[21] In commenting on community organization as an approach to health promotion and prevention in minority neighborhoods, Fisher[22] and colleagues emphasize the need for cultural sensitivity if such programming is going to make a real difference. Dimensions of community organization particularly relevant to African-American communities are identified as:

- Social support: Interpersonal peer-to-peer tactics can be used for promoting change.
- Informal networks: Informal networks of family and friends provide sources and channels of information and assistance.
- Multiple-change tactics: Use of multiple channels of assistance improves the odds that individuals isolated from one source of information or assistance will have access to others.

Fisher proposes that community organization strategies hold particular promise for addressing the health problems of African-American communities. Empowerment and local ownership inherent in community-organization approaches increase the likelihood of participation in and enthusiasm for health promotion and risk-reduction programs in African-American neighborhoods.

An excellent example of community-based programming is offered by the Healthy Cities initiative in Europe and the United States. Recognizing that the health of individuals and families is determined by a broad range of social, economic, environmental, and political factors, the healthy cities idea was identified as a means to achieve health for all within a context of equity and social justice. Healthy Cities is directed toward developing healthy public policies, creating supportive environments, strengthening community action, developing personal skills of community citizens, and reorienting health care services. For case studies of six cities participating in Healthy Cities Indiana, the reader is referred to the work of Flynn.[23] In describing the Indiana initiative, which is based in the School of Nursing at Indiana University, Flynn emphasizes the importance of a broad-based community committee to coordinate such an effort. It is critical that top city officials and leaders be publicly committed to this effort and so indicate in a wide array of media. Cities conduct comprehensive community assessments, provide data-based information to policy makers, seek consultation, conduct workshops and networking sessions, set priorities and goals, hire staff technical support, and secure resources for programming. Development of the power base to support change and community participation to bring about change are critical to the success of cities in becoming healthy places to live, learn, and work.

A minimal-contact community health-promotion campaign is described by Maibach et al.[24] The campaign targeted increasing self-efficacy (belief in ability to perform various behaviors) as the primary means of bringing about behavior change. This program was one element of the Stanford Five Cities Project, designed to reduce risk of heart disease by increasing exercise, losing weight, modifying diets, quitting smoking, and taking measures to better control blood pressure. All materials were produced using social cognitive theory as the framework. The primary strategies used throughout the materials included: encouraging participants to establish a behavioral goal, using community members as models of appropriate behavior change, using credible health experts to give advice on behavior change, and focusing on developing skills needed to make behavior changes. The campaign had four major components: five bimonthly newsletters; five self-help behavior change kits (weight loss, jogging, walking, nutrition, and smoking cessation) that were provided at no cost; contests, competitions, lectures, special radio and television programs; and print and electronic media campaigns to promote these materials and activities. Each of the five minicampaigns focused on one heart disease risk factor. The minicampaigns were conducted throughout the year. Approximately 5000 community residents were registered as participants. Measurements assessed self-efficacy, campaign exposure, and health behaviors. In a comparison of baseline and follow-up data, participants showed significantly increased exercise self-efficacy, healthy food consumption, and walking. Unhealthy food consumption decreased significantly. Exposure to the campaign increased self-efficacy. Positive changes in self-efficacy appeared to result in greater participation in health-promoting behaviors. In turn, improvements in health behaviors appeared to increase feelings of self-efficacy. This study provided evidence that a minimal-contact community campaign can achieve a degree of change in health behaviors.

The Boston Codman Square Community Partnership[25] for Health Promotion was an attempt to design a program that would avoid the failure of traditional health promotion approaches in reaching poor communities. Codman Square is a minority community whose residents are of low socioeconomic status. High rates of social and health problems exist, fostered by poverty, substandard housing, social isolation, poor self-esteem, lack of interpersonal skills, and hopelessness. The project adopted a health-promotion strategy that directly addressed the environmental, social, and behavioral consequences of poverty that affect the health of the population. In the program, a variety of models were used—community participation, community organization, empowerment education, and community-oriented primary care. The program used local residents trained as lay health workers to deliver home-based health services and to create partnerships, linkages, and communication networks to foster reorganization and reorientation of the community to better address health problems. The objectives of the program focus on:

1. Making health services more responsive to community health needs and concerns
2. Increasing capacity of community organizations to work on health issues
3. Increasing residents' control over and satisfaction with life in the community
4. Creating ongoing community-health professional partnership to plan and implement community health initiatives
5. Recruiting and training 10 community residents as lay health workers to provide home-based health education and referral services to every household
6. Developing an ongoing health data collection system for use in program planning, evaluation, and research

The effectiveness of this program will be evaluated over time. The use of multiple models of community and behavior change optimizes the chances of success for this program in a concerned but impoverished community.

A review of major community-based cardiovascular disease prevention programs is provided by Shea and Basch.[26] Results from these studies indicate that community approaches to improving the health of populations are cost-effective. Research to date on community prevention and health-promotion efforts needs to be carefully examined to glean valuable information about what works with differing population groups and what does not.

• DIRECTIONS FOR RESEARCH ON SETTINGS FOR HEALTH PROMOTION

Health promotion efforts are increasingly being established in multiple settings. The interface among these efforts is critical to achieving synergy and cumulative effects. Health scientists need to address both the content and process of interventions but also broader issues of designing and evaluating seamless, coordinated health-promotion and disease-prevention services for diverse populations throughout the life span. Suggested directions for research include:

1. Explicating health-promotion and disease-prevention beliefs and practices in diverse families and communities as a basis for effective and culturally sensitive programming

2. Developing uniform methods for assessing health outcomes and cost savings across a range of programs and communities
3. Determining the synergistic effects of worksite, school, family, and community health-promotion efforts on population health outcomes
4. Identifying the interactive effects of unhealthy lifestyles and exposure to unhealthy environments
5. Identifying the short-term and long-term effects of poverty on the wellness potential of youth and their families, and testing school, worksite, and community strategies for optimizing health for individuals and families in the presence of adverse circumstances
6. Identifying the characteristics of health-strengthening environments in families, schools, worksites, and communities
7. Tracking the health care outcomes of families and communities receiving care from multiservice nursing centers with major emphasis on health promotion and prevention

• SUMMARY

Multiple settings offer the opportunity for provision of health-promotion services. Nurses, particularly nurses with an understanding of community health issues and problems, are ideally suited to provide leadership in the design, development, implementation, and evaluation of health-promotion programs in schools, worksites, nursing centers, and other community settings. Financial support for such programs should be sought from a variety of public and private sources. Quality of life for populations as well as length of life is emerging as a major concern. Nurses are critically needed to work with communities and with populations of all ages to improve the quality of their lives and of their environments so that present and future generations have a "bright future" in health.

REFERENCES

1. Gilliss CL. Why family health care? In: Gilliss CL, Highley BL, Roberts BM, et al, eds. *Toward a Science of Family Nursing.* Menlo Park, Calif: Addison-Wesley Publishing Co.; 1989.
2. Knutsen SF, Knutsen R. The Tromso Survey: The family intervention study—the effect of intervention on some coronary risk factors and dietary habits, a 6-year follow-up. *Prev Med.* 1991;20:197–212.
3. Baranowski T, Simons-Morton B, Hooks P, et al. Center-based program for exercise change among black American families. *Health Educ Q.* 1990;17(2);179–196.
4. Bomar PJ, eds. *Nurses and Family Health Promotion.* Baltimore, Md: Williams & Wilkins; 1989.
5. Hawkins JD, Catalano RF. Broadening the vision of education: schools as health promoting environments. *J School Health.* 1990;60:178–181.
6. Perry CL, Murray DM. Enhancing the transition years: the challenge of adolescent health promotion. *J School Health.* 1982;5:307–311.

7. Dryfoos JG. *Full Service Schools: A Revolution in Health and Social Services for Children, Youth and Families.* San Francisco, Calif: Jossey-Bass Inc. Publishers; 1994.
8. Uphold CR, Graham MV. Schools as centers for collaborative services for families: a vision for change. *Nurs Outlook.* 1993;41(5):204–211.
9. Millstein SG, Nightingale EO, Petersen AC, et al. Promoting the healthy development of adolescents. *JAMA.* 1993;269:1413–1415.
10. Igoe J. Empowerment of children and youth for consumer self-care. *Am J Health Prom.* 1991;6(1):55–64.
11. Moberg DP, Piper DL. An outcome evaluation of project model health: a middle school health promotion program. *Health Educ Q.* 1990;17(1):37–51.
12. Dryfoos JG. Adolescents at risk: a summation of work in the field—programs and policies. *J Adolesc Health.* 1991;12:630–637.
13. Cohen WS. Health promotion in the workplace: a prescription for good health. *Am Psychol.* 1985;40:213–216
14. Sorensen G, Rigotti N, Rosen A, et al. Effects of a worksite nonsmoking policy: evidence for increased cessation. *Am J Public Health.* 1991;81:202–204.
15. Jeffrey RW, Forster JL, French SA, et al. The Healthy Worker Project: A work-site intervention for weight control and smoking cessation. *Am J Public Health.* 1993;83:395–401.
16. Erfurt JC, Foote A, Heirich MA, et al. Improving participation in worksite wellness programs: comparing health education classes, a menu approach, and follow-up counseling. *Am J Health Prom.* 1990;4(4):270–278.
17. McCauley MJ, Mirin E. Employee-sponsored health promotion: why and how to make it a family affair. *Occup Med.* 1990;5:771–787.
18. Pelletier KR. A review and analysis of the health and cost-effective outcome studies of comprehensive health promotion and disease prevention programs at the worksite: 1991-1993 update. *Am J Health Prom.* 1993;8(1):50-62.
19. Weiss S. Community health promotion demonstration programs: introduction. In: Matarazzo JD, Weiss SM, Herd JA, et al, eds. *Behavioral Health: A Handbook of Health Enhancement and Disease Prevention.* New York, NY: John Wiley and Sons; 1984:1137–1139
20. Wickizer TM, Von Korff M, Cheadle A, et al. Activating communities for health promotion: a process evaluation method. *Am J Public Health.* 1993;83:561–567.
21. Eng E, Salmon ME, Mullen F. Community empowerment: the critical base for primary care. *Fam Community Health.* 1992;15(1):1–12.
22. Fisher EB, Auslander W, Sussman L, et al. Community organization and health promotion in minority neighborhoods. *Ethn Dis.* 1992;2:252–272.
23. Flynn BC. Healthy cities: a model of community change. *Fam Community Health.* 1992;15(1):13–23.
24. Maibach E, Flora JA, Nass C. Changes in self-efficacy and health behavior in response to a minimal contact community health campaign. *Health Communication.* 1991;3(1):1–15.
25. Schlaff AL. Boston's Codman Square Community Partnership for health promotion. *Public Health Rep.* 1991;106(2):186–191.
26. Shea S, Basch CE. A review of five major community-based cardiovascular disease prevention programs, II: interventions strategies, evaluation methods, and results. *Am J Health Prom.* 1990;4(4):279–287.

5

Empowerment for Self-Care

- The Role of the Professional Nurse
- Self-Care Education Throughout the Life Span
  - A. Self-Care for Children and Adolescents
  - B. Self-Care for Young and Middle-Aged Adults
  - C. Self-Care for Older Adults
- Goals of Health Education for Self-Care
- The Process of Self-Care Education
  - A. Mutually Assessing Self-Care Competencies and Needs
  - B. Determining Learning Priorities
  - C. Identifying Long-Term and Short-Term Objectives
  - D. Facilitating Self-Paced Learning
  - E. Using Positive Reinforcement to Increase Perceptions of Competence and Motivation for Learning
  - F. Creating a Supportive Environment for Learning
  - G. Decreasing Barriers to Learning
  - H. Evaluating Client Progress Toward Health Goals
- Other Important Considerations in Self-Care Education
- Directions for Research on Self-Care
- Summary

Individuals, families, and communities expend a great deal of energy in self-care activities. Self-care, a universal requirement for sustaining and enhancing life and health, is both an ongoing activity for individuals and groups and an area of competence to be developed. Self-care directed toward health protection and health promotion can be defined as "activities initiated or performed by an individual, family, or community to achieve, maintain, or promote maximum health.[1] Care of self and dependent others to maximize health includes actions directed toward minimizing threats to personal health, self-nurturance, self-improvement, and personal growth. Active involvement in self-care is widely acknowledged as an important strategy for achieving national health goals. According to Stoto and his colleagues, "There is a need to involve the general public in health promotion and prevention, in order to enable individuals to determine for themselves the means to achieve optimal health. . . . The (national health) objectives should go well beyond health professionals and health agencies and develop consumer roles and outreach programs that are more conducive to achieving the objectives and reaching the population in greatest need."[2]

Self-care within the medical model has been primarily defined as self-care in illness, compliance with therapeutic regimens, and active participation in rehabilitative activities to minimize the sequelae of illness. Self-care for health promotion goes beyond self-care in illness and requires that clients gain knowledge and competencies that can be used to **maintain** and **enhance** health. In both prevention and health promotion, self-care is primary, with professional care—in the form of active protection (immunization) against disease, education, or guidance—secondary. Woods[3] proposed a health-oriented conceptual model of self-care using the four models of health proposed by Smith[4]: the clinical, role performance, adaptive, and eudaemonistic models. In the clinical domain, self-care focuses on symptom detection, monitoring, evaluation, and response. The role performance domain emphasizes self-care as maximizing functional capacities to perform familial and social roles as well as activities of daily living in an acceptable manner. In the

TABLE 5–1. RELATIONSHIPS AMONG MODELS OF HEALTH, CONCEPTS, STRATEGIES, AND OUTCOMES IN SELF-CARE

MODEL OF HEALTH	CONCEPTUAL ORIENTATIONS	SELF-CARE STRATEGIES	OUTCOMES
Clinical	Illness behavior Health-deviation self-care requirements Early detection of illness	Symptom perception and monitoring, evaluation, and response, including discretionary nonaction, use of prescription and nonprescription medication, lay consultation, and formal health services	Morbidity Mortality Use of health services Cost of health care
Role performance	Universal self-care requirements Developmental self-care requirements	Normalizing strategies Rehabilitation programs to promote performance of activities of daily living	Role performance Functional capacity in activities of daily living: independence
Adaptive	Models for coping with stress Self-management	Stress-management programs Self-management programs	Behavioral change Stress-related symptoms Self-efficacy
Eudaemonistic	Health-promotion models	Health-promotion programs	Well-being, harmony, fitness

(From Woods N[3] p. 6, with permission.)

adaptive domain, stress management and optimal adjustment to transient and permanent life changes constitute the focus for self-care. The eudaemonistic domain emphasizes self-care as the exercise of competencies necessary to promote well-being, harmony, and overall fitness for vigorous living. This framework for conceptualizing self-care is presented in Table 5–1. Woods emphasized the need to better link self-care strategies to measurable health outcomes, since little attention has been given to this link in health literature. Consideration of self-care approaches and their outcomes should go beyond strategies in the province of medicine, nursing, and other health professions to consideration of strategies that lie outside the province of traditional healing. Such explorations would constitute a grass roots approach to investigating self-care and might well lead to new understandings of the boundaries and strengths of self-care throughout the life span.

• THE ROLE OF THE PROFESSIONAL NURSE

Professional nurses have a major responsibility for enhancing clients' capacity for self-care. Nurses have long recognized the right of individuals and families to be both informed and active participants in their care.

Orem[5] describes three types of self-care requisites: universal, developmental, and health-deviation self-care requisites. Universal self-care requisites include:

1. Maintenance of sufficient air
2. Maintenance of sufficient water
3. Maintenance of sufficient food
4. Provision of care associated with elimination processes and excrement
5. Maintenance of a balance between activity and rest
6. Maintenance of a balance between solitude and social interaction
7. Prevention of hazards to human life, human function, and human well-being
8. Promotion of human functioning and development within social groups in accord with human potential

Developmental self-care requisites fit into two categories:

1. Maintenance of living conditions that support life processes, promote development, or human progress toward higher levels of organization of human structure and maturation
2. Provision of care either to prevent the occurrence of deleterious effects of conditions that can affect human development or to mitigate or overcome these effects from various conditions

The nurse focusing on health promotion is primarily concerned with universal and developmental requisites, although health-deviation requisites (needs for knowledge and skills to care for self in illness) must be promptly attended to if they arise.

Orem has developed a Self-Care Nursing Model that describes three systems within professional nursing practice: a compensatory system, a partially compensatory system, and an educative-developmental system. In compensatory care, the nurse provides total care for the client. Such care is most common in intensive-, acute-care settings within hospitals during severe illness. Partially compensatory care is implemented when the nurse and the client share the responsibility for care. Care during rehabilitation from illness or in advanced chronic illness is partially compensatory. In contrast to the preceding two types of care, the **educative-developmental** nursing system gives the client primary responsibility for personal health, with the nurse functioning in a consultative capacity. It is this third nursing system that is most appropriate for health protection and health promotion.

With increasing emphasis on primary care in the United States and throughout the world, the educative-developmental component of nursing practice is viewed with renewed interest as a reimbursable service by health payors, including managed care organizations. This broadened perpective on value-added to health care by educative-developmental services is long overdue. Major areas of educative-developmental nursing for self-care include enhancing clients' capacities for exercise and physical fitness, nutrition and weight control, stress management, multimodal risk reduction, maintenance of family and other social support systems, avoidance of injurious and violent behaviors, and environmental modifications in homes, schools, worksites, and the community to reduce hazards to health and strengthen health-enhancing features. Education, counseling, and environmental interventions directed to these ends should be paid for with health care dollars.

Broad-based efforts directed at activating the general public for self-care should be spearheaded by nurses in collaboration with communities and other health professionals. These efforts should also be supported by public health monies. Activation of health care consumers to "take charge" of their health is based on the assumptions that they should be:

1. Actively involved in health problem solving
2. Making rational and informed choices regarding health and health care
3. Developing competencies and skills that foster creativity and adaptivity amid changing life circumstances
4. Striving for greater mastery of environmental conditions that impact health and well-being
5. Promoting public policy making to undergird healthy lifestyles in diverse communities
6. Advocating for the development of health financing plans that provide payment for a range of self-care education services for all people

The ideas of individual, family, and community empowerment for self-care are closely related. It is only as people work in concert that advances will be achieved to make self-care a coherent social movement with a significant impact on the quality and cost of health care delivery. The multiple self-care organizations and programs throughout the United States are primarily self-pay or free and each is directed at a particular health-related need. Careful examination should be given to existing programs and their outcomes. Successful programs should be integrated throughout the educational and health care sectors nationally, with tailoring to fit local needs.

• SELF-CARE EDUCATION THROUGHOUT THE LIFE SPAN

Self-Care for Children and Adolescents

Childhood and adolescence are developmental periods during which social and cognitive skills for autonomous decision making and responsible self-care are developed. Approaches to enhancing self-care behaviors of children and adolescents must focus on both families and peer groups. This dual approach is critical, since values, attitudes, beliefs, and behaviors of families and peers influence children's lifestyles. Parents, in providing physical care for children and promoting cultural adjustment, serve as powerful role models of health and health-related behaviors. They depict family health care functions and various approaches to linking with the broader health care resources in the community. The rapid developmental changes that occur for children and adolescents and the emerging yet malleable behavioral patterns that will carry into adulthood make the preschool and school-age years an ideal time to enhance self-care skills for preventive and health-promotive behaviors.

Igoe[6] has aptly described the need for activating and empowering children and youth for self-care, including optimal use of health care services. She and her colleagues have developed programs to promote active involvement of children of all ages in primary care encounters using HealthPACT (Participatory and Assertive Consumer Training). HealthPACT is a role-development program for health consumers of school age. The program prepares children and adolescents with the knowledge and skills to engage in health-promoting behaviors and to assume a more active and responsible role in use of health care services. Children are taught their basic consumer rights to be informed, to choose, to be heard, and to be safe. For use during appointments with health care providers, they are provided with a memory cue that encourages and supports them in being active participants in their own health care. For example, the acronym TLADD (talk, listen and learn, ask, decide, do) serves as a memory cue for desired behaviors during an appointment for health care. The instructional process for HealthPACT includes role modeling of TLADD behaviors, participatory social skills training, and rehearsal with peers of TLADD behaviors and other social skills for heightening participation with the health care provider. The program also works with health care providers in the community to modify office routines and protocols to enhance children's opportunities for participation in their health care encounters. To implement the HealthPACT program, there must be upfront planning with the adults who are significant in the lives of children (parents, teachers, school health personnel) and community health care providers. Manuals are available to help adults follow through in encouraging TLADD behaviors. Evaluation studies indicate that the program has been successful in increasing knowledge about health consumerism, changing attitudes toward health care providers, changing health habits, and increasing health locus of control. This program should be an integral part of all comprehensive health education programs in elementary and secondary schools in the United States.

Peer groups play a critical role in molding lifestyles for school-aged children, particularly adolescents. When peers reinforce the active health consumer role, peer pressure becomes a positive force. An increasing number of school health programs today are giving considerable attention to lifestyle education that increases children's health and resilience, teaches skills for modifying peer group affiliations and resisting the pressure of peers who encourage health-damaging behaviors, and fosters community caring and involvement to improve the health of others, including peers and the less fortunate members of the community.

Peer group affiliation and risk behaviors were explored among early adolescents by Dolcini and Adler.[7] They found that characteristics of the crowd that adolescents "hung out" with determined the likelihood of abandoning constructive self-care for risky behaviors. In their study, the identified crowds were the "Smarts," "Elites," and "Popular Blacks." The Smarts exhibited behaviors that meet traditional adult expectations of high scholastic achievement and being well-behaved and unlikely to engage in risky behaviors. The Elites and Popular Blacks were very similar. Both had the personal strengths of being socially and athletically competent but were more likely than Smarts to be using alcohol and drugs and engaging in sexual behavior. A group of students outside the main social structure, Outsiders, also reported a high level of drug use and engagement in sex. Group membership appears to facilitate risky behaviors by both peer pressure and providing alcohol and drug availability. Changing peer norms and perceptions of peer norms represents an important approach to fostering responsible self-care among youth. Peer discussions and action projects focused on health promoting self-care can create a climate more supportive of emerging healthful lifestyles in school-age youth and less supportive of health-damaging behaviors.

An important group to attend to for self-care education are children and youth who have dropped out of school or are homeless. Self-care education sessions for these children may have to be held in parks, food kitchens, or homeless shelters. Special sensitivity to the lack of resources for daily living and to low levels of motivation on the part of some for self-care and self-preservation is critical.

Self-Care for Young and Middle-Aged Adults

Young and middle-aged adulthood is the time in the life cycle when many persons are intensely involved in careers and child rearing. The momentum of everyday life and the demands of dependent others may leave little time for focusing on health in the absence of an illness crisis. The strengthening of intrafamilial support for self-care is particularly important at this time when adults need to accept responsibility for modeling and teaching younger and older children competent self-care; increasing family knowledge and expertise with health-promotion skills; and learning how and when to use health care resources for the family. Adult learners bring a great deal to self-care education including a background of life experiences, self-direction in learning, problem- or interested-centered (as opposed to subject-centered) learning needs, and interest in immediate application. Caporael-Katz[8] has described self-care education for adults as consisting of the following components:

1. Provision of a period of time for expression of feelings
2. Reinforcement of client self-esteem
3. Provision of open access to health information
4. Practice of self-care skills that could be applied immediately

5. Presentation of alternative views on health issues
6. Critical evaluation of both traditional medicine and alternative therapies

Adults tuned in to their own needs for self-care may be effective in reducing the stress inherent in multiple societal roles, including familial and work responsibilities that many young and middle-age adults fulfill. Systematically planning health-promotion activities into daily routines at work or with family members can both enhance health in a busy lifestyle and model healthy lifestyles to family members. Adequate attention to self-care during the young and middle-aged years promotes optimal productivity and life satisfaction and lays the groundwork for a healthy and productive retirement and old age rather than one fraught with discomfort, disability, and compromised quality of life.

Self-Care for Older Adults

Self-care for older adults focuses on maximizing independence, vigor, and life satisfaction. Adequate self-care education must take into account the physical, sensory, mobility, sexual, and psychosocial changes that currently characterize the aging process. Interestingly, while not all changes of aging can be slowed or reversed, aggressive self-care can maintain or increase cardiac and pulmonary functioning as well as physical fitness. Weight control can enhance mobility. Research has indicated that exercise can enhance the self-esteem of older adults and in some cases decrease depression and anxiety.

Personality and coping styles do not appear to change significantly with age. Thus, persons who develop positive coping skills early in life can meet social demands in later years, find meaning in life, and direct ample energy to appropriate self-care activities.

Retirement is a significant life event for which appropriate self-care in the form of anticipatory planning must take place to maximize ease of adjustment. Gioiella[9] has identified the following self-care actions that facilitate healthy retirement:

1. Planning ahead to insure adequate income
2. Developing friends not associated with work
3. Decreasing time at work in the last years before retirement by taking longer vacations, working shorter days, or working part-time
4. Developing routines, including adequate physical activity, to replace the structure of the work day
5. Relying on other people and groups in addition to spouse to fill leisure time
6. Developing leisure time activities before retirement that are realistic in energy and monetary cost
7. Preparing for exhilaration followed by ambivalence before satisfaction with one's retirement lifestyle develops
8. Assessing living arrangements, and if relocation is necessary, expending time in developing new social networks
9. Expecting role loss to have a short-term impact on self-esteem and one's marital relationship

Older adults often have more discretionary time available for pursuit of personal wellness than younger adults. They should be challenged to use this time productively and counseled concerning resources available within the community to facilitate such efforts.

The fastest growing segment of the population in the United States is the old-old, comprising individuals over 85 years of age. These individuals need safe, health-enhancing communities as well as support services to assist them in continuing health-promotion activities, including exercise, social support, and healthy nutritional practices. With adequate support from families and health professionals, most older adults would choose to remain in their own home throughout their old age. The nation must address the scope of health-protection and health-promotion services needed by the elderly to support their self-care capabilities. Cost-effective and efficient methods for developing these services using new, user-friendly communication technologies to augment personal contact warrants exploration. More attention must be given to promoting the health and well-being of older adults, a growing segment of the US citizenry.

GOALS OF HEALTH EDUCATION FOR SELF-CARE

While education of the public for self-care is an integral part of a number of federal documents and policies, including *Healthy People 2000: National Health Promotion and Disease Prevention Objectives,*[10] it has yet to become a highly viable and visible focus for federal health expenditures. Only a small percentage of the federal budget is actually spent on health-education activities. Within the federal government, the Office of Disease Prevention and Health Promotion (ODPHP), the Office on Smoking and Health (OSH); the Office of Women's Health, the Office of Minority Health, and the Centers for Disease Control and Prevention are examples of major agencies focused on meeting the health-education needs of the public. National goals for health education for self-care are not well articulated in a single document but can be implied from numerous documents addressing various self-care issues, from hypertension to good nutrition. Recommended goals in the public and private sectors for self-care education directed toward health protection and health promotion include:

1. Raise the consciousness of the American people regarding major threats to health that they can prevent or ameliorate and provide the individual, group, and environmental means to do so.
2. Change the dominant definition of health to include not only the absence of illness but high-level wellness among individuals, families, and communities.
3. Create conditions facilitating empowerment of communities for self-care to address the social and environmental ills that blight the lives of the community and its inhabitants.
4. Create financial and other incentives to foster active health-information seeking and change to more positive health practices.
5. Assist people in developing the requisite knowledge and skills to successfully implement health-protecting and health-promoting behaviors.
6. Disseminate culturally and socioeconomically appropriate health-enhancing techniques and strategies to the population.
7. Provide the educational base in preschool, elementary, and secondary schools to undergird healthy living throughout the life span.

To achieve these goals, health policy makers and health professionals must be particularly sensitive to the extent to which problems of literacy and poverty present barriers to health education. This is not a problem to be taken lightly. Approaches to self-care education that use indigenous community workers and communication media such as radio that do not require reading but are accessible to a vast majority of the population must be considered as an important means of educating populations about self-care needs and strategies. Competent self-care must also be economically plausible to individuals and families living in poverty. This requires coordination of public, private, and volunteer services to provide coherent self-care education and options to facilitate responsible yet low-cost follow-through.

• THE PROCESS OF SELF-CARE EDUCATION

Responses of individuals and groups to the process of health education for self-care are multidimensional and complex. The client brings to the learning situation a unique personality and learning style, established social interaction patterns, numerous group affiliations, cultural norms and values, proximal and distal environmental influences, and a given level of readiness to adopt self-care behaviors. The nurse also comes with intact personality characteristics, values, and social circumstances that affect the nature of the interaction. The self-care education process as a collaborative endeavor between client and nurse is depicted in Figure 5–1. The interaction for self-care education brings the professional expertise of nurses and other health care professionals together with the health care knowledge and goals of the client, either individual or group. Mutual assessment of health care competencies and strengths as well as needs by the client and nurse will determine what learning priorities are set, the pace of learning (long-term and short-term objectives), and the interpersonal and environmental support needed for learning. Barriers to learning and implementing self-care behaviors should be identified and directly addressed with clients. Failure to identify and realistically deal with barriers can result in frustration and a lack of satisfaction for clients when they evaluate progress toward their self-care goals. Specific components of the self-care education process are described below.

Mutually Assessing Self-Care Competencies and Needs

The client often comes to the encounter with health care professionals with certain self-care goals in mind. Competencies related to these goals can be assessed through informal discussion, health-knowledge checklists (Fig. 5–2), or structured tests of knowledge in specific content areas. The first approach is recommended for low-literacy clients or those uncomfortable with paper-and-pencil tasks. Observation of actual behavior can also provide useful insights, if this is possible at the school or worksite.

The activated client shows evidence of motivation in aggressively seeking health information that will assist in self-care. The existence of apathy, lack of interest, and inattention should alert the nurse to a lack of motivation on the part of the client. Reasons for lack of interest should be explored so that the nurse can knowledgeably intervene to increase motivation.

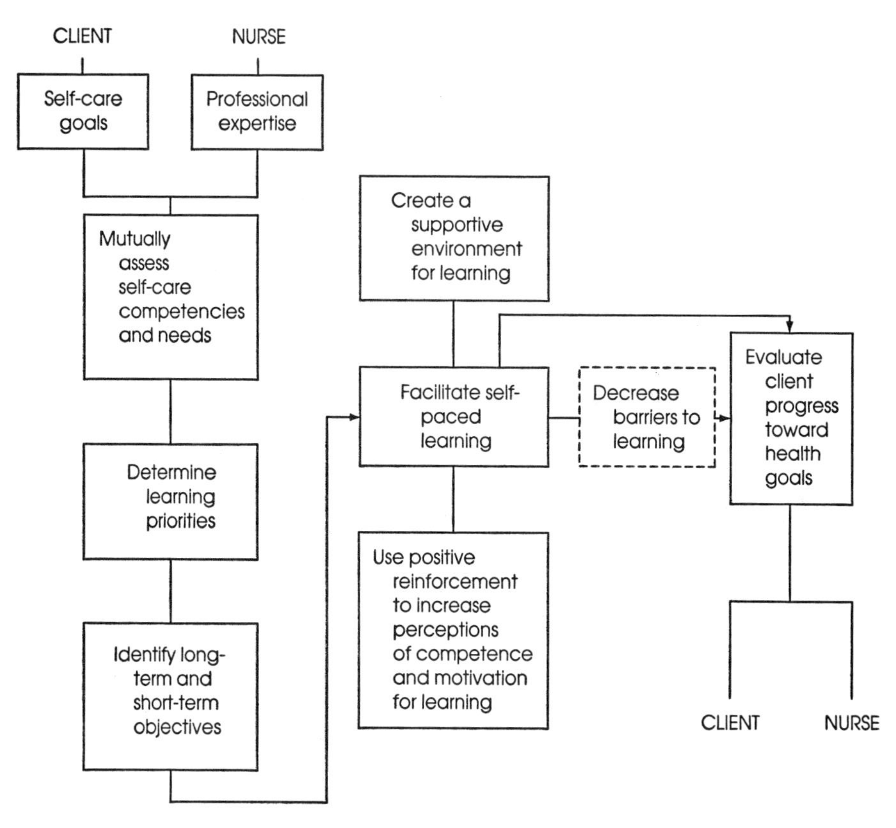

Figure 5–1. The self-care education process.

Determining Learning Priorities

Deciding where to begin is often a dilemma for the nurse when the client needs information about a variety of different health topics. Clients have definite ideas about what they wish to know and what is important to them. Sometimes interest may not lie in the area that poses the greatest threat to personal health. As an example, a client may smoke but be more interested in starting to exercise than in quitting smoking. While the nurse may believe that smoking constitutes a more serious threat to the health of the client than a sedentary life-style, it is obviously better to be a physically active smoker than an inactive smoker, since risks are synergistic. If the nurse assists the client to develop an exercise program, the client may also develop a heightened awareness of the negative impact of smoking on lung capacity and physical endurance. At that point, the client may exhibit readiness to discuss approaches to smoking cessation based on concrete experiences with the health- and activity-compromising effects of smoking.

Identifying Long-Term and Short-Term Objectives

Identification of long- and short-term objectives is important in self-care education. Long-term objectives guide large segments of learning. Short-term objectives fit under a

In the list below, please check those behaviors that you are comfortable in performing for yourself without assistance from others.

- ____________ Counting my pulse at the wrist for 1 minute
- ____________ Counting my pulse at the neck for 1 minute
- ____________ Selecting comfortable and appropriate shoes for brisk walking or jogging
- ____________ Selecting appropriate clothing for walking or jogging activities
- ____________ Planning a progressive schedule of exercise to meet my personal needs
- ____________ Indicating the ideal weight range for my height
- ____________ Calculating my maximal heart rate during exercise
- ____________ Planning time for exercise that is convenient and possible
- ____________ Describing warm-up exercises that I could do before brisk walking or running
- ____________ Describing procedures for cooling down after vigorous exercise
- ____________ Exercising intensively at least four times a week for 30 minutes
- ____________ Integrating physical-fitness activities with my recreational interests
- ____________ Maintaining a record of my progress in physical fitness over a period of several months
- ____________ Eating appropriately before or after vigorous exercise
- ____________ Explaining how stress is released through physical exercise
- ____________ Describing how to avoid injuries during exercise

Figure 5–2. Health-knowledge checklist for exercise and physical fitness.

specific long-term objective and identify the specific content or activities that must be progressively mastered. The objectives should be realistic, neither too easy, resulting in boredom, nor too hard, resulting in discouragement. An example of a goal and objectives identification form is presented in Figure 5–3. Use of the form allows the client to check off each objective as it is attained and maintain awareness of the desired behavioral and health outcomes. Both the nurse and the client should retain a copy for continuing reference and update.

Facilitating Self-Paced Learning

The pace at which a client will learn depends on personal motivation, assertiveness, perseverance, skill, and learning style. The pace of learning may also vary with age, health status, and educational level. Self-pacing is important to allow the client to be self-

Health Goal: Increased Physical Fitness	
Long-term Objective: To take a brisk walk for 45 minutes four times a week	
Related Short-term Learning Objectives	**Objectives Attained**
1. Demonstrate how to check my pulse at the neck by counting beats for 10 seconds and multiplying by six 2. State heart rate that I should achieve during exercise 3. Demonstrate two warm-up exercises to use before walking 4. Demonstrate two cool down exercises to use after brisk walking 5. Construct a weekly schedule for brisk walking 6. Map out three different and interesting routes to take when walking	

Figure 5–3. Goal and objectives identification form.

directed and maintain control over the learning process. The pace at which the client meets each short-term objective will vary, and expectations of both the client and the health professional should be adjusted accordingly. The important factor is not how rapidly knowledge or skill is attained but the extent of mastery.

The nurse must be realistic about teaching and learning and accept both good and bad days in clients of all ages. Sometimes the nurse and client will be elated with the results, sometimes discouraged. When efforts are less rewarding than anticipated, the pace of learning should be reviewed carefully. It is possible that expanding the time frame for learning will result in increased success for the client. This is especially true for young children and adolescents, who have less experience to draw on in the learning process than do adults.

Using Positive Reinforcement to Increase Perceptions of Competence and Motivation for Learning

In education for self-care, the client, the nurse, and the family of the client all play important roles in reinforcement. The nurse should be attuned to small steps in client progress and use positive reinforcement such as praise and compliments frequently to enhance the client's feelings of success in developing competence in self-care. Cues should be used to facilitate successful responses and immediate feedback provided to correct errors in performance. When cues and error feedback are intermingled with positive reinforcement, they are helpful, nonthreatening, and enhance intrinsic motivation of the client. Immediate and consistent reinforcement facilitates rapid learning and assists the client in deriving satisfaction from learning. Once learning has occurred, intermittent reinforcement of the desired response strengthens the behavior, making it more resistant to extinction.

Family members need to learn to serve as sources of support for one another in developing health behaviors. For example, achievement of a specific goal may be rewarded by a family outing in the park or by the family spending time together in a favorite activity at home. By providing mutual support, a sense of healthy interdependence rather than crippling dependence is created within the family.

Clients should be made aware of the importance of self-reward or self-reinforcement in the health education process. It is important that they learn to reward their own efforts and achievements, since much of the time, contingent reinforcement for self-care cannot be supplied by others. A schedule of rewards can be tailored by the client to personal preferences. However, use of foods as reinforcement should be discouraged. It is important that the client also learn to use internal self-reinforcement such as self-praise and self-compliment. Learning to use internal self-reward in an appropriate manner permits the client to be less dependent on the availability of tangible objects to facilitate the learning process.

Creating a Supportive Environment for Learning

The environment in which health education for self-care is provided is vitally important to the success of educational efforts. If a clinic is used for health education, the rooms in which self-care is taught should be warm, comfortable, and informal. A desk should not be placed in the room; instead, tables and chairs or sofa and chairs should be placed in a conversational setting. Walls should be pleasant in color with pictures and textured materials used to create a homelike, supportive, and nonthreatening climate. Visual aids in flip-chart form on an easel at a comfortable height for the nurse to use while seated in a chair are ideal. If very young children are present during the self-care education sessions, an area with attractive toys and books may need to be provided for their use. This will minimize distraction of the parents. If children are old enough to be included in the sessions, they should be actively involved. Often, use of bright colors and interesting figures or designs on flip charts will amuse children and maintain their interest. Children can play an important role in reinforcing learning or in reminding parents and other family members to engage in the recommended behaviors.

To the extent possible, actual materials available in the home should be used in teaching. If a client is expected to use a booklet on low-cholesterol foods at home in preparing meals, the booklet to be used should be the basis for instruction. If the client is learning relaxation techniques, audiotapes and videos for practice must be usable in the client's home. They should be demonstrated in the clinic and questions answered regarding their use. Well-illustrated materials should be supplied liberally to the client to take home to provide reinforcement of knowledge and skills gained during health-education sessions.

Since the minimal time needed for most health instruction is 15 to 30 minutes, the nurse must determine whether individual or small-group teaching methods are to be used. If health education is provided to groups, the groups should be kept small to facilitate interaction and attention to the specific needs of group members. A combination of group and individual instruction may also be helpful. This combined approach allows for efficient use of professional time yet meets the unique educative-developmental needs of clients.

Decreasing Barriers to Learning

Barriers to learning can result from various sources: personal values, beliefs, and attitudes; lack of motivation; poor self-concept; or inadequate cognitive or psychomotor skills. Whatever the source, if the client exhibits lack of progress, barriers within the individual as well as within the family, relevant social groups, and the environment should be explored. Barriers must often be identified and attenuated or eliminated before progress can continue.

Approaches to dealing with obstacles to healthy behavior should be an integral part of the health-education plan. In this way, problems are addressed systematically, and progress in dealing with the barriers can be periodically assessed. The client may be unaware of what is inhibiting progress or reluctant to share such information with the nurse. A climate of trust will facilitate communication between the client and the nurse concerning obstacles to learning and performance.

Evaluating Client Progress Toward Health Goals

Evaluation is a process by which the nurse and client in collaboration judge to what degree long- and short-term objectives and health goals have been attained. All evaluation involves direct or indirect observation of behavior. The major source of error in direct measurement is inadequate sampling of the target behaviors during brief clinic or home visits. A source of error in indirect measurement is that self-observation skills of clients may be inadequately developed, or clients may ascribe a "halo effect" to themselves, seeing performance of health behaviors as more frequent or more intensive than they actually are.

A combination of methods should be used in evaluating client progress. These may include: checklists of objectives (see Fig. 5–3), client progress notes, laboratory measurements, paper-and-pencil tests, verbal questioning, and direct observation. The primary purpose of evaluation is to provide an accurate picture for clients of where they stand in attaining their health goals. The desired outcome from self-care education is a sustained effect of the self-care education intervention that permanently changes lifestyle or behavior.

• OTHER IMPORTANT CONSIDERATIONS IN SELF-CARE EDUCATION

Each client's desire for efficacy or competence in self-care must be assessed by the nurse. The fact cannot be ignored that some individuals do not want to be responsible for their own self-care but instead wish to function within society in a highly dependent role. Their desire for competence may have been frustrated by a health care system that makes people feel infantile and helpless. It is critical that the nurse assess very early in interactions with clients the extent to which they desire to assume responsibility for their own care once they are given the requisite knowledge and skills to do so. Interdependency of roles within each family must be considered before making decisions about how self-care education will be targeted. Often, an optimal approach can be to include family members in self-care education.

Clients' conceptualization of health will also determine the content that they view as meaningful in self-care education. When health is defined as maintaining stability or avoiding overt illness, health-protecting behaviors such as immunization, self-examination for signs of cancer, and periodic multiphasic screening may be most important to the client. When health is defined as self-actualization or exuberant well-being, the emphasis of health education may be placed on relaxation techniques, enhancing self-awareness, environmental appreciation during outdoor physical activity, or developing aspects of self that represent untapped potential.

The success of self-care education depends on thoughtful consideration of culture and its dimensions including race, ethnicity, socioeconomic class, sexual orientation, age, and gender. Increasingly, health personnel provide care to people of varying backgrounds and life circumstances. In working with individuals and families who live in poverty areas, nurses must realize that it is not possible to have effective self-care without altering the environmental factors that affect poverty-level families. These factors include high rates of unemployment, poor housing, inadequate child-care facilities, and prevalence of violent behavior. A major aspect of health initiatives with poverty-level clients is group (churches, schools, community organizations) empowerment to enable change.

An expanding volume of literature is available to assist health professionals in understanding diverse cultures and in appropriately tailoring health education for self-care to incorporate traditional cultural beliefs. A word of caution is in order concerning transcultural use of published health education materials. It is often supposed that simply translating materials into the language of another culture provides appropriate audiovisual teaching aids and pamphlets for client education. Such is often not the case, however. The sense of modesty among women of Hispanic origin may make pictures and illustrations of human anatomy offensive to them. In the Navajo culture, questions directed at finding out information about another's personal problems and habits are considered rude and inappropriate behavior. Thus, assessment of self-care competency has to be approached in an indirect manner or modified to accommodate reluctance for personal disclosure. Within the Navajo culture, the family plays a central role in advice giving and decision making. Consequently, failure to involve the family in education for self-care can greatly decrease the impact of such efforts.[11] Materials for educational use in specific cultures should be prepared by people within the target culture or in consultation with them. Furthermore, it is important for practitioners of Western medicine to interact with traditional healers in a culture to find innovative ways in which several healing systems may together reinforce positive self-care practices.[12]

• DIRECTIONS FOR RESEARCH ON SELF-CARE

Although self-care has been practiced for centuries, it has only become the focus of research for health professionals within the last two decades. Theoretical work by Orem has been the primary driving force in nursing for empirical work on the various dimensions of self-care and related nursing care systems. Directions for research in self-care to broaden our understanding of this widely occurring but little understood phenomenon include:

1. Identify developmental changes in self-care agency across the life span.
2. Determine how peers affect self-care practices of preadolescents and adolescents.
3. Critically analyze the health care outcomes of self-care.
4. Study self-care practices outside the domains of traditional health care.
5. Test culturally appropriate interventions to enhance self care among individuals and families.

Further work is needed both in instrumentation and in prospective studies to provide a basis for intervention studies to test the usefulness of empirically based self-care strategies.

• SUMMARY

In self-care education, it is important to emphasize the competencies of clients for self-direction and self-responsibility in planning and managing self-care activities. In addition, environmental constraints impairing self-care must be addressed and resolved to optimize client success. The content and pace of learning experiences should be controlled by the client. The nurse's primary role is that of consultant. Educative-supportive care provided by the nurse should enable clients to achieve those health goals that they have set for themselves. The nurse, in functioning as a resource person, enhances the success of clients in acquiring knowledge and skills in self-care. Further research on the dimensions of self-care within the context of health protection and health promotion will provide important information for facilitating optimum self-care across diverse populations.

REFERENCES

1. Steiger NJ, Lipson JG. *Self-care Nursing: Theory and Practice.* Bowie, Md: Brady Communications; 1985:12.
2. Stoto M, Behrens R, Rosemont C, eds. *Healthy People 2000: Citizens Chart the Course.* Washington, DC: National Academy Press; 1990;21.
3. Woods N. Conceptualization of self-care: towards health-oriented models. *Adv Nurs Sci.* 1989;12(1):1–13.
4. Smith J. The idea of health: a philosophical inquiry. *Adv Nurs Sci.* 1981;3(3):43–50.
5. Orem DE. *Nursing: Concepts of Practice.* 3rd ed. New York, NY: McGraw-Hill Inc; 1985.
6. Igoe JB. Empowerment of children and youth for consumer self-care. *Am J Health Prom.* 1991;6(1):55–64.
7. Dolcini MM, Adler NE. Perceived competencies, peer group affiliation, and risk behavior among early adolescents. *Health Psychol.* 1994;13:496–506.
8. Caporael-Katz B. Health, self-care and power: shifting the balance. *Top Clin Nurs.* 1983;5:31–41.
9. Gioiella EC. Healthy aging through knowledge and self-care. *Aging Prev.* 1983;3(1):39–51.
10. *Healthv People 2000: National Health Promotion and Disease Prevention Objectives.* Washmgton, DC: US Public Health Service; 1991. US Dept of Health and Human Services publication PHS 91-50212.
11. Hammonds TA. Self-care practices of Navajo Indians. In: Riehl-Sisca J., ed. *The Science and Art of Self-Care.* Norwalk, Conn: Appleton-Century-Crofts; 1985;171–180.
12. Earls F. Health promotion for minority adolescents: cultural considerations. In: Millstein SG, Petersen AC, Nightingale EO, eds. *Promoting the Health of Adolescents.* New York, NY: Oxford University Press; 1993:58–72.

III

PART THREE

Planning for Prevention and Health Promotion

6

Assessment of Health, Health Beliefs, and Health Behaviors

- Assessment of the Individual Client
  - A. Nursing Frameworks for Health Assessment
  - B. Physical Fitness Evaluation
  - C. Nutritional Assessment
  - D. Health-Risk Appraisal
  - E. Life-Stress Review
  - F. Spiritual Health Assessment
  - G. Social Support Systems Review
  - H. Health-Beliefs Review
  - I. Lifestyle Assessment
  - J. Further Assistance with Assessment
- Assessment of the Family
- Assessment of the Community
- Directions for Research
- Summary

A thorough assessment of health, health beliefs, and health behaviors is the foundation for tailoring a health-protection–promotion plan to a given client. Assessment provides the database for making clinical judgments concerning the client's health strengths, health problems, nursing diagnoses, and desired health or behavioral outcomes, as well as the interventions likely to be effective. This information determines the nature of the client–health-professional encounter. The portfolio of assessment tools to be used depends on characteristics of the client, including developmental stage and cultural orientation. In this chapter, the primary focus is on assessment of the individual. However, approaches for assessing families and communities are also discussed.

• ASSESSMENT OF THE INDIVIDUAL CLIENT

Assessment of the individual client in the context of health promotion expands beyond physical assessment to also include a comprehensive examination of other client health parameters, health beliefs, and health behaviors. The components of health assessment focusing on individual clients are (1) functional health patterns, (2) physical fitness evaluation, (3) nutritional assessment, (4) health risk appraisal, (5) life stress review, (6) spiritual health assessment, (7) social support systems review, (8) health beliefs review, and (9) lifestyle assessment.

Nursing Frameworks for Health Assessment

Health assessment as performed by the nurse is a collaborative process with the client, which promotes mutual input into decision making and planning to improve the client's health and well-being. The desired outcomes of health assessment are to: (1) identify health assets, (2) identify health-related lifestyle strengths, (3) determine key health-related beliefs, (4) identify health beliefs and health behaviors that put the client at risk, and (5) determine how the client wants to change to improve the quality of life. The initial assessment provides a valuable baseline against which subsequent assessments can be compared.

Several guides for nursing assessment and diagnosis are currently available. These taxonomies are gradually being expanded to include diagnoses appropriate to aspects of wellness as well as illness. Current diagnostic systems in nursing focus primarily on the individual. Taxonomies that address families and communities (eg, Omaha System) still need to be developed or incorporated widely into the assessment and diagnostic activities of the discipline. I am confident that nursing will expand its taxonomies guiding clinical judgment to further undergird wellness activities. Rapidly increasing knowledge about health promotion and health protection will continue to fuel this effort.

At this point, it is important to differentiate between nursing assessment and diagnosis as they are used in this book. **Nursing assessment** is systematic collection of data about client health status, beliefs, and behaviors relevant to developing a health-protection–promotion plan. **Nursing diagnosis** is a clear specification of areas for improvement to maximize health status.

The North American Nursing Diagnosis Association (NANDA) provides a nursing diagnosis taxonomy developed in collaboration with the American Nurses Association (ANA) and the International Council of Nurses (ICN), *Nursing Diagnoses: Definitions & Classification: 1995–1996.*[1] The taxonomy is structured around the nine human response patterns of exchanging, communicating, relating, valuing, choosing, moving, perceiving, knowing, and feeling. Examples of diagnoses relevant to health protection and health promotion include the following: Altered nutrition: Potential for more than body requirements (exchanging), risk for altered parent/infant/child attachment (relating), potential for enhanced spiritual well-being (valuing), risk for activity intolerance (moving), and situational low self-esteem (perceiving).[1(pp8–11)] The NANDA defining characteristics of each diagnosis, as well as related factors and risk factors, provide guidance as to what the critical assessment areas are in relation to that diagnosis. This taxonomy, although heavily focused on the alterations, dysfunctions, and impairments of illness, has gradually expanded to include more diagnoses relevant to risk reduction and health promotion. Following health assessment, the NANDA classification provides one means for clearly labeling some of the issues and problems identified.

Gordon's[2] functional health patterns presented in the *Manual of Nursing Diagnosis: 1993–1994* offers a related classification system. Gordon offers a typology of 11 functional health patterns for classifying nursing diagnoses: health perception–health management, nutritional–metabolic, elimination, activity–exercise, sleep–rest, cognitive–perceptual, self-perception–self-concept, role–relationship, sexuality–reproductive, coping–stress tolerance, and value–belief.[2(pp 2–5)] The actual list of diagnoses contains those accepted by NANDA as well as additional diagnoses. Gordon states: "Functional health patterns of clients, whether individuals, families or communities, evolve from client-environment interaction. Each pattern is an expression of biopsychosocial integration. No one pattern can be understood without knowledge of the other patterns. . . . Dysfunctional health patterns (described by nursing diagnoses) may occur with disease; dysfunctional health patterns may also lead to disease."[2(p 2)] All patterns must be assessed to provide a comprehensive basis for the development of a useful plan of care. The judgment about the function or dysfunction of a pattern is based on comparison of the target client to his or her own baseline as well as identified gender, developmental, social, and cultural norms. A major strength of Gordon's work is the provision of guidelines for the conduct of a nursing history and examination to assess clients' functional health patterns. As assessment proceeds, diagnostic hypotheses are generated to direct targeted or more detailed data collection. The reader should refer to the *Manual of Nursing Diagnoses: 1993–1994* for the recommended formats for assessment of functional health patterns in adults, infants, and young children, families, and communities.[2(pp10–30)]

Nursing Diagnosis for Wellness: Supporting Strengths[3] is the published guide most focused on assessment of client strengths related to health promotion. This guide incorporates some of the NANDA diagnostic categories but expands to include wellness diagnoses organized according to the functional health patterns proposed by Gordon. Examples of wellness nursing diagnoses (client strengths) include: nutrition, adequate to meet or maintain body requirements (nutrition–metabolic); exercise level, appropriate to maintain wellness state (activity–exercise); and spiritual strength (value–belief). Case studies and sample care plans illustrate how diagnostic statements can provide direction for health-protection–promotion care planning.

A description of assessment areas that have special relevance for health promotion and protection follows.

Physical Fitness Evaluation

Physical fitness is an important part of personal health status that is discussed in detail in Chapter 9. Because of the sedentary lifestyles that, for many individuals, begin early in childhood and continue into adulthood, evaluation of physical fitness is a critical part of any nursing assessment. It is applicable to clients of all ages, with restrictions on some areas of testing for individuals who are physically compromised. It is important to differentiate between **skill-related physical fitness** and **health-related physical fitness.** Skill-related fitness is defined by those qualities that contribute to successful athletic performance: agility, speed, power, and reaction time. Health-related fitness includes qualities found to contribute to one's general health, including cardiorespiratory endurance, muscular strength and endurance, body composition, and flexibility, which are briefly discussed below.[4] For more comprehensive information, the reader should consult other sources.[5]

Cardiorespiratory Endurance

This aspect of fitness reflects the ability of the circulatory and respiratory systems to efficiently adjust to and recover from exercise. There are a number of approaches to assessing cardiorespiratory endurance. Two approaches are presented here. For children and adolescents between the ages of 9 and 18 years, a **1-mile walk/run test** can be used. This consists of having the individual walk or run 1 mile at the fastest pace possible. One mile can be measured out on either an outdoor or indoor track. Youths should be encouraged to practice the run the day before and warm up just before the run.[4(p 103)] Health fitness standards indicate that a 9-year-old should complete the mile in 13 minutes or under and an 18-year-old in 10:30 minutes or under.[6]

The **step test** is a field version of the laboratory stress test for adults. If the step test is conducted in a clinic setting, the electrocardiogram may be monitored. The availability of a physician for emergency backup is suggested if the client is over 40 years of age, obese, or has a history of cardiovascular difficulties. The step test is not as physiologically stressful as the laboratory stress test, but caution should be exercised in testing individuals with high-risk profiles for cardiovascular disease. For the step test, a step 16 to 17 inches high is recommended. The step rate should be 24 steps per minute for men and 22 steps per minute for women. Each step consists of the following sequence: left foot up; right foot up; left foot down; right foot down. Apical or carotid pulse rates are measured after stepping for 3 minutes at the prescribed cadence. With the client comfortably seated in a chair following step testing, pulse rates are counted for 15 seconds from 5 to 20 seconds into recovery and multiplied by 4 to obtain recovery heart rate. In the 95th percentile, recovery rate will be 140 for women and 124 for men. In the 10th percentile ranking, recovery rate will be 184 for women and 178 for men.[7]

Muscular Strength and Endurance

As a test of muscular strength and endurance, bent-knee sit-ups (Fig. 6–1) can be used. The number of **sit-ups per minute** is counted. Older subjects or those with cardiovascular disorders must be observed carefully for fatigue during strength and endurance testing. Sit-ups should be terminated if signs of distress occur in the client. Between 36 and 45 years old, men are rated as excellent if they can perform 42 or more sit-ups, women if they can perform 39 or more sit-ups. Men and women are below average if they can only perform 21 and 12 respectively. For over 46 years of age, men are rated excellent if they can perform 38 or more sit-ups, women if they can perform 24 or more sit-ups. Men and women are below average if they can perform only 18 and 11 respectively.[8]

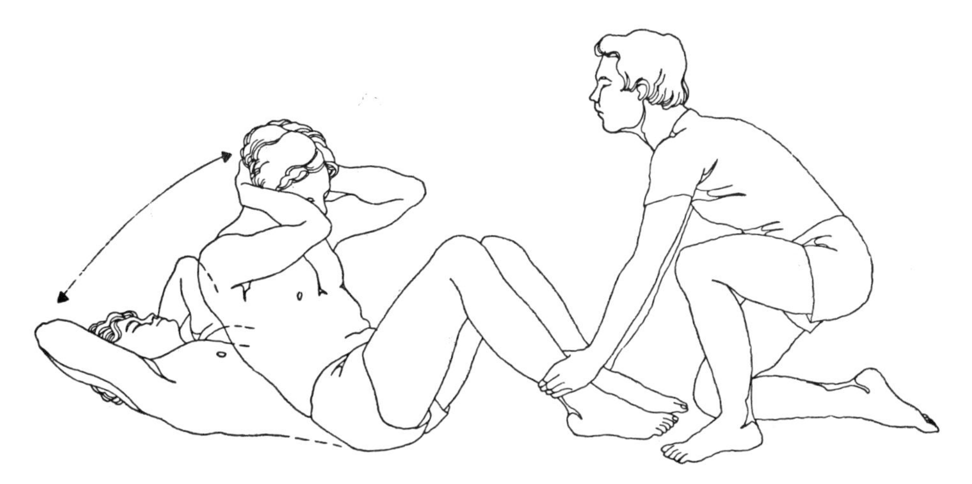

Figure 6–1. Bent-knee sit-ups.

Body Composition

Hydrostatic weighing underwater is considered the "gold standard" of indirect body fat estimates. However, because of the complex equipment needed and the time and potential anxiety involved, it is seldom used in the clinical setting. Anthropometry is used most frequently to assess body composition by measuring skin folds. A quality pair of skin-fold calipers is needed, and measures should be taken at the triceps and subscapular sites as shown in Figure 6–2. Three measures should be taken at each of the sites and the median values summed. For young adults, at the 50th percentile, the sum of skin folds is 21 for men or 9.4% body fat; the sum of skin folds for women is 30 or 22.8% body fat.[4(p130)] Marked deviation above or below these values should alert the health care provider to assess for either too much or too little nutrient intake for body requirements.

Flexibility

Flexibility is also an important component of physical fitness. It is the ability to move muscles and joints through their maximum range of motion. Flexibility may decrease with age or as a result of chronic illness. The lack of ability to flex or extend muscles or joints often reflects poor health habits, such as sedentary lifestyle, inappropriate posture, or faulty body mechanics. Loss of flexibility greatly decreases the client's ability to move about with ease and comfort.

Trunk flexion measures the client's ability to stretch back and thigh muscles. The client sits on a floor mat or on a flat examining table with legs fully extended and feet flat against a box (Fig. 6–3). Arms and hands are extended forward as far as possible and held for a count of three. With a ruler, the distance that the client can reach beyond the proximal edge of the box can be measured in inches. If the client cannot reach the edge, the distance of the fingertips from the edge is measured and reported as a negative number. Norms for trunk flexion vary among men and women. The range for men is −6 to

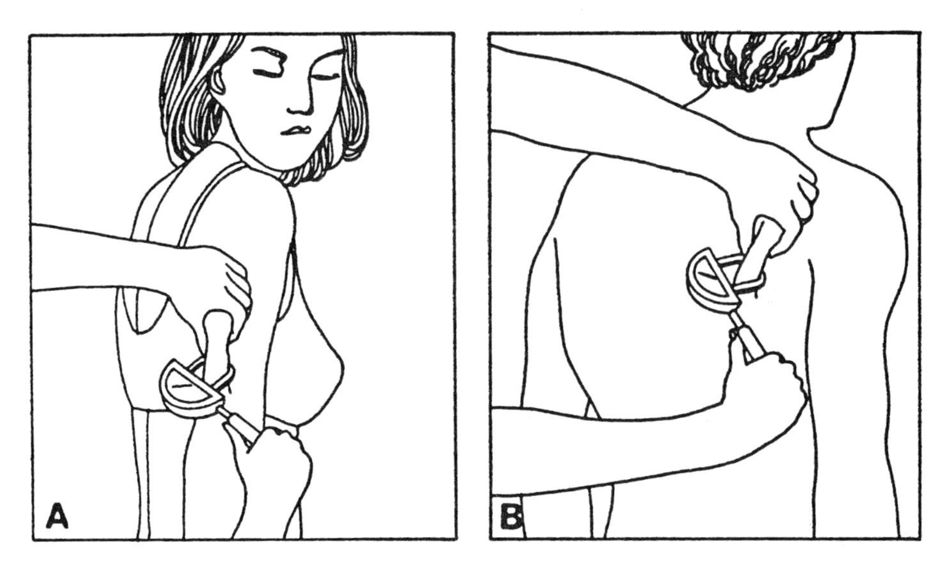

Figure 6–2. Skin-fold sites **A.** Triceps. **B.** Subscapula.

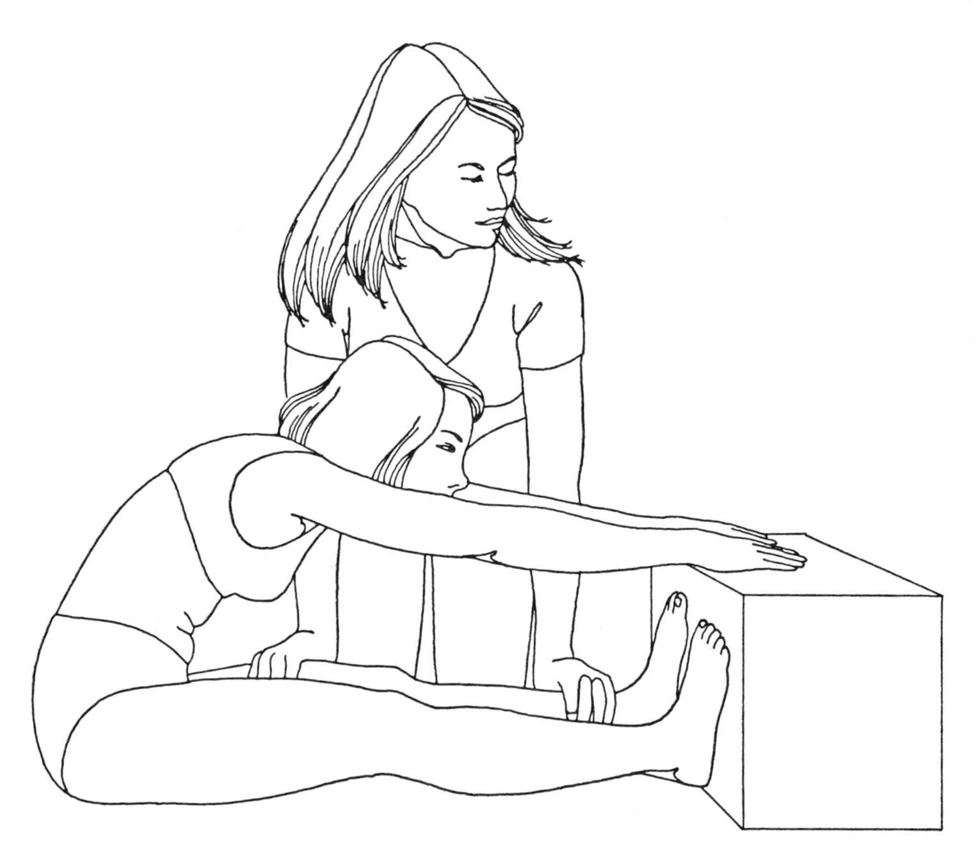

Figure 6–3. Trunk flexion.

+8 inches; for women, −4 to +10 inches. The average (mean) for men is +1 inch; for women, +2. The desired range for men is +1 to +5 inches; for women, +2 to +6.

The data collected during physical fitness evaluation can be used to assist the client in planning an appropriate exercise or physical activity program. Careful attention to assessment will optimize the fit of the exercise prescription to the physical capabilities of the client.

Nutritional Assessment

Effective planning for health promotion requires evaluation of the nutritional status of clients. Comprehensive nutritional assessment requires the use of four different types of assessment tools: anthropometric, biochemical, clinical, and dietary.[9] Anthropometric assessment (see above) includes height and weight measures as well as skin-fold thicknesses to be compared with standard values. Height and weight tables for adults are presented in Table 6–1. Height should be measured wearing 1-inch heels. Weight should be taken with lightweight clothing. In addition to body weight, skin-fold measurements provide a simple criterion for obesity. Triceps skin fold thicknesses indicative of obesity for children, adolescents, and men and women of differing age groups are presented in Table 6–2. Deviations from any of the norms on the measurements should be noted by the nurse and recorded as a part of the nutritional assessment.

Biochemical assessment can be conducted through blood or urine analyses to identify nutritional deficiencies. In addition to laboratory tests for cholesterol, triglycerides, glucose, and high-density lipoproteins, tests for protein (creatinine index, serum protein, serum albumin, total lymphocyte count, blood urea nitrogen, and uric acid), for serum or plasma vitamin levels (water-soluble, fat-soluble), and for minerals (calcium, sodium, potassium, iron, phosphorus, and magnesium) may be used to assess nutritional status.[9(pp240–241)]

Clinical examination can detect physical signs in skin, muscular and skeletal systems, eyes, tongue, etc, that suggest malnutrition. For an overview of physical signs suggestive of malnutrition, refer to *Nutrition in Health Maintenance and Health Promotion for Primary Care Providers,* by Y.M. Gutierrez.[9(pp242–244)]

Clients' current dietary patterns should be assessed. Clients should be instructed to keep a record of everything eaten for 5 to 7 days during the week prior to their clinic appointment or home visit. The record can be kept on a food diary form that allows the listing of the types of foods and amounts consumed during regular meals and snacks. When such a diary is kept accurately, daily food choices can be compared with the *Food Guide Pyramid* from the US Department of Agriculture's Human Nutrition Information Service (presented in Chapter 10) or analyzed using published daily food guides or the many computerized dietary analysis packages available. The nurse should be prepared to explain the *Food Guide Pyramid* to the patient as a basis for dietary planning. Once the usual dietary patterns of the client have been identified, the nurse can provide needed nutritional assistance to the client (see Chapter 10). Further, the nurse should work with nutritionists to prepare materials that inform the client about the latest thinking in use of nutritional supplements, including vitamins and minerals (calcium, iron, etc) as well as protein or complex carbohydrates.

Poor eating patterns, obesity, and malnutrition occur in **all** socioeconomic classes. In

TABLE 6–1. WEIGHT TABLE ACCORDING TO HEIGHT AND FRAME

HEIGHT		WEIGHT IN POUNDS (FRAME)		
Feet	Inches	Small	Medium	Large
Adult men				
5	2	128–134	131–141	138–150
5	3	130–136	133–143	140–153
5	4	132–138	135–145	142–156
5	5	134–140	137–148	144–160
5	6	136–142	139–151	146–164
5	7	138–145	142–154	149–168
5	8	140–148	145–157	152–172
5	9	142–151	148–160	155–176
5	10	144–154	151–163	158–180
5	11	146–157	154–166	161–184
6	0	149–160	157–170	164–188
6	1	152–164	160–174	168–192
6	2	155–168	164–178	172–197
6	3	158–172	167–182	176–202
6	4	162–176	171–187	181–207
Adult Women				
4	10	102–111	109–121	118–131
4	11	103–113	111–123	120–134
5	0	104–115	113–126	122–137
5	1	106–118	115–129	125–140
5	2	108–121	118–132	128–143
5	3	111–124	121–135	131–147
5	4	114–127	124–138	134–151
5	5	117–130	127–141	137–155
5	6	120–133	130–144	140–159
5	7	123–136	133–147	143–163
5	8	126–139	136–150	146–167
5	9	129–142	139–153	149–170
5	10	132–145	142–156	152–173
5	11	135–148	145–159	155–176
6	0	138–151	148–162	158–179

Derived from data of the Build Study, 1979.

TABLE 6–2. TRICEPS SKIN-FOLD THICKNESS INDICATING OBESITY (mm)

AGE (yr)	MALES	FEMALES
5	≥12	≥15
10	≥13	≥17
15	≥15	≥20
20	≥16	≥28
25	≥20	≥29
30 and above	≥23	≥30

addition, dietary risk factors for chronic disease are widespread in the American population. Therefore, assessment of nutritional status and dietary habits is a critical part of comprehensive health assessment for all clients including individuals, families, and specific target groups (high-schoolers, pregnant women, the elderly, etc).

Health-Risk Appraisal

The purpose of health-risk appraisal is to provide clients with an estimate of health threats to which they may be particularly vulnerable because of biologic makeup, family history, and lifestyle.[10] Personal risk profiles are determined for clients using information from their health history, laboratory diagnostics, physical fitness evaluation, nutritional assessment, and lifestyle assessment. Risk factors can generally be classified according to the categories in Figure 6–4.

It is assumed that providing information concerning mortality risk (estimated probability of death from a particular disease within the next 10 years) prior to the development of signs and symptoms of disease will stimulate individuals to change their lifestyles to avert illness. The assumptions underlying risk appraisal are: (1) each person is faced with certain quantifiable health hazards as a member of a specific group, (2) the client's risk is comparable to the average risk or mortality experience for a group with similar characteristics, and (3) knowledge of risk and related anxiety or concern are the sources of motivation for health-behavior change.

The usefulness of health-risk appraisal is currently limited to those diseases that have high resultant mortality rates. It is an accepted fact that the risk of developing any disease generally increases the greater the number of risk factors present and the greater their intensity. Through health-risk appraisal, clients are given an indication of what might **on-average** occur if they have the health experience of their current referent group (personal risk age) and what improvements they could make in their mortality profile (achievable or target risk age) if they adopted more positive behaviors of other groups (eg, stopping smoking, using seat belt, decreasing alcohol use, exercising, decreasing saturated fat intake).

The accuracy of mortality predictions from this method have been questioned, since population data do not accurately reflect the risk profile for a specific individual. Smith et al[11] reported that health-risk appraisal (HRA) overestimates the probability of mortality from coronary heart disease. Further, risk appraisal in and of itself is unlikely to result in reductions in risk. If clients are to alter behavior significantly, risk appraisal must be linked to behavior-change programs and other appropriate community health resources. It

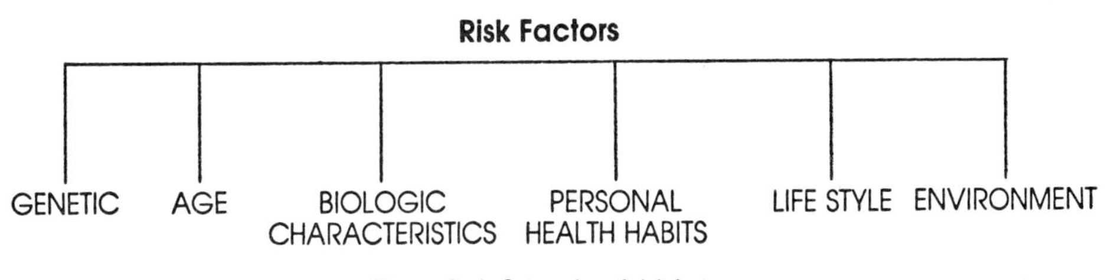

Figure 6–4. Categories of risk factors.

is unethical to apprise individuals of their risk level without providing supportive counseling and resources to facilitate behavior-change efforts. The lifestyle changes to be made should be arrived at collaboratively by the nurse and the client. Weiss[12] has commented on the possible adverse effects of risk appraisal. Predictions of premature death or shortened life expectancy may cause anxiety and depression in older adults who believe that it is too late to change risk status. Thus, in the decision to use risk appraisal with clients, both the advantages and disadvantages of this assessment tool must be considered.

Paper-and-pencil as well as computerized forms of HRAs are available from several commercial sources. Most appraisals also provide computerized analysis of individual risk based on national mortality data for selected health problems. These health problems usually include one or more of the 10 leading causes of death, with increasing attention being given to the social morbidities, such as death from violence and depression leading to suicide. Examples of risk-appraisal instruments include those focused on a single disease, such as the Cardiac Risk Factor Questionnaire developed by the Executive Health Group[13] and those focused on a number of health problems, such as the University of Minnesota Health Risk Appraisal developed by Raines and Ellis.[14(appB)] The Health Risk Appraisal (37-item questionnaire) available from the Centers for Disease Control and Prevention is the most commonly used format.[15]

Many companies use HRA as the "starter" for their health-promotion and risk-reduction program. Occupational health nurses often identify risk factors such as obesity, smoking, and high blood pressure, which are precursors of serious diseases and premature death. Through subsequent interventions, nurses aim to decrease employee illness, absenteeism, and disability and thus decrease health care costs for the company.[16] In one study of 55 employees in a public utility company, when risk assessment was combined with health-promotion education, the following behaviors reportedly improved over a 13-month period: limiting daily caloric intake to less than 2000 calories, limiting cholesterol to less than 300 milligrams, limiting saturated fat in the diet, reducing sodium intake, 20 minutes of vigorous conditioning exercise weekly, walking 1 continuous mile or climbing 10 flights of stairs daily, use of seat belts, obtaining examination of rectum or colon during last year, and obtaining physician breast examination and Pap smear (women).[17] The use of a weak one-group pretest/posttest design was a major limitation of the study. More research is needed to further understand the positive behavioral effects as well as the potential negative effects of HRA.

Life-Stress Review

Stress has been identified as a potential threat to mental health and physical well-being and has been associated with the occurrence of illness (heart disease, cancer, gastrointestinal disorders, etc) in numerous studies. Psychoneuroimmunology as a field focuses on understanding the disruptive effects of stress on the neural and immune systems. Because of its apparent centrality to health, life stress should be evaluated as a part of comprehensive health assessment. The Life-Change Index[18] is frequently used to evaluate stress in adults. Instruments to measure stress in youth have also been developed and include the Adolescent Perceived Events Scale,[19] the Life Events Scales (LES-C for 5- to 12-year-olds; LES-A for 13- to 18-year-olds),[20,21] and the Adolescent Life Change

Scale.[22] In contrast, the Hassles and Uplifts Scales measure day-to-day stressing or destressing experiences rather than major life events.[23] The State-Trait Anxiety Inventory[24] is a tool for assessing the extent of acute and chronic tension and anxiety that clients experience, whereas the Stress Warning Signals Inventory[13(p182)] provides clients with information about how they respond to stressful events so that they can break the stress cycle early on and save wear and tear on their bodies and minds. Stress Charting assists clients to pinpoint what aspects of their lives may be most stressful. Several of these instruments are described below.

Life-Change Index

Holmes and Rahe developed a tool to measure the extent of life change in the recent past. Life changes are defined as dramatic and taxing events requiring significant readjustment. The number of changes occurring within any given 2-year period has been shown to be weakly to moderately predictive of subsequent illness. Some studies have shown that stressful life events may precede a number of health problems, such as acute infections, coronary heart disease, and cancer. It is proposed that either compromise of immunocompetence or deterioration of healthy lifestyle habits account for this relationship. The original Life-Change Index is presented in Figure 6–5. Other life-change scales are available for different age groups. The Life-Change Index can be administered to the client in a short period of time and scored by adding up the "scale of impact" values for all life events checked. The extent of life stress can be evaluated using the scale for scoring presented in Table 6–3.

Hassles and Uplifts Scales

Hassles are defined as the irritating, frustrating, distressing demands that to some degree characterize everyday life (traffic jams, losing things, arguments). Uplifts, the counterparts of hassles, are defined as the positive experiences or joys of life, such as getting a good night's rest, receiving a letter from a friend, or spending time with a pet. It has been proposed that assessment of daily hassles and uplifts may be a better approach to the prediction of health or illness outcomes than the usual assessment of life events. If negatively toned stressors such as hassles cause neuroendocrine changes that predispose to illness, positively toned experiences such as uplifts may buffer stress disorders.[23(pp20–23),25]

Kanner and Feldman explored the effects of hassles and uplifts, as well as perceived control of those events, among a group of 140 adolescents in relation to the experience of depression. Fewer hassles and more uplifts were related to less depression. Further, those adolescents who felt they had control over hassles and uplifts in their lives were less depressed than those who reported less control.[26] In a study of Navajo Indians, major life events and daily hassles were measured among adults presenting for either inpatient or outpatient care at a selected US Indian Health Service facility. The number of outpatient visits and hospital admissions were monitored during the subsequent 2 years. Both major life events and daily hassles increased risk of hospital admission, whereas daily hassles were also predictive of increased use of outpatient services. These findings support the potential cross-cultural validity of the impact of daily hassles on health status and related health care use.[27] Hassles and uplifts scales have been developed for both children and adults.[26(pp190–191),23(pp33–39)]

Please check those life changes that you have experienced personally during the past *two years.*

Life Event	Scale of Impact	
Death of Spouse	100	______
Divorce	73	______
Marital separation	65	______
Jail term	63	______
Death of close family member	63	______
Personal injury or illness	53	______
Marriage	50	______
Fired at work	47	______
Marital reconciliation	45	______
Retirement	45	______
Change in health of family member	44	______
Pregnancy	40	______
Sex difficulties	39	______
Gain of new family member	39	______
Business readjustment	39	______
Change in financial state	38	______
Death of close friend	37	______
Change to different line of work	36	______
Change in number of arguments with spouse	35	______
Mortgage over $20,000	31	______
Foreclosure of mortgage or loan	30	______
Change in responsibilities at work	29	______
Son or daughter leaving home	29	______
Trouble with in-laws	29	______
Outstanding personal achievement	28	______
Spouse begins or stops work	26	______

Figure 6–5. Life-change index.

Life Event	Scale of Impact	
Begin or end school	26	______
Change in living conditions	25	______
Revision of personal habits	24	______
Trouble with boss	23	______
Change in work hours or conditions	20	______
Change in residence	20	______
Change in schools	20	______
Change in recreation	19	______
Change in church activities	19	______
Change in social activities	18	______
Mortgage or loan less than $20,000	17	______
Change in sleeping habits	16	______
Change in number of family get-togethers	15	______
Change in eating habits	15	______
Vacation	13	______
Christmas (if approaching)	12	______
Minor violations of the law	11	______
Total		______

Figure 6–5. (continued). (From Holmes T, Rahe E,[18(p213)] with permission.)

TABLE 6–3. SCORING THE LIFE-CHANGE INDEX

SCORE RANGE	INTERPRETATION
0–150	No significant problems, low or tolerable life change
150–199	Mild life change (approximately 33% chance of illness)
200–299	Moderate life change (approximately 50% chance of illness)
300 or over	Major life change (approximately 80% chance of illness)

(From Holmes T, Rahe E,[18(p213)] with permission.)

State-Trait Anxiety Inventory

Another instrument suggested for use as part of the life-stress review is the State-Trait Anxiety Inventory, which consists of 20 items pertaining to the amount of tension or anxiety the client feels at that moment (state), and 20 items concerning the way the client generally feels (trait). Sample questions from the inventory are presented in Figures 6–6 and 6–7. Clients respond by rating themselves on a 4-point scale for each item.[24] A State-Trait Anxiety Inventory for Children, "How I Feel Questionnaire," has also been developed. Children respond by rating themselves on a 3-point scale.[28] Both instruments and administration manuals are available from Mind Garden, Palo Alto, California. The State-Trait Anxiety Inventories provide an efficient yet reliable means for assessing feelings of tension or stress experienced by child and adult clients.

Stress Warning Signals Inventory

In order to assist clients in understanding how they respond to stress, they must be made aware of the symptoms that provide personal feedback concerning an elevated stress level. Once clients are aware of their own stress signals, they can use stress-management techniques presented in Chapter 11 more effectively. Symptoms of stress may be physical, behavioral, emotional, or cognitive as shown in Figure 6–8.

Stress Charting

The Menninger Foundation Biofeedback Center, in their stress management seminar, uses a stress-charting exercise that allows clients to list sources of stress. After listing as many stressors as possible, the client is instructed to write the number associated with each stressor in the section of the circle that describes the area of life in which the stressor occurs. If it is a stressor that is particularly troublesome, the client should place the

Directions: Statements that people have used to describe themselves are given below. Read each statement and then blacken in the appropriate circle to the right of the statement to indicate how you *feel* right now, that is, *at this moment.* There are no right or wrong answers. Do not spend too much time on any one statement but give the answer which seems to describe your present feelings best.

① = Not at All; ② = Somewhat;
③ = Moderately So; ④ = Very Much So

I feel at ease	①	②	③	④
I feel upset	①	②	③	④
I feel nervous	①	②	③	④
I am relaxed	①	②	③	④
I am worried	①	②	③	④

Figure 6–6. Sample items from the self-evaluation questionnaire: State Anxiety Inventory. (From Spielberger C, Gorsuch R, Lushene R, The State-Trait Anxiety Inventory, copyright © 1968, with special permission.)

Directions: A number of statements that people have used to describe themselves are given below. Read each statement and then blacken in the appropriate circle to the right of the statement to indicate how you generally feel. There are no right or wrong answers. Do not spend too much time on any one statement, but give the answer that seems to describe how you generally feel.

① = Not at All; ② = Somewhat;
③ = Moderately So; ④ = Very Much So

I wish I could be as happy as others seem to be	①	②	③	④
I am "calm, cool, and collected"	①	②	③	④
I feel that difficulties are piling up so that I cannot overcome them	①	②	③	④
I am inclined to take things hard	①	②	③	④
I am content	①	②	③	④

Figure 6–7. Sample items from the self-evaluation questionnaire: Trait Anxiety Inventory. (From The State-Trait Anxiety Inventory, Spielberger C, Gorsuch R, Lushene R, copyright © 1968, with special permission.)

number closer to the center of the circle. The center of the circle represents the client. The stress-charting exercise appears in Figure 6–9. After completion of this portion of the life-stress review, the client should be aware of (1) the stresses that he or she is experiencing in daily living, (2) the areas of life in which multiple stressors are occurring, and (3) the personal closeness or distance of each stressor from the self.

In the 1990s, instruments were developed that focus on measuring coping strengths and mastery of stress in children and adults. Ryan-Wenger developed the Schoolager's Coping Strategies Inventory to measure the type, frequency, and effectiveness of children's stress-coping strategies. Children between 8 and 12 years of age were asked in group discussions to identify the kinds of things that they do when they are experiencing stress. The resulting instrument and its psychometric evaluation are described by the developer.[29] Younger[30] reports on the development and testing of an instrument to measure mastery of stress in adults. Mastery is defined as a human response to difficult or stressful circumstances in which a person gains competence and control over the experience of stress. This 89-item instrument yields both a stress score and mastery score and is appropriate for administration to adults 19 years of age or older.

Life-stress assessment, as well as assessment of mastery of stress and coping strategies, provides information valuable in planning effective stress-management interventions with the client. Increased self-awareness resulting from this component of health assessment facilitates the use of stress-management and relaxation techniques described in Chapter 11.

Spiritual Health Assessment

Spiritual health is the ability to develop one's spiritual nature to its fullest potential, including the ability to discover and articulate one's basic purpose in life, to learn how to

Stress Warning Signals

PHYSICAL SYMPTOMS

- ☐ Headaches
- ☐ Indigestion
- ☐ Stomachaches
- ☐ Sweaty palms
- ☐ Sleep difficulties
- ☐ Dizziness
- ☐ Back pain
- ☐ Tight neck, shoulders
- ☐ Racing heart
- ☐ Restlessness
- ☐ Tiredness
- ☐ Ringing in ears

BEHAVIORAL SYMPTOMS

- ☐ Excess smoking
- ☐ Bossiness
- ☐ Compulsive gum chewing
- ☐ Attitude critical of others
- ☐ Grinding of teeth at night
- ☐ Overuse of alcohol
- ☐ Compulsive eating
- ☐ Inability to get things done

EMOTIONAL SYMPTOMS

- ☐ Crying
- ☐ Nervousness, anxiety
- ☐ Boredom—no meaning to things
- ☐ Edginess—ready to explode
- ☐ Feeling powerless to change things
- ☐ Overwhelming sense of pressure
- ☐ Anger
- ☐ Loneliness
- ☐ Unhappiness for no reason
- ☐ Easily upset

COGNITIVE SYMPTOMS

- ☐ Trouble thinking clearly
- ☐ Forgetfulness
- ☐ Lack of creativity
- ☐ Memory loss
- ☐ Inability to make decisions
- ☐ Thoughts of running away
- ☐ Constant worry
- ☐ Loss of sense of humor

Do any seem familiar to you?

Check the ones you experience when under stress. These are your stress warning signs.

Are there any additional stress warning signals that you experience that are not listed? If so, add them here.

____

____

____

____

____

Figure 6–8. Stress Warning Signals. (From Benson & Stuart,[13] with permission.)

experience love, joy, peace, and fulfillment, and how to help ourselves and others achieve their fullest potential.[31] In a holistic approach to health assessment, it is critical to appraise the spiritual health of clients, because spiritual beliefs to which individuals subscribe affect their interpretations of life events. Assessing spirituality goes beyond inquiring about a client's membership in a particular religion and taps deeper beliefs and

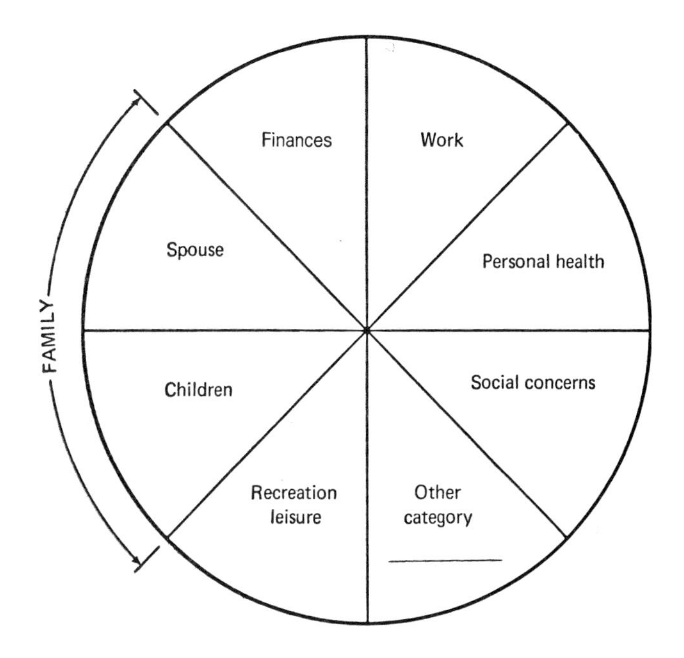

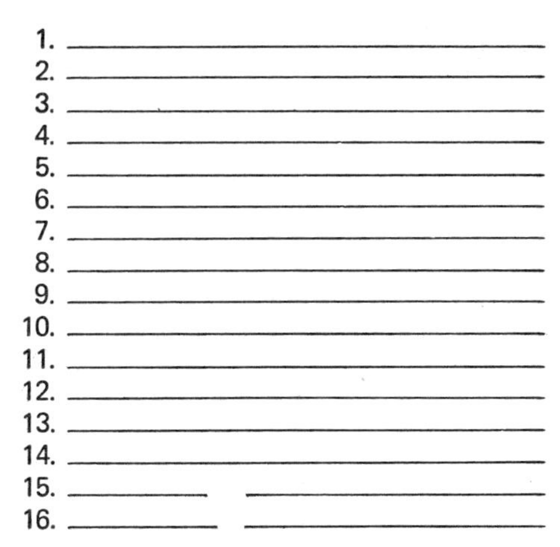

Figure 6–9. Stress charting. (Adapted with permission from D Walters, Biofeedback Center, The Menninger Foundation, Topeka, Kan.)

feelings about the meaning of life, love, hope, forgiveness, and life after death.[32] Connectedness is an important part of spirituality and includes being connected with one's inner self including getting in touch with one's feelings and values, being connected with others in meaningful relationships, and being connected with a larger purpose in life. Religious or philosophical beliefs such as commitment to humankind or trust in God put life in perspective and provide a reason for living.[33]

Areas of spirituality to be assessed include relationship with a higher being, relationship with self, and relationships with others.[31(pp12–17)]

I. Relationship with a higher being
   A. The importance of God or a higher being in the client's life
   B. Use of prayer and spiritually oriented readings as a means of dealing with life situations
   C. Belief in life after death or continuing spiritual existence
   D. Participation in individual or group worship activities
II. Relationship with self
   A. Existence of personal life goals that give meaning to life
   B. Spiritual beliefs that engender hope and zest for living
   C. Awareness of life priorities
   D. Commitment to spiritual growth
III. Relationships with others
   A. Extent of concern about the spiritual well-being of others
   B. Openness to sharing thoughts, feelings, and spiritual beliefs with others
   C. Respect for other individuals as spiritual beings

Questions related to spiritual assessment are usually asked toward the end of the interview when the client and nurse are more at ease with each other. Clients should be informed that assessing their spiritual well-being is integral to evaluating their overall health.

Social Support Systems Review

A number of instruments for reviewing social support systems are presented in Chapter 12 and so are not presented again here. Social support configuration can be analyzed using the support systems review as in Figure 12–3 or depicted using support diagramming as in Figure 12–4. Stewart[34] provides an overview of instruments that have been developed by nurse scientists to measure social support. Some of these instruments can also be used effectively in clinical settings, as well as in research.

Health-Beliefs Review

Health-belief measures can be classified as health-specific or behavior-specific. The health beliefs selected for assessment with any given client will depend on the areas of health and health behavior of most concern to the client. Although many health-belief measures of potential clinical use exist, only a few examples are identified here. The constructs in Table 6–4 have been shown through research to be related to actual performance of health-protecting or health-promoting behaviors in various populations. The

TABLE 6–4. HEALTH-BELIEF MEASURES AND EXAMPLES OF INSTRUMENTS

MEASURE	INSTRUMENT
HEALTH-SPECIFIC BELIEFS	
Health locus of control	The multidimensional health locus of control scale (MHLC)* Assesses beliefs in internal, chance, and powerful others locus of control of health
Health care competence	Perceived health competence rating scale† Assesses perceived capability to care for one's own health
Definition of health	Laffrey health conception scale‡ Assesses one's conception of health in form domains: clinical, role performance, adaptive, and eudaimonistic
Intrinsic motivation for health behavior	Health self-determinism index§ Health self-determinism index for children** Assesses active, independent decision making regarding health behavior and the self-satisfaction that the behavior engenders
BEHAVIORAL-SPECIFIC BELIEFS	
Exercise self-efficacy	Exercise self-efficacy scale** Assesses confidence in ability to continue exercise on a regular basis
Exercise benefits and barriers	Exercise benefits/barriers scale‡‡ Expected outcomes and barriers to exercise§§ Assesses perceptions of the "pros" or positive outcomes of exercise as well as the barriers, hurdles, or constraints to exercise
Social support for exercise	Exercise social support scale*** Assesses the emotional and instrumental support for exercise provided by mother, father, brothers, sisters, and friends

*Wallston et al[35]
†Smith et al[36]
‡Laffrey[37]
§Cox[38]
**Cox[39]
††A Baudura, personal communication,1992.
‡‡Sechrist et al[40]
§§Steinhardt et al[41]
***A Garcia, MA Broda, personal communication.

behavior-specific measures almost always are more powerful than the health-specific measures in explaining and predicting the occurrence of health behaviors.

Clients' scores on a personally tailored portfolio of health-belief measures can provide an indication of readiness and motivation to engage in particular health behaviors. The health beliefs to be assessed should be determined through preliminary discussions between the nurse and client.

Lifestyle Assessment

Increasing evidence indicates that there is a great deal that individuals can do to maintain and enhance their well-being and prevent the early onset of disabling health problems by engaging in a health-promoting lifestyle. A thoughtful review of health habits with subsequent follow-up counseling and education can greatly increase the motivation and competence of clients to care for themselves in a responsible manner.

Health-Promoting Lifestyle Profile II (HPLP-II)

In the context of health, lifestyle is defined as discretionary activities with significant impact on health status that are a regular part of one's daily pattern of living.[42] Health-promoting behavior is an expression of the human actualizing tendency that is directed toward optimal well-being, personal fulfillment, and productive living. The 52-item HPLP-II, a revision of the original instrument, consists of six subscales, which are intended to measure major components of a healthy lifestyle: health responsibility, physical activity, nutrition, interpersonal relations, spiritual growth, and stress management. Means can be derived for each subscale separately or a mean obtained on the total instrument as a measure of overall health-promoting lifestyle.[43] Although this instrument is frequently used in research, it can provide important information about a client's lifestyle when used in primary health care. The instrument, scoring instructions, and psychometric information can be obtained from Dr. Susan Noble Walker, College of Nursing, University of Nebraska Medical Center. Sample items for each of the subscales appear in Table 6–5.

The profile of means on the HPLP-II can provide information useful in developing an individualized health-promotion plan that identifies lifestyle strengths and resources as well as areas for further growth. There is a need for development of additional lifestyle assessment tools that are appropriate for children, adolescents, and families. An adolescent version is being designed.

Stage-of-Change Assessment

In relation to any given behavior change, clients may be at one of several stages. Based on various studies of behavioral changes from smoking cessation to exercise adoption, recurring stages seem to emerge. Prochaska and colleagues propose in the transtheoretical model that the stage of behavior change will determine the behavioral plan for interven-

TABLE 6–5. HEALTH-PROMOTING LIFESTYLE PROFILE II SUBSCALES AND SAMPLE ITEMS

SUBSCALE	SAMPLE ITEM
Health responsibility	Read or watch TV programs about improving my health. Question health professionals in order to understand their instructions.
Physical activity	Exercise vigorously for 20 or more minutes at least 3 times a week (brisk walking, bicycling, aerobic dancing, using a stair climber). Get exercise during usual day activities (such as walking during lunch, using stairs instead of elevators, parking car farther away from destination and walking).
Nutrition	Choose a diet low in fat, saturated fat, and cholesterol. Eat 2–4 servings of fruit each day.
Interpersonal relations	Spend time with close friends. Settle conflicts with others through discussion and compromise.
Spiritual growth	Feel connected with some force greater than myself. Am aware of what is important to me in life.
Stress management	Take some time for relaxation each day. Pace myself to prevent fatigue

tion that is likely to be most effective. Stages of change for positive health behaviors can be assessed with the True-False questions presented in Table 6–6.[44]

Following completion of Lifestyle Assessment, the interest of the client in making various changes can be assessed as well as the stage of the client in relation to each behavior. Prochaska and colleagues propose that "staging" a client in relation to various health behaviors will allow for more precise tailoring of interventions.

Further Assistance with Assessment

The assessment process described in this section of the chapter provides the nurse with important information for working with the client to develop individually tailored plans for protective-promotive care. A number of the tools presented could be used with older children and adolescents as well as with adults of all ages. Some of the tools cited have been developed specifically for youth. The nurse should assess the cultural appropriateness of the various tools for target populations before using them. Additional assessment instruments that are applicable to the clinical setting as well as to research are described by Frank-Stromborg.[45] Assessment tools are presented for areas such as functional status, coping, information-seeking behaviors, and self-care activities. Nursing clinics, community health centers, and primary care centers should maintain an up-to-date resource file of assessment tools so that the assessment portfolio for any given client can be customized.

• ASSESSMENT OF THE FAMILY

Assessment of the family, as well as assessment of the individual, is critical to successfully planning for health behavior change. The family is the primary social structure for health promotion within society. It is within the context of the family that health behaviors are learned and the rudiments of health-enhancing or health-damaging lifestyles emerge. The family acts as a powerful mediating factor in determining how its members cope with a wide range of health concerns and challenges.[46] Thus, the family is a logical unit of assessment and intervention for health promotion, since it has the primary responsibility for: (1) developing self-care and dependent-care competencies of the family, (2) fostering resilience of family members, (3) providing social and physical resources to the family group, and (4) promoting healthy individuation while maintaining family cohesion. Although women generally carry the major responsibility for health decision

TABLE 6–6. QUESTIONS FOR ASSESSING STAGES OF BEHAVIOR CHANGE

1. I currently do not (specify exact behavior, eg, exercise 30 minutes three times a week, eat 2–4 servings of fruit daily) and do not intend to start in the next 6 months. (Precontemplation)
2. I currently do not (specify behavior), but I am thinking about starting to do so in the next 6 months. (Contemplation)
3. I have tried several times to (specify behavior) but am seriously thinking of trying again in the next month. (Planning)
4. I have (specify behavior) regularly for less than 6 months. (Action)
5. I have (specify behavior) regularly for more than 6 months. (Maintenance)

making and health education for the family, the task of fostering health and healthy behaviors should be "mainstreamed" as an integral part of family functioning.

In assessment of the family, the varying family forms that exist today, such as one-parent families and blended families, must be taken into consideration. The milieu for the promotion of health is likely to differ significantly across families, depending on their composition, structure, socioeconomic status, living environment, and cultural context. Healthy family traits can be expressed in many different ways. There is no one correct way to spend quality time together, promote physically active families, or express affection. Family strengths can have many different modes of expression. When conducting a family health assessment, the nurse must be attuned to this wide range of variation among families as well as variations produced by developmental transitions in family life.[47] Several approaches to assessment that can be used in all types of families are described briefly here.

Using a systems approach, Whall proposed health assessment guidelines for families. She suggested that the following categories be assessed: (1) individual subsystems (developmental, biologic, psychologic, and social characteristics), (2) interactional patterns (relationships, communication patterns, roles, and attachment patterns), (3) unique characteristics of the whole (group psyche, capacity for change, belief systems, group dynamics, developmental needs, typologic actions, and economics), and (4) environmental interface synchrony (reciprocal effects of family and community). The full-length assessment tool appears in Whall's original work.[48]

Friedman has described a structural-functional approach to family assessment.[49] Within this framework, the family is viewed as a system with the following features: value structure, role structure, power structure, communication patterns, affective function, socialization function, health care function, and family coping function. This approach to assessment is based on systems theory and provides insight concerning the internal processes of the family as well as the relationship of the family to the environment and larger social system. Family decision-making patterns in relation to health are identified in assessing power structure and health care function.

Wright and Leahey[50] provide a thorough description of the Calgary Family Assessment Model (CFAM), which they have adapted specifically for nurses to use when assessing families. Their model for assessment consists of the following major categories: family structural assessment, family developmental assessment, and family functional assessment.

In structural assessment, the family is analyzed in terms of both its internal and external structure. Aspects of the internal structure include family composition, rank order, subsystem, and boundary. Components of the external structure are culture, religion, social class status and mobility, environment, and extended family.

Through family developmental assessment, the nurse appraises the current stage of the family in relation to family developmental history.[50(p38)] Wright and Leahey's assessment of family development focuses primarily on the traditional family developmental cycle, but they also discuss assessment of alterations in the family developmental life cycle brought about by separation, divorce, single parenthood, and remarriage by divorced persons.

Family functional assessment is dichotomized as instrumental functioning and expressive functioning. *Instrumental functioning* refers to the routine activities of everyday living, while *expressive functioning* is elaborated as emotional communication, verbal communication, nonverbal communication, circular communication, problem solving, roles, control, beliefs, and alliances and coalitions.[50(p54)] The reader is referred to Wright and Leahey's book for a detailed discussion of the family assessment model that they propose.

Mischke-Berkey et al[51] propose a family health assessment scheme that focuses on assessment of tensions and stress created by situations in normal family life and on family health issues. The Neuman Health-Care Systems Model provides the blueprint for this assessment tool. Flexible and normal lines of defense as well as lines of resistance are important concepts in this assessment framework.

The Darlington Family Interview Schedule and Darlington Family Rating Scale have been described in detail by Wilkinson.[46(pp171–196)] The interview explores the family's view of health issues or problems; children's health, development, emotional behavior, relationships and conduct; parent's physical and psychologic health, marital harmony (if two-parent family), social support, and parenting skills; parent-child relationships in terms of care and control; and family functioning in terms of closeness, power hierarchies, emotional atmosphere and rules, developmental stage, and strengths. A rating scale is used to summarize the data as a basis for developing a strategy for care. The rating scale provides a succinct presentation of child, parent, and family information.

An excellent compilation of approximately 20 measures of family functioning that is potentially useful in practice has been prepared by Sawin et al.[52] Examples of instruments described in this compilation are: Feetham Family Functioning Survey, Family Adaptability and Cohesion Scale, and the Family Hardiness Index. These instruments can be used in health assessment of families as a basis for developing a health protection-promotion plan. Information provided on each instrument includes description with sample items, psychometric properties, cross-cultural uses, gender sensitivity, applicability to variant family structures, list of selected studies using the instrument, critique, and source for accessing the tool. The reader is referred to this excellent resource for further information on family assessment tools developed by nurses and other professionals.

A major gap in family assessment tools is the lack of an instrument that measures family dimensions of health-related lifestyle. Nurse scientists need to direct their attention to the development of valid and reliable tools to assess families' aggregate health behaviors. Areas suggested for assessment in such an instrument appear in Table 6–7.

In summary, family assessment complements individual assessment; thus, the two should be considered as interrelated processes. To provide further guidance to nurses in working with families, a format for developing a family health protection-promotion plan is presented in Chapter 7.

• ASSESSMENT OF THE COMMUNITY

A third essential component of health assessment is community analysis or appraisal. Community analysis is the process of assessing and defining needs, opportunities, and re-

TABLE 6–7. SUGGESTED AREAS FOR ASSESSMENT OF FAMILY HEALTH-RELATED LIFESTYLE

Nutrition
1. Meals prepared in the home are generally consistent with the food guide pyramid.
2. Healthy snacks are consumed in the home.
3. Knowledge about healthy eating habits is shared among family members.
4. Mutual assistance occurs among family members for maintenance of recommended weights and avoidance of overweight and underweight.
5. Family members praise each other for healthy eating.
6. Family members encourage each other to drink 6–8 glasses of water per day.
7. Family members base purchase decisions on nutritional labels on food.

Physical Activity
1. Many family outings consist of vigorous or moderate physical activity.
2. Exercise equipment is available within the home.
3. Use of home exercise equipment is part of "family time."
4. Family members expect each other to be physically active.
5. A family membership is held in recreational facilities or programs.
6. Time together is seldom spent watching television or playing video games.
7. Family prefers to spend as much time out-of-doors as possible.

Stress Control and Management
1. Family manages time well to minimize stressful demands on members.
2. Family often relaxes, shares stories, and laughs together.
3. Emotional expression is encouraged within the family.
4. Family members share stressful experiences with each other.
5. Family members offer each other assistance with difficult tasks.
6. Family members seldom "get on each other" about their faults.
7. Periods of relaxation and sleep are considered important by the family.

Health Responsibility
1. A schedule for preventive care visits is maintained by the family.
2. Family often discusses news and articles about health topics.
3. Family members are encouraged to seek health care early if a problem develops.
4. Personal responsibility for health is encouraged by the family.
5. Family feels a sense of responsibility for the health of the family and each member.
6. Health professionals are consulted about health promotion as well as care in illness.
7. Appropriate protective behaviors are openly discussed and encouraged (abstinence, use of condoms, hearing protection, eye protection, sunscreen).

Family Resilience and Resources
1. Worship or spiritual experiences are a regular part of family activities.
2. Family members share a sense of "togetherness" despite difficult life events.
3. Family has a common sense of purpose in life.
4. Family members encourage each other to "keep going" when life is difficult.
5. Growth in positive directions is mutually encouraged within the family.
6. Health is nurtured as a positive family resource.
7. Personal strengths and capabilities are nurtured.

Family Support
1. Family has a number of friends or relatives that they see frequently.
2. Family is involved in community activities and groups.
3. Family members frequently praise each other.
4. In times of distress, the family can call on a number of other families or individuals for help.
5. Disagreements are settled through discussion rather than verbal abuse or physical violence.
6. Family members model healthy habits for each other.
7. Professional support services are sought when needed.

sources involved in initiating community health action programs. It is critical to recognize that analysis is done **with** the community, not **on** the community. Local citizens and organizations must be involved in the assessment process in order to have "ownership" of the program and to build widespread commitment to community action.[53] It is important to recall at this point that *Healthy People 2000: National Health Promotion and Disease Prevention Objectives* are essentially community-oriented. All sectors of the community must be activated to achieve the broad national goals set for the year 2000: increase the span of healthy life for Americans, reduce health disparities among Americans, and achieve access to preventive services for all Americans. Objectives focused on violence and abusive behaviors, educational and community-based programs, occupational safety and health, environmental health, and maternal and infant health all require community assessment and intervention.[54]

A community is a social system that encompasses the collective human energies of individuals, families, and nonfamilial groups. It is the context in which aggregates and individuals either "bloom" or lie dormant. The community is a system with complex relationships among interdependent subsystems. Clark specifies the critical attributes of a community as: group orientation in which the group's goals take priority over those of individual members; common bonds between members such as lifestyle, ethnicity, or culture; and significant social interaction among individuals that make up the community.[14] Communities have both health strengths and resources as well as health issues or problems. Communities must be competent in meeting their responsibilities to provide for the highest level of well-being of their members. Characteristics of the community must be assessed to determine what the community health assets and challenges are.

Goeppinger[55] has identified five approaches to collecting data about communities: informant interviewing (directed conversation with community members); participant observation (sharing in community life activities); mobile survey (observation while driving about); secondary analyses (use of preexisting data); and community surveys (organized data collection efforts). Since community citizens constitute a critical primary data source, informant interviewing should always be used as one approach to data collection. An assessment methodology that combines at least three to four of these data collection methods is more likely to provide a holistic picture of the community than an assessment that relies on only one or two approaches.

One approach to community assessment is to collect information about the following community subsystems and their interrelationships: (1) values and culture, (2) politics, (3) education, (4) recreation, (5) transportation, (6) religion, (7) communications and media, (8) welfare, (9) economics, (10) utilities, (11) business and labor, (12) social life, (13) safety and protection, and (14) health. In assessing the health subsystem, population growth patterns, functional activity status, nutritional status, dominant lifestyle patterns, coping ability, community stressors, goal setting and achievement capabilities, and risk factors need to be assessed in addition to traditional indices of morbidity, mortality, and accessibility of health care resources.

The nature of the assessment should be determined by the time available and the way in which the data will be used. Spradley describes a continuum of assessment important for the nurse to consider to economize on time and effort. In a comprehensive assessment, all relevant information about the community is synthesized from existing documents and primary data collection. This approach is costly and time-consuming so should not be undertaken unless such a comprehensive study is absolutely essential before high-priority program goals can be addressed. A familiarization assessment is much more efficient and provides a broad rather than in-depth overview of the community at large. Problem-oriented assessment begins with a single problem and assesses the community in terms of that problem, for instance, neighborhood violence. Aspects of the community relevant to that health issue are assessed to determine their contributory, ameliorative, or preventive effects. Subsystem assessment is focused on a particular sector of the community and permits an in-depth assessment of that sector. For example, the subsystem might be education to determine the impact of educational programs on the health and productivity of the community.[56]

Data collection methods are numerous and varied. Existing records should be mined for as much data as possible before primary data collection is instituted. Key informants knowledgeable about the community provide another important data source. When primary data collection is necessary, focus group interviewing often is the method of choice because of the rich interactive data that can be obtained using this method. Survey data can also be important as information from a large segment of the population on key assessment questions is provided.

TABLE 6–8. COMPONENTS OF COMMUNITY ASSESSMENT

Human Biology
1. Composition of population by age, gender, and race
2. Population patterns of longevity
3. Genetic inheritance patterns by gender and race
4. Disease incidence and prevalence compared to prior years, and to state and national statistics
5. Health status indicators (immunization levels, nutritional status, mobility)

Environment
1. Physical environment (urban/rural/suburban, housing, water supply, parks and recreation, climate, topography, size, population density, aesthetics, natural or manmade resources, goods and services, health risks)
2. Psychologic environment (productivity level, cohesion, mental health status, communication networks, intergroup harmony, future orientation, prevalence of stressors)
3. Social environment (income and education levels, employment, family composition, religious affiliations, cultural affiliations, language(s) spoken, social services, organization profile, leadership and decision-making structures)

Community Lifestyles
1. Consumption patterns (eg, nutrition, alcohol)
2. Occupational groups
3. Leisure pursuits
4. Community health attitudes and beliefs
5. Patterns of health-related behaviors in aggregates
6. History of paticipation in community health action

Health System
1. Health care services available (health promotion, prevention, primary care, secondary care, tertiary care, mental health)
2. Accessibility of promotive and preventive care (low income, homeless, varying racial and ethnic groups)
3. Financing plans for health care

(Adapted from Clark MJ,[14,appJ] with permission.)

Community assessment provides the data regarding a community's health status from which community diagnoses are derived. Thus, community assessment is a primary building block for planning, implementing, and evaluating community health-promotion and prevention programs. The components of a community assessment have been identified by Clark and have been organized and further expanded by this author in Table 6–8.

Assessment of communities is a complicated and time-consuming task. It requires collaboration on the part of many individuals in the community besides health professionals. However, such assessment is critical to the identification of community strengths and resources as well as to the diagnosis of community problems or deficits. Successful implementation of community health-promotion and prevention programs depends in large part on accurate assessment of community characteristics.

• DIRECTIONS FOR RESEARCH

Research that develops and tests new measurement and assessment tools for the health, health beliefs, and health behaviors of individuals and aggregates from diverse racial, cultural, and socioeconomic backgrounds is of high priority. The tools used in both clinical practice and research must be reliable and valid. Assessment tools should be based on theoretical or conceptual frameworks that provide the infrastructure for development of individual items and scales.

• SUMMARY

Health assessment can be carried out at the individual, family, or community level. Because assessment is time-intensive for the nurse and the client, tools for use must be carefully selected according to the client's characteristics and presenting health issues. The nurse and client should determine what assessments are needed and combine them into a portfolio for that particular client.

Information technology will increasingly make computerization of assessment tools possible. Thus, clients may be able to complete self-assessments at home as time allows, with transmission of the information via computer in advance of health care visits.

REFERENCES

1. North American Nursing Diagnosis Association. *Nursing Diagnoses: Definitions & Classification 1995–1996.* Philadelphia, Pa: NANDA; 1994.
2. Gordon M. *Manual of Nursing Diagnosis: 1993–1994.* St Louis, Mo: Mosby Year Book; 1993.
3. Houldin AD, Saltstein SW, Ganley KM. *Nursing Diagnosis for Wellness: Supporting Strengths.* Philadelphia, Pa: JB Lippincott Co; 1987.
4. Barrow HM, McGee R, Tritschler KA. *Practical Measurement in Physical Education and Sport.* 4th ed. Philadelphia, Pa: Lea & Febiger; 1989.
5. American College of Sports Medicine. *Guidelines for Exercise Testing and Prescription.* 4th ed. Philadelphia, Pa: Lea & Febiger; 1991.

6. American Alliance for Health, Physical Education, Recreation and Dance. *Health-related Physical Fitness: Test Manual.* Reston, Va: AAHPERD; 1980.
7. Katch FI, McArdle WD. *Nutrition, Weight Control and Exercise.* 3rd ed. Philadelphia, Pa: Lea & Febiger; 1988.
8. Golding LA, Myers CR, Sinning WE. *The Y's Way to Physical Fitness.* Champaign, Ill: Human Kinetics; 1982.
9. Gutierrez YM. *Nutrition in Health Maintenance and Health Promotion for Primary Care Providers.* San Francisco, Calif: University of California, San Francisco School of Nursing; 1994.
10. Gazmararian JA, Foxman B, Yen LT, et al. Comparing the predictive accuracy of health risk appraisal: the Centers for Disease Control versus Carter Center program. *Am J Public Health.* 1991;81:1296–1301.
11. Smith KW, McKinlay SM, Thorington BA. The validity of health risk appraisal instruments for assessing coronary heart disease risk. *Am J Public Health.* 1987;77:971–974.
12. Weiss SM. Health hazard-health risk appraisals. In: Matarazzo JD, Weiss SM, Herd JA, et al, eds. *Behavioral Health: A Handbook of Health Enhancement and Disease Prevention.* New York, NY: John Wiley & Sons; 1984:275–276.
13. Benson H, Stuart EM. *The Wellness Book.* New York, NY: Birch Lane Press; 1992:379.
14. Clark MJ. *Nursing in the Community.* Stamford, Conn: Appleton & Lange; 1996.
15. Centers for Disease Control. *CDC Health Risk Appraisal User Manual.* Atlanta, Ga: CDC Division of Health Education; 1984. US Govt Printing Office publication 746-011/15233.
16. Sherman Z. Health risk appraisal at the worksite. *American Association of Occupational Health Nursing Journal.* 1990; 38(1):18–24.
17. Bamberg R, Acton RT, Goodson L, et al. The effect of risk assessment in conjunction with health promotion education on compliance with preventive behaviors. *J Allied Health.* 1989;18:271–280.
18. Holmes T, Rahe R. The social readjustment rating scale. *J Psychosom Res.* 1967;11:213.
19. Compas BE, Davis GE, Forsythe CJ, et al. Assessment of major and daily stressful events during adolescence: the Adolescent Perceived Events Scale. *J Consult Clin Psychol.* 1987;55:534–541.
20. Coddington RD. The significance of life events as etiologic factors in the disease of children, I: a survey of professional workers. *J Psychosom Res.* 1972;16:7–18.
21. Coddington RD. The significance of life events as etiologic factors in the diseases of children, II: a study of a normal population. *J Psychosom Res.* 1972;16:205–213.
22. Yeaworth RC, York J, Hussey MA, et al. The development of an adolescent life change event scale. *Adolescence.* 1980;15:91–97.
23. Kanner AD, Coyne JC, Schaefer C, et al. Comparison of two modes of stress measurement: daily hassles and uplifts versus major life events. *J Behav Med.* 1981;4:1–39.
24. Spielberger CD, Gorsuch RL, Lushene R, et al. *Manual for State-Trait Anxiety Inventory.* Palo Alto, Calif: Consulting Psychologists Press Inc; 1983.
25. DeLongis A, Coyne JC, Dakof G, et al. Relationship of daily hassles, uplifts, and major life events to health status. *Health Psychol.* 1983;1:119–136.
26. Kanner AD, Feldman SS. Control over uplifts and hassles and its relationship to adaptational outcomes. *J Behav Med.* 1991;14:187–201.
27. Zyzanski SJ, Wright AL. Life events and daily hassles and uplifts as predictors of hospitalization and outpatient visitation. *Soc Sci Med.* 1992;34:763–768.
28. Spielberger CD, Edwards CD, Lushene RE, et al. *State-Trait Anxiety Inventory for Children—Preliminary Manual.* Palo Alto, Calif: Mind Garden; 1973.

29. Ryan-Wenger NM. Development and psychometric properties of The Schoolagers' Coping Strategies Inventory. *Nurs Res.* 1990;39:344–349.
30. Younger JB. Development and testing of The Mastery of Stress Instrument. *Nurs Res.* 1993;42:68–73.
31. Chapman LS. Developing a useful perspective on spiritual health: love, joy, peace and fulfillment. *Am J Health Prom.* 1987; 12–17.
32. Carson VB. *Spiritual Dimensions of Nursing Practice.* Philadelphia, Pa: WB Saunders Co; 1989.
33. Bellingham R, Cohen B, Jones T, et al. Connectedness: some skills for spiritual health. *Am J Health Prom.* 1989;4(1):18–24,31.
34. Stewart MJ. Social support instruments created by nurse investigators. *Nurs Res.* 1989;38:268–275.
35. Wallston KA, Wallston BS, DeVellis R. Development of the multidimensional health locus of control (MHLC) scales. *Health Educ Monogr.* 1978;6:161–170.
36. Smith MS, Wallston KA, Smith CA. The development and validation of the Perceived Health Competence Scale. *Health Educ Res.* 1995;10(1):51–64.
37. Laffrey SC. Development of a health conception scale. *Res Nurs Health.* 1986;9:107–113.
38. Cox C. The Health Self-Determinism Index. *Nurs Res.* 1985;34:177–183.
39. Cox C. The Health Self-Determinism Index for children. *Res Nurs Health.* 1990;31:237–246.
40. Sechrist KR, Walker SN, Pender NJ. Development and psychometric evaluation of the Exercise Benefits/Barriers Scale. *Res Nurs Health.* 1987;10:357–365.
41. Steinhardt MA, Dishman RK. Reliability and validity of expected outcomes and barriers for habitual physical activity. *J Occup Med.* 1989;31:536–546.
42. Wiley JA, Camacho TC. Lifestyle and future health: evidence from the Alemeda County study. *Prev Med.* 1980;9:1–21.
43. Walker SN, Sechrist KR, Pender NJ. The health-promoting lifestyle profile: development and psychometric characteristics. *Nurs Res.* 1987;36(2):76–81.
44. Prochaska JO, Velicer WF, Rossi JS et al. Stages of change and decisional balance for 12 problem behaviors. *Health Psychol.* 1994;13(1):39–46.
45. Frank-Stromborg M. *Instruments for Clinical Nursing Research.* Boston, Mass: Jones & Bartlett; 1992.
46. Wilkinson IM. *Family assessment: a basic manual.* New York, NY: Gardner Press Inc; 1993.
47. Gershwin MW, Nilsen JM. Healthy families: forms and processes. In: Gilliss CL, Highley BL, Roberts BM, et al, eds. *Toward a Science of Family Nursing.* Menlo Park, Calif: Addison-Wesley Publishing Co Inc; 1989:77–91.
48. Whall AL. Nursing theory and assessment of families. *J Psychiatr Nurs.* 1981;19:30–39.
49. Friedman MN. *Family nursing: theory and assessment.* 2nd ed. New York, NY: Appleton-Century-Crofts; 1985.
50. Wright LM, Leahey M. *Nurses and Families: A Guide to Family Assessment and Intervention.* Philadelphia, Pa: FA Davis Co; 1984.
51. Mischke-Berkey K, Warner P, Hanson S. Family health assessment and intervention. In: Bomar PJ, ed. *Nurses and Family Health Promotion: Concepts, Assessment, and Interventions.* Baltimore, Md: Williams & Wilkins; 1989:139–154.
52. Sawin KJ, Harrigan MP, Woog P. *Measures of Family Functioning for Research and Practice.* New York, NY: Springer; 1995.
53. Haglund B, Weisbrod RR, Bracht N. Assessing the community: its services, needs, leadership, and readiness. In: Bracht N, ed. *Health Promotion at the Community Level.* Newbury Park, Calif: Sage Publications Inc; 1990:91–108.

54. *Healthy People 2000: National Health Promotion and Disease Prevention Objectives.* Washington, DC: US Public Health Service; 1991. US Dept of Health and Human Services publication PHS 91-50212.
55. Goeppinger J. Community as client: using the nursing process to promote health. In: Stanhope M, Lancaster J, eds. *Community Health Nursing: Process and Practice for Promoting Health.* St. Louis, Mo: CV Mosby Co; 1984:379–404.
56. Spradley BW. *Community Health Nursing: Concepts and Practice.* 3rd ed. Glenview, Ill: Scott, Foresman/Little, Brown; 1990.

7

Developing a Health-Protection–Promotion Plan

- Guidelines for Preventive Services
- The Health-Planning Process
  - A. Review and Summarize Data from Assessment
  - B. Reinforce Strengths and Competencies of the Client
  - C. Identify Health Goals and Related Behavior-Change Options
  - D. Identify Behavioral or Health Outcomes
  - E. Develop a Behavior Change Plan
  - F. Reiterate Benefits of Change
  - G. Address Environmental and Interpersonal Facilitators and Barriers to Change
  - H. Determine a Time Frame for Implementation
  - I. Commit to Behavior-Change Goals
- Revisions of the Health-Protection–Promotion Plan
- Directions for Research
- Summary

Clients should be active participants in interpreting the assessment data and in health care planning. Client collaboration with the nurse in planning for care promotes positive perceptions of worth and affirms the ability of individuals, families, or communities to self-regulate and function on their own behalf in improving health and creating conditions supportive of healthy lifestyles. The role of the nurse is to **assist** clients with health planning rather than to **control** the process. During assessment, the nurse and client develop a mutual understanding of (1) the health and risk status of the client; (2) current health-behavior patterns of the client; (3) attitudes and beliefs that affect health and health-related behaviors of the client; (4) expectations of important referent groups; (5) behavioral options potentially available to the client; (6) the interaction of social-ethnic-cultural background with health practices; (7) potential or actual barriers to health-protecting and -promoting self-care; and (8) existing support systems for health-promoting behaviors. Developing a systematic plan for behavior change provides an opportunity for the client to express stabilizing and actualizing tendencies in purposeful ways directed toward increasing wellness and enhancing life satisfaction.

Health planning is a dynamic process in which flexibility to meet the changing needs of clients is critical. The plan systematically lends direction but does not dictate goals that must be attained or behaviors that must be learned. The health-protection–promotion plan should be reasonable both in terms of demands on the client and the time frame allocated for accomplishment of desired health or health-related goals. Knowledge, skills, and strengths of the client should be utilized in the planning process. Capitalizing on positive health practices currently a part of personal or family lifestyle creates a sense of competence or efficacy as well as the behavioral control essential to successful behavior change. The nurse and the client should together assess the stage of change (precontemplation, contemplation, preparation, action, maintenance) for behaviors the client wishes to modify. The client can then discuss with the nurse strategies for change that are likely to be most effective. The plan should be revised as needed to make behavior change a positive growth experience for clients. The ultimate goal of health planning and implementation is to make health protection and health promotion a way of life that individuals, families, and communities can manage and enjoy.

Innovative developments in information technology increasingly allow personalization of assessment and intervention protocols to the unique characteristics and needs of individual clients. Nurses should be actively involved in the design of health-assessment and health-planning software that is interactive and client-friendly.

• GUIDELINES FOR PREVENTIVE SERVICES

With increasing emphasis on the prevention of disease, varying sets of guidelines for the delivery of preventive services to individuals and families throughout the life span have been developed. These guidelines, for the most part, focus on clinical care directed toward protection from specific diseases such as AIDS or behavioral morbidities such as substance abuse. Nurses in all settings where primary care is delivered should become familiar with the following sets of guidelines to make sure that their clients benefit from "state-of-the-science" preventive services: *Guide to Clinical Preventive Services,*[1] *Clinician's Handbook of Preventive Services,*[2] *AMA Guidelines for Adolescent Preventive Services,*[3] and *Bright Futures: Guidelines for Health Supervision of Infants, Children, and Adolescents.*[4] These publications provide recommendations and rationale for a wide array of preventive maneuvers.

• THE HEALTH-PLANNING PROCESS

The process for developing a health-protection–promotion plan is outlined below, with each step in the process discussed separately. These nine steps actively involve both the client and the nurse in the health-planning process:

1. Review and summarize data from assessment.
2. Reinforce strengths and competencies of the client.
3. Identify health goals and related behavioral change options.
4. Identify behavioral or health outcomes that will indicate that the plan has been successful from the client's perspective.
5. Develop a behavior change plan based on the client's preferences, stages of change, and on "state-of-the science" knowledge about effective interventions.
6. Reiterate benefits of change and identify incentives for change from the client's perspective.
7. Address environmental and interpersonal facilitators and barriers to behavior change.
8. Determine a time frame for implementation.
9. Commit to behavior change goals and to structure the support needed to accomplish them.

Specific approaches that can be used to initiate and sustain behavioral change will be discussed in Chapter 8.

Review and Summarize Data from Assessment

During assessment, a wealth of information is shared between nurse and client. The reduction of this information to manageable proportions is accomplished by summarizing qualitative data and calculating scores and subscores on the various instruments employed in assessment of a specific client. From assessment activities, the nurse and client should have information available in the following domains as a basis for planning and action:

1. Physical health status
2. Status in relation to functional health patterns
3. Physical fitness
4. Nutritional status
5. Major health risks
6. Sources of life stress
7. Spirituality
8. Social support
9. Key health beliefs
10. Health-related lifestyle
11. Family health beliefs and practices
12. Environmental and community supports or constraints for health behaviors

Clients can be guided through the data summary process by the nurse during one or more clinic appointments or home visits. Both nurse and client should retain a copy of the assessment summary for continuing reference during the health-planning process.

Reinforce Strengths and Competencies of the Client

Each individual or family seen by the nurse already has in place a system of health-care practices compatible with their cultural orientation. Thus, the nurse and client should achieve consensus on areas in which the client is already taking informed and responsible health action as well as on areas for further development of self-care competencies.

Designed for: James Moore

Home Address: 714 George

Home Telephone Number: 222-3333

Occupation (if employed): building services supervisor

Work Telephone Number: 445-6666

Cultural Identification: African-American

Birth Date: 3/14/55 Date of Initial Plan: 8/3/95

Client strengths:	Satisfactory peer relationships, spiritual strength, adequate sleep pattern
Major risk factors:	Elevated cholesterol, mild obesity, sedentary lifestyle, moderate life change, multiple daily hassles, few reported uplifts
Nursing diagnoses: (derived from assessment of functional health patterns)	Diversional activity deficit; altered nutrition: more than body requirements; caregiver role strain (elderly mother)
Medical diagnoses: (if any)	Mild hypertension
Age-specific screening recommendations: (derived from Guide to Clinical Prev. Services)	Blood pressure, cholesterol, fecal occult blood, malignant skin lesions, depression
Desired behavioral and health outcomes:	Become a regular exerciser (3xs/week), lower my blood pressure, weigh 165 lbs.

Figure 7–1. Example of an Individual Health-Protection–Promotion Plan.

Personal Health Goals (1 = highest priority)	Selected Behaviors to Accomplish Goals	Stage of Change	Strategies/ Interventions for Change
1. Achieve desired body weight	Begin a progressive walking program	Planning	Counter-conditioning Reinforcement management Patient contracting
	Decrease caloric intake while maintaining good nutrition	Action (eating 2 fruits and 2 vegetables daily; using low-fat dairy products for last 2 months)	Stimulus control Cognitive restructuring
2. Decrease risk for hypertension-related disorders	Change from high to low sodium snacks	Contemplation	Consciousness raising Learning facilitation
3. Learn to manage stress effectively	Attend relaxation classes and use home relaxation tapes	Contemplation	Consciousness raising Self-reevaluation Simple relaxation therapy
4. Increase leisure-time activities	Join a local bowling league	Contemplation	Support system enhancement

Figure 7–1. (continued). Example of an Individual Health-Protection–Promotion Plan.

Clients bring unique strengths to the health-planning task. These assets should be identified, acknowledged, and reinforced by the nurse. Since clients will carry out health behaviors in ways that fit their cultural beliefs, preferences, and current levels of knowledge and skill, existing cultural practices supportive of health should be integrated into the overall health plan. The client's sense of cultural or ethnic pride should be reinforced during the health-planning process.

Through teaching, guidance, and support, the nurse nurtures and enhances existing competencies to meet health needs. Self-care requirements and resources of individuals will vary according to age, gender, developmental stage, and health status. The self-care needs of families may vary by family composition, developmental tasks being confronted, and role demands. While clients will differ in their requirements for self-care and in their competencies for self-management, it is important that the nurse emphasize to all clients their own importance as "primary self-care agent." Promoting client responsibility

Designed for (family name): The Marshalls

Home Address: 1718 Green St.

Home Telephone Number: 777-4444

Occupations of Employed Members of Household: Mother-Dental assistant

Work Telephone Number: 883-7777

Family Form: One-parent family

Cultural Identification: Asian-American

Family Members:	Position in Family	Birth Date	Occupation/ Student/Retired
	Joan (Mother)	9/65	Dental assistant
	Dana (Daughter)	4/79	Student
	Tiffany (Daughter)	7/85	Student
	Eric (Son)	1/89	Student

Date of Initial Plan: ________________

Family strengths:	Open communication patterns, intrafamily cooperation, healthy snacks consumed at home
Major risk factors:	Mother recently divorced, oldest daughter has driver's license, high life change for family, minimal family physical activity
Nursing diagnoses:	Family coping: potential for growth
Medical diagnoses for family members:	None
Desired behavioral and health outcomes:	Active family outings, avoidance of early sexual activity and binge drinking among adolescent family members, injury prevention for children, adjustment to new family form

Figure 7–2. Example of a Family Health-Protection–Promotion Plan.

Family Health Goals (1 = highest priority)	Selected Behaviors to Accomplish Goals	Stage of Change	Strategies/ Interventions for Change
1. Healthy adjustment to single-parent family status	Realign family responsibilities	Action (divorced 3 mo)	Social liberation Family process maintenance Caregiver support
	Increase spiritual resources (increase church attendance)	Contemplation	Spiritual support Helping relationships
	Discuss life purpose and goals among family members	Planning	Self-reevaluation Self-esteem enhancement Anticipatory guidance
2. Develop more active family lifestyles	Plan active family outings (biking, recreation center)	Planning	Exercise promotion Environmental reevaluation Modeling
3. Foster healthy sexuality among preadolescent and adolescents	Provide age-appropriate information	Action	Anticipatory guidance Parent education: adolescent
	Enhance self-esteem through praise, expression of affection, and assistance with skill development	Maintenance	Self-esteem enhancement Helping relationships

Figure 7–2. Example of a Family Health-Protection–Promotion Plan. (continued).

4. Encourage adolescents to avoid alcohol use	Hold family meetings to discuss binge drinking, drinking and driving, use of nonalcoholic alternatives	Contemplation	Parent education: adolescent Self-responsibility facilitation Substance use prevention

Figure 7–2. Example of a Family Health-Protection–Promotion Plan. (continued).

for health does not negate the importance of the nurse's working to change the larger social infrastructure to make health-promoting options more available to communities. Personal change and social change are both essential for effective health protection and promotion.

A sample health-protection–promotion plan for an individual client is presented in Figure 7–1 and one for a family in Figure 7–2. In both planning tools, sections in which client strengths can be identified are provided.

• IDENTIFY HEALTH GOALS AND RELATED BEHAVIOR-CHANGE OPTIONS

The next step in the planning process is to identify personal or family health goals, prioritize them, and review related behavior-change options. Systematically reviewing the range of changes that are possible to achieve important health goals can assist clients in making informed choices concerning the behavioral changes on which they will focus in the initial health-protection–promotion plan. Providing relevant information but letting the client determine priorities for change constitutes educative-supportive care by the nurse. Clients should not be made to feel guilty or inadequate in regard to current health practices. During health counseling sessions the nurse should create enthusiasm and excitement about growth in positive directions and about enjoyment of new health-related experiences.

Many clients will initially place high priority on areas of health protection in which the threat of illness is tangible and easily understood. Decreasing risk for specific chronic health problems fits the medical orientation to which most Americans have been socialized. A high level of client interest in risk reduction indicates to the nurse that health protection is likely the most meaningful area for emphasis in early health planning. Mastery of specific health-protection measures will often motivate clients to consider making additional lifestyle changes directed toward health promotion in order to experience a higher level of health and well-being.

Clients often give important emotional cues concerning the behaviors they wish to change. Examples of such cues include:

"I hate myself when I gorge on fattening foods!"
"I get mad at myself for being so uptight!"
"I feel very sad when I think of how little time our family spends together."

The more open an individual or family is in discussing health concerns with the nurse, the higher the probability of developing a meaningful health-protection–promotion plan. Often areas that the client is reluctant to discuss, such as marital relationships, human sexuality, spirituality, and family cohesiveness, are the most crucial areas for behavior change in order to enhance well-being. A "safe" climate should be created in which the client can discuss health issues of highest personal concern with assurance that communication will remain confidential.

Identify Behavioral or Health Outcomes

It is critical that the nurse and client together determine the desired health outcomes from implementation of the health-protection–promotion plan. Clear identification of outcomes both energizes and guides the client in health behaviors. The client's perceptions concerning the outcomes desired should determine the criteria that will be used to evaluate whether the plan and its implementation has been successful. Have I reached my goal or made significant progress toward it? is a critical question that must be asked periodically by the client to evaluate the viability of the health-protection–promotion plan.

Research literature that supports the link between particular interventions and desired outcomes should inform the nursing process and the plan that is developed. For example, the factors or strategies that have been shown to affect the likelihood of maintaining a healthy diet should be integrated into the plan for persons wishing to address nutritional issues. The nurse should be cautious about the outcomes selected. For example, a behavioral goal of eating only at meals may be easier to attain than a goal of losing a certain number of pounds. Weight will most likely be lost if the plan is followed, but tangible behaviors are more under the control of the client and thus easier to reinforce and manage. Long-term outcomes can be set but achieved through a progressive set of short-term outcomes that move the client toward the desired end points.

Develop a Behavior Change Plan

A constructive program of change is based on the client taking "ownership" of those behavior changes selected for implementation within everyday life. The client should be assisted in examining major value–behavior inconsistencies that exist. Alternative actions that are both healthful and enjoyable to the client need to be substituted for the behaviors that are inconsistent with personal values. It is unfortunate that what individuals and families have learned to prefer or value within the American lifestyle frequently can be detrimental to health.

At this point, clients should select from all the behavioral options available those behaviors that are appealing and that they are willing to try. This brings clients full circle from assessing current health status and lifestyle, through considering health goals and behavioral options, to actually identifying those behavior changes they are willing to adopt in order to accomplish desired goals and achieve health outcomes. The client's priorities for behavior change will reflect personal values, activity preferences, estimates of cognitive and psychomotor skills, affective responses to the various behavioral options, expectations for success in learning and carrying out the various behaviors, and ease with which the selected behaviors can be integrated into lifestyle. The stage of change of the client in relation to each of the selected behaviors should be assessed.

Appropriate strategies and interventions to facilitate behavior change can be identified from the *Nursing Interventions Classification,*[5–8] from transtheoretical model literature,[9] or from the extensive literature in the behavioral sciences on behavior change. The nurse should develop expertise with implementing behavior-change interventions, including the activities that constitute the intervention and the appropriate sequencing of those activities. As the expert health care provider with skill in behavior-change facilitation, the nurse can then assist the client in gaining the self-change skills needed for the adoption and maintenance of positive health behaviors.

Reiterate Benefits of Change

Although clients are aware of the changes they want to make and the benefits of change, these benefits need to be frequently reiterated by both the nurse and the client. The client should keep a list of benefits from the changes being made in a highly visible place so that they can be reviewed frequently. This may be on the refrigerator, the bathroom mirror, the dashboard of the car, or the computer at the workplace. Keeping health benefits "in front" of the client is a reminder that the behaviors in the health-promotion plan are personally worthwhile and directed toward important life goals.

The benefits of change may include both health-related and non–health-related outcomes anticipated by the client. Although nurses tend to think in terms of health benefits, sensitivity to non–health-related benefits of change is important as these may be central to the client's motivation to engage in health-protection–promotion planning and implementation.

Address Environmental and Interpersonal Facilitators and Barriers to Change

Environmental features and interpersonal relationships that support positive change should be used to bolster the client's efforts to modify lifestyle. Facilitators can be used to counter barriers to change and encourage the client when problems occur in the behavior-change process. Both instrumental and emotional support from their social network are important in encouraging clients to persist with change efforts when the going gets difficult or competing demands or preferences vie for attention.

All individuals and families experience barriers to changing behavior. Although some obstacles cannot be anticipated, others can be planned for and their potential negative impact considerably weakened. If the client is aware of possible barriers and has formulated plans for dealing with them if they arise, successful behavior change is more likely to occur.

Barriers to effective health behavior can arise from inside clients themselves, from significant others, or from the environment. Internal barriers to change may be lack of motivation, fatigue, boredom, giving up, lack of appropriate skills, or disbelief that behavior can be successfully changed. Family members can impose considerable barriers if they encourage continuation of health-damaging behaviors or if they actively discourage attempts at behavior change. Environmental barriers that may inhibit positive change include lack of space or appropriate setting in which to carry out the selected activity; dangers within the immediate environment, such as heavy traffic or high crime rate; or inclement weather. The client should be assisted by the nurse in dealing with these environmental barriers or in locating another setting appropriate for health activities.

Determine a Time Frame for Implementation

Progress toward healthier lifestyles needs to be made over a period of time in order to allow new behaviors to be learned well, integrated into one's lifestyle, and stabilized. Attempting to change or initiate a number of new behaviors all at once may result in confusion, discouragement, and the client's abandonment of the health-protection–promotion plan. Whether the client is attempting to reduce risk for chronic diseases or to enhance health status, gradual rather than abrupt change is desirable. Just as health education for self-care must proceed at the pace of the learner rather than at that of the nurse, changes in behavior must be sequenced in reasonable steps appropriate for the client.

Developing a time plan for implementation allows appropriate knowledge and skills to be mastered before a new behavior is implemented. For example, it is difficult to warm up before brisk walking or jogging if the client has no idea of what appropriate warm-up exercises are. The time frame for developing a given behavior may be several weeks or several months. If the client is rewarded for accomplishing short-term goals, this provides encouragement for continuing pursuit of long-term goals and desired outcomes. A meaningful plan requires that deadlines be set for accomplishing specific goals. Adherence to deadlines should be encouraged, with changes made only when the time frame must be shortened or lengthened to make it more conducive to permanent behavior change.

Commit to Behavior-Change Goals

Through identification of new behaviors that the client is willing to try, a verbal commitment is made to change. However, the client may be more motivated to follow through with selected actions if the personal commitment is formalized. A commitment to change can be formalized in a number of ways: (1) nurse–client contract agreements like those that appear in Figures 7–3 and 7–4, (2) self-contracts such as those shown in Figures 7–5 and 7–6, (3) public announcements to family members and friends of intentions to engage in new behaviors, (4) integration of new health behaviors into daily or weekly calendar, and (5) purchase of necessary supplies (eg, low-fat foods, relaxation audiotapes) and equipment (eg, exercise bike, walking shoes).

Behavioral contracts contain specific information about (1) the change to be made, (2) the way the change is to be accomplished, (3) the individual or family members who are to engage in the change, (4) the time frame for behavior change, and (5) the consequences of meeting or not meeting the terms of the agreement. A **nurse–client contract** provides direction for the helping relationship through identification of mutual objectives and responsibilities of each party to the contract. Contracts allow clients to participate actively in their own care by choosing goals that can be realistically accomplished. Generally, the client is responsible for carrying out certain behaviors, while the nurse is responsible for providing information, training, counseling, or specific reinforcement rewards. The nurse, as the health care professional involved in the contract, bears the additional responsibility of providing helpful input and continuing feedback to the client con-

Nurse–Client Contract and Agreement

Statement of Health Goal: *Decreased feelings of stress and tension*

I *Jim Johnson* (client) promise to *use progressive relaxation techniques (four-muscle groups) upon arriving home from work each day* (Client Responsibility)

for a period of *one week*, whereupon,

Kathy Turner (nurse) will provide *a copy of Herbert Benson's book, Relaxation Response* (Nurse Responsibility)

on *Saturday, March 7th* (date) to me.

If I do not fulfill the terms of this contract in total, I understand that the designated reward will be withheld.

Signed: ______________________ (client)

______________________ (date)

______________________ (nurse)

______________________ (date)

Figure 7–3. Sample nurse–client contract for an individual client.

cerning the adequacy of performance of activities identified in the contract. It is also critical that the nurse be consistent and conscientious in managing the reinforcement-reward contingencies of the contract. Failure in fulfilling this commitment will destroy the trust and confidence placed in the nurse by the client.

In a nurse–client contract with a family, the agreement may be made to brisk-walk, jog, or bicycle together two to three times each week or to modify their nutritional prac-

Nurse–Client Contract and Agreement

Statement of Health Goal: *Improve eating habits*

We *The Nichols* (family) promise to eat two servings of *vegetables and two servings of fruit daily* (family responsibility)

for a period of *one week* whereupon,

Lana Buxton (nurse) will provide *four movie theater tickets at the Strand Theater* (nurse responsibility)

on *Friday, April 10th* (date) to us.

If we do not fulfill the terms of this contract in total, We understand that the designated reward will be withheld.

Signed: ______________________ (family representative)

______________________ (date)

______________________ (nurse)

______________________ (date)

Figure 7–4. Sample nurse–client contract for a family.

tices, such as increasing vegetables in their diet to three to four servings per day. Family members, because of their continuing contact and emotional connectedness, can serve as important sources of encouragement, reinforcement, and reward for one another.

The extent to which the contract has worked must be evaluated. Did the client accomplish the goal fully, partially, or not at all? If failure occurred, what were the reasons?

Self-Contract

Personal Health Goal: ___*Change Dietary Habits*___

I ___*Doris Downs*___ promise myself that I will ___*follow*___

___*the sample menus for a 1200 calorie diet for breakfast, lunch, and*___

___*dinner*___ for a period of ___*two days*___,

whereupon I will ___*buy myself a new pair of earrings*___

on ___*Wednesday, June 8th*___ .

Signed ________________________

Date ________________________

Figure 7–5. Sample individual self-contract.

Self-Contract

Family Health Goal: ___*Get more exercise*___

We ___*The Stones*___ promise each other that we will ___*go*___

___*swimming at the "Y" once a week*___ for a period of ___*three weeks*___

whereupon we will ___*buy the newest version of Trivial Pursuit*___

on ___*Friday, February 10th*___ .

Signed: ________________________

____

____

Date ________________________

Figure 7–6. Sample family self-contract.

Behavior: Learn to Use Progressive Relaxation as One Approach to Handling Stress	
Component of Behavior	**Reward or Reinforcement**
Attend first class session at 9 A.M. Saturday at the county health department	Watch the football game in the afternoon on TV
Use relaxation audiotape at home for 20 minutes of practice Sunday	Call John and visit for a while
Monday	Spend an hour at the driving range
Tuesday	Buy a new paperback novel
Wednesday	Praise myself for having practiced relaxation each day thus far
Thursday	Invite Harry and Jim over to play pool
Friday	Take my family to a movie
Attend second class session at 9 A.M. Saturday at the County Health Department	Take an orange juice break afterwards with Bret, a class member
Practice relaxation techniques for 20 minutes providing my own cues rather than using the tape Sunday	Go for a short drive and enjoy the scenery
Monday	Spend 30 minutes reading my new novel
Tuesday	Buy myself a new bottle of aftershave lotion
Wednesday	Praise myself for persistence and successful practice
Thursday	Allow myself to linger in a warm shower longer than usual
Friday	Go to stock car races with the family
Keep my weekly record of relaxation practice	The nurse will provide a copy of *Relaxation Response* by Herbert Benson

Figure 7–7. Reward-reinforcement plan.

How could the contract be reorganized so that the probability of successful completion is high? Does the contract need to be renegotiated? Should the contract be terminated? Careful analysis of the contracting process and evaluation of subsequent outcomes will permit the nurse and client to design contracts that successfully move clients toward desired health goals.

In a **self-contract** the client is responsible for both the behavioral commitment and for reinforcement of identified behaviors. Self-contracting is an effective approach for enhancing the client's control over behavior, thus creating a sense of independence, competence, and autonomy. The client does not become overly dependent on the nurse for reinforcement but instead serves as the source of rewards for positive health behaviors. Rewards can be extrinsic such as tangible objects (magazine, cosmetics), or experiences (warm bath, telephone call to a friend) or intrinsic (self-praise, feelings of pride). Rewards selected should be highly desirable to the client in order to have reinforcement value. A reward-reinforcement plan can be developed as illustrated in Figure 7–7. Use of rewards for behavior and lifestyle change are discussed in more detail in Chapter 8.

Success in fulfilling the agreements in the contract enhances the client's self-esteem and problem-solving abilities. The client gains increased confidence in meeting future health needs. In reality, it is the client who must learn to manage a self-reward system that is supportive of emerging positive health practices.

Publicly announcing intentions to engage in a new behavior to family members and close friends is still another way of solidifying commitment to a particular course of action. The expectations of significant others that the client will follow through with the designated behavior can trigger personal encouragement and emotional and instrumental support on the part of significant others that enhance motivation for behavior.

Integrating new behaviors into one's calendar is an important way of building them into daily routines. For example, exercise time can be scheduled during the lunch hour and the appointment for exercise kept just like an appointment with one's boss or coworker. Lack of time is a frequent excuse for being unable to follow through with newly adopted behaviors. When time is actually scheduled to accomplish health behaviors, the probability of their occurrence is significantly enhanced.

Purchasing necessary supplies and equipment is still another way of making a commitment to behavior change. When equipment is purchased and a monetary investment is made, clients are much more likely to follow through with the desired behavior. For example, people who have exercise equipment and exercise videos in their home are more likely to be active than persons who do not.

• REVISIONS OF THE HEALTH-PROTECTION–PROMOTION PLAN

A schedule for periodic review of the health-protection–promotion plan should be established. Revisions should be carried out during counseling sessions, with both the client and the nurse contributing to the process. Impetus for changes in the plan may result from mastery of target behaviors, changes in client's values and priorities, or awareness of new options available to the client. Outdated plans fail to provide impetus or direction for change and thus become uninteresting and meaningless to the client. Periodic revision and updating of the health plan provides a systematic approach for movement of the client toward higher levels of health behavior and health.

• DIRECTIONS FOR RESEARCH

Many nursing research questions relative to planning for health protection and health promotion can be identified. Nurses are in a pivotal position to address these questions and create new knowledge about the behavior-change process. Questions to be addressed include:

1. How can face-to-face and computerized feedback from health assessment be combined to optimize level of motivation for health-protection and -promotion planning?
2. To what extent do nurses reinforce clients' positive cultural health practices during health counseling?
3. During what stages of change for a given health behavior is intrinsic motivation likely to be more effective than extrinsic motivation?
4. What factors affect the tempo of behavior change at different life stages?
5. To what extent does successful behavior change increase beliefs concerning self-esteem, self-efficacy, and behavioral control?

• SUMMARY

The health-protection–promotion plans presented in this chapter provide individuals and families with a systematic approach to improving health practices and lifestyle. All clients should be provided with a health portfolio that contains a summary of their health assessment, their health-protection–promotion plan and other relevant health records. It is imperative that clients take home all the information and planning documents needed to follow through successfully with their desired behavior changes. Focusing on outcomes desired by the client will energize and direct implementation of the plan. Adjusting the plan as needed to ensure client success is vital to effective health-protective and -promotive care.

REFERENCES

1. US Preventive Services Task Force. *Guide to Clinical Preventive Services: An Assessment of the Effectiveness of 169 Interventions.* Baltimore, Md: Williams & Wilkins, 1989.
2. US Public Health Service. *Clinician's Handbook of Preventive Services: Put Prevention into Practice.* Waldorf, Md: American Nurses Publishing; 1994.
3. American Medical Association. *AMA Guidelines for Adolescent Preventive Services: Recommendations and Rationale.* Baltimore, Md: Williams & Wilkins; 1994.
4. Green M, ed. *Bright Futures: Guidelines for Health Supervision of Infants, Children, and Adolescents.* Arlington, Va: National Center for Education in Maternal and Child Health, 1994.

5. McCloskey JC, Bulecheck GM, eds. *Nursing Interventions Classification (NIC): Iowa Intervention Project.* St Louis, Mo: Mosby Year Book; 1992.
6. Daly JM, ed. *NIC Interventions Linked to NANDA Diagnoses: Iowa Intervention Project.* Iowa City, Iowa: University of Iowa; 1993.
7. Craft MJ, Denehy JA. *Nursing Interventions for Infants and Children.* Philadelphia, Pa: WB Saunders Co; 1990.
8. Maas M, Buckwalter KC, Hardy M. *Nursing Diagnoses and Interventions for the Elderly.* Menlo Park, Calif: Addison-Wesley Publishing Co; 1991.
9. Prochaska JO, Velicer WF, DiClemente CC, et al. Measuring processes of change: application to the cessation of smoking. *J Consult Clin Psychol.* 1988;56:520–528.

IV
PART FOUR

Strategies for Prevention and Health Promotion: The Action and Maintenance Phases

8

Modification of Health-Related Lifestyle

Individuals and groups have tremendous plasticity and potential for change. Development of unique resources and realization of human potential are achieved through progressive, planned change that is guided by goals highly relevant and meaningful to the clients themselves. Because of human beings' capacity for self-knowledge, self-regulation, decision making, and creative problem solving, self-directed change is possible. Self-change can be defined as new behaviors that clients willingly undertake to achieve self-selected goals or desired outcomes. The power and skill to change health behaviors or modify health-related lifestyles are within the domain of clients. The expertise to provide educative-developmental care facilitative of behavior change and to foster environmental conditions supportive of healthy behaviors are within the domain of the professional nurse. The nurse promotes a positive climate for change, serves as a catalyst for change, assists the client with various steps of the change process, and develops the client's capacity to maintain change.

To best promote behavior change, the nurse must have positive regard for the client and sensitivity to the client's cultural heritage. Nurses and clients should be matched, whenever possible, so that the nurse is competent in the "culture of origin" of the client. Cultural competence enables the nurse to better understand the particular life situation of the client and to facilitate the client's efforts to make lifestyle changes that fit with cultural beliefs and lifeways. Health behaviors with "cultural fit" are more likely to be maintained over time as an integral aspect of lifestyle. Maintenance of positive behavior change over an extended period of time is critical if clients are to gain significant health benefits from the changes made.

Attempts of individuals and families to change may be focused on the cessation of a health-damaging behavior such as smoking or alcohol misuse, or on the acquisition of a healthy behavior such as consumption of a nutritious diet or learning positive family communication skills. Often both kinds of changes will be made at the same time. It is imperative that the nurse have a theoretically based understanding of the change process so that she or he provides appropriate care during each stage of change. Various stages of change have been identified in the literature, the most common being the stages of adoption and maintenance. It has been widely assumed that different professional interventions are needed during each stage. Currently, the dominant paradigm in the literature to explain the process of behavior change is the transtheoretical model.

THE TRANSTHEORETICAL MODEL OF BEHAVIOR CHANGE

The transtheoretical model was developed by Prochaska and DiClemente, based on their extensive research on smoking cessation among adults.[1] They propose that health-related behavior change progresses through five stages, regardless of whether the client is trying to quit a health-threatening behavior or adopt a healthy behavior. These stages are: precontemplation, contemplation, planning or preparation, action, and maintenance.

- Precontemplation: A client is not thinking about quitting or adopting a particular behavior, at least not within the next 6 months (not intending to make changes).
- Contemplation: A client is seriously thinking about quitting or adopting a particular behavior *in the next 6 months* (considering a change).
- Planning or Preparation: A client who has tried to quit a negative behavior or adopt a positive behavior in the past year is seriously thinking about engaging in the contemplated change *within the next month* (making small or sporadic changes).
- Action: This phase covers the period of 6 months during which the client has made the behavior change and it has persisted (actively engaged in behavior change).
- Maintenance: This is the period beginning 6 months after action has started and continuing indefinitely. This stage involves continuation and stabilization of the change (sustaining the change over time).[2]

Interestingly, Prochaska and DiClemente do not have a sixth stage of "relapse" consistent with the theory of relapse prevention (see Chapter 2). They appear to interpret relapse as immediate return to one of the former stages in the model.

An attempt has been made to integrate various core concepts from other models of behavior change into the transtheoretical model. In particular, the concept of **decisional balance** from Janis and Mann's decision-making model[3] is integral to the theory. The Janis and Mann model is a conflict model that assumes sound decision making involves comparison of all potential gains and losses, which are entered into a balance sheet. The behavior should occur when the potential gains of engaging in the behavior outbalance the losses. Janis and Mann categorize the potential gains and losses into four categories: (a) personal gains or losses, (b) gains or losses for significant others, (c) self-approval or disapproval, and (d) approval or disapproval from significant others. Prochaska and colleagues have combined these four categories into two: pros and cons of engaging in the behavior. Decisional balance has been shown to have particular patterns across behavior-change stages. In fact, Prochaska proposed two principles about the relationship between pros and cons across stages that have held up in his examination of 12 health-related behaviors. The first principle states that progression from precontemplation to action is a function of approximately a one-standard-deviation increase in the pros of a health behavior change. The second principle states that progression from precontemplation to action is a function of approximately a one-half-standard-deviation decrease in the cons of a health behavior change.[4] Cross-sectional studies of 12 health behaviors showed that during precontemplation, the cons of changing the behavior were higher than the pros. During either contemplation or preparation, depending on the behavior, the pros increase was followed by a decrease in the cons so that there was a crossover in decision balance. That is, for the majority of behaviors studied, the balance between the pros and cons had reversed before action occurred. During the maintenance stage, the pros of engaging in the desirable behavior or not engaging in the undesirable behavior continued to outweigh the cons.[2(pp43–44)] These principles are an interesting attempt to quantify the dose-response relationship between a cognitive shift and a behavioral change.

In two other studies, it appeared that another concept, self-efficacy, could be integrated into the transtheoretical model. Self-efficacy shifted in a predictable way across the stages of behavior change, with clients progressively becoming more efficacious.[5,6] Prochaska and his colleagues have suggested that, rather than test two different models of behavior change to see if one outpredicts or outperforms a competing model, we test the ability of one model of behavior change to integrate empirically the core constructs of an alternative model.[2(p45)] Given the overlap of some of the concepts in the health-behavior models currently in the literature, Prochaska's suggestion may prove fruitful as an approach to structuring nursing interventions for behavior change.

A number of studies have shown that although the transtheoretical model was developed on a health-damaging behavior, smoking, the stages of change are applicable to positive health behaviors such as exercise.[7–9]

Prochaska's research has suggested that different processes are emphasized at the various stages of change. Processes of change are covert or overt activities that people engage in to modify their experiences and their environments in order to modify behavior. The 10 processes of change presented in Table 8–1 were identified in multiple studies and have their roots in various therapy systems (behavioral, cognitive, existential, experiential, humanistic, etc). They are categorized in the transtheoretical model as either experiential or behavioral processes or strategies.

TABLE 8–1. PROCESSES OF CHANGE

PROCESS	DEFINITION
Experiential Processes	
Consciousness raising	Efforts by the individual to seek new information and to gain understanding and feedback about the problem
Dramatic relief	Affective aspects of change, often involving intense emotional experiences related to the problem behavior
Environmental reevaluation	Consideration and assessment by the individual of how the problem affects the physical and social environments
Self-reevaluation	Emotional and cognitive reappraisal of values by the individual with respect to the problem behavior
Social liberation	Awareness, availability, and acceptance by the individual of alternative lifestyles in society
Behavioral processes	
Counterconditioning	Substitution of alternative behaviors for the problem behavior
Helping relationships	Trusting, accepting, and utilizing the support of caring others during attempts to change the problem behavior
Reinforcement management	Changing the contingencies that control or maintain the problem behavior
Self-liberation	The individual's choice and commitment to change the problem behavior, including the belief that one *can* change
Stimulus control	Control of situations and other causes that trigger the problem behavior

(From Marcus BH, Rossi JS, Selby VC, et al. The stages and processes of exercise adoption and maintenance in a worksite sample. Health Psychol. *1992;11:387. With permission.)*

According to Prochaska, experiential processes are much more important than behavioral processes for understanding and predicting progress in the early stages of change. Behavioral processes are much more important for understanding and predicting transition from preparation to action and from action to maintenance. Once an individual's stage has been assessed using the transtheoretical model, the nurse can select appropriate processes to help the client progress from stage to stage.[10] When a nurse is working with an individual or with a family, one particular technique may be chosen or several different techniques may be combined in a more complex behavior-change program. It is critical that both nurse and client be involved in decisions concerning approaches to be used at each stage of the process.

Although the transtheoretical model has been selected as the framework for this chapter, the nurse should explore other theories of behavior change. These can be found primarily in the psychologic, sociologic, and political science literature.

• PROCESSES FOR CHANGE

A number of experiential and behavioral strategies for change are described here, including several identified in Table 8–1. Experiential processes are to a large extent internally focused on behavior-linked emotions, values, and cognitions. Behavioral processes focus directly on behavioral change. Because of the major responsibility of the nursing profession for promoting lifestyle change, experiential and behavior strategies for doing so have become an integral part of the nursing profession's taxonomy of interventions. The reader should refer to the Nursing Interventions Classification (NIC) for further information on the following behavior change interventions discussed in this book: self-modification assistance, cognitive restructuring, calming techniques, and progressive muscle relaxation.[11]

Experiential Processes

Consciousness Raising

Seeking and processing information, observing others, and interpreting information in light of one's personal situation are the primary activities reported most frequently during the contemplation stage.[12] The client should be provided with materials that discuss the health-related issues being confronted including the short- and long-term consequences for the individual and for significant others of engaging in a healthy behavior or continuing an unhealthy behavior. Risk-appraisal and risk-reduction counseling can be used to raise consciousness concerning how changing behavior can lower risk for chronic illness. Self-awareness and self-development counseling can emphasize the possibilities for actualizing health potential through behavior change. "Headliners" from national newspapers and magazines focused on the benefits of change or the negative consequences of not changing may be particularly effective during the contemplation stage because of the "eye-catching" format in which the information is presented. The client should be given a list of potential information resources and encouraged to become an active participant in information gathering.

A wide range of "consciousness-raising" media should be used including posters, audiocassettes, videos, and computer-based programs. Furthermore, the materials used need to be culturally specific to the client to optimize impact. Individuals with whom the client can identify who depict the behaviors the client is considering adopting can provide testimonials of successful change. These changes may be in level of exercise, in family communication patterns, or in risky behaviors such as smoking or alcohol use. The enhancement of self-efficacy, an important determinant of behavior, can begin during consciousness raising. Persons who have successfully changed their behavior can reassure and persuade clients that they can accomplish the same goals. This input can enhance the clients' perceptions of capabilities to make the desired changes in behavior (self-efficacy).

Family members can be engaged in conversations regarding how they perceive the target behavior and how they would like to see the client change. The extent to which family members would actively assist the client in making desired changes and how they would provide assistance can be explored. This feedback can increase the client's awareness of the interpersonal support that will potentially be available. Membership in self-help or self-change groups can be critical at this point, as the group can provide input to the client on the process of change, the barriers or environmental constraints likely to be encountered in making changes, and various means of overcoming these constraints. Learning from the reported experiences of others or directly observing their coping behaviors can further increase clients' perceptions of self-efficacy and lower perceived barriers to successful behavior change. Focusing attention through consciousness raising on the area(s) for health-behavior change can bring about increasing identification with the values, beliefs, and emotions associated with change.

Self Reevaluation

Toward the end of the contemplation stage and into the preparation and action stages, clients direct energies toward reevaluating themselves, their self-standards and their values. The client may ask questions such as, Will I like myself better or be more accepting of myself as a nonsmoker, exerciser, or thinner person?[12(p99)] Do I view myself as someone who can capably manage stress?

Personal values and beliefs are internalized early in life from the values and beliefs of significant others. Internalized beliefs provide standards of conduct by which the self is evaluated. Adherence to standards that we set for personal behavior enhances self-concept through feelings of pride and self-satisfaction, whereas violation of self-standards for behavior result in negative feelings of guilt and self-censure. Threats to the self-concept through violation of internalized values and standards can decrease feelings of self-esteem. When a contradiction exists between the personal values and beliefs central to the self-concept and current behavior, it can most directly be resolved by engaging in behavior change. Further, the more clients perceive that they are the kind of persons that engage in a particular behavior, the more likely they are to intend to perform the behavior consistent with self-standards. Strong intentions to meet personal standards should lead to actual performance of the behavior.[13]

Self-reevaluation, sometimes called self-confrontation, is an intervention technique based on the premise that change results from the arousal of an affective state of dissatisfaction within the client as a result of recognition of disturbing inconsistencies between self-standards (values, beliefs) and behaviors. It is assumed that once significant dissatisfaction is experienced, the person will be motivated to make behavioral changes to achieve consistency.[14] Inconsistencies of most concern to the client rather than to the nurse should be the focus for intervention, as the motivation and energies for change reside within the client.

Another strategy for reevaluating or confronting the self is to have the client examine personal self-standards and behaviors in comparison to individuals or groups that the client admires. For example, what are the standards and behaviors of persons who exercise regularly, consume healthy diets, or deal effectively with day-to-day stressors. Seeing specific differences between self and "models" or important reference groups can be the impetus for clients to make personal changes in behavior consistent with a reorientation in self-standards and values. Research to determine normative attitudes and values of individuals who routinely practice health-protecting and health-promoting behaviors would provide meaningful information on which to base self-reevaluation nursing interventions.

The client can also use self-reevaluation to contrast the personal behavioral consequences of continuing a health-damaging behavior with the consequences of discontinuing the behavior. For example, the nurse can ask the client to list several activities that would be possible if smoking were discontinued, then predict likely restrictions on behavior if smoking behavior were not changed. This analysis of the consequences of two opposing behaviors can create a sense of disequilibrium in the client by contrasting "what is or will be" with "what could be." With the perception of a threat to the self-system from behavior change, the client may respond with denial of the need to change or with anxiety. In using self-reevaluation techniques, the nurse must evaluate the extent to which the client can tolerate disequilibrium as a stimulus for behavior change. Support and encouragement should be provided to lessen resultant anxiety so that constructive health behaviors can be developed.[14]

Self-reevaluation as a counseling technique is based on the premise that since individuals function holistically, a change in self-standards will result in subsequent changes in behavior. A change in one part of the system results in a modification of the whole to attain equilibrium. The mechanisms whereby self-reevaluation results in behavior change still need to be studied further and clarified.

Cognitive Restructuring

Cognitive restructuring focuses on clients' thinking, imagery, and attitudes toward the self and self-competencies as they affect the change process. The basic assumption behind this approach to behavior change, commonly referred to as rational-emotive therapy,[15] is that the way that individuals evaluate a specific situation and their ability to cope with it determines their emotional reaction to it (positive or negative). The critical factor in determining an individual's response is not the actual situation as much as what the person says internally (eg, appraisals, attributions, and evaluations in the form of self-statements or self-generated images) and associated emotions before or during the target event. The self-statement is an important concept in cognitive restructuring. It can be defined as a covert verbalization that elicits emotional reactions. Self-statements are assumed to be the mediating link between internal or external stimulus and behavior response. The task of the nurse is to help clients recognize the messages they give themselves about their health and health-related behaviors and to help them correct problematic patterns of thinking and dysfunctional beliefs.[16] Often dysfunctional beliefs lead to low levels of perceived self-efficacy and subsequent inability to adopt or maintain a desired health behavior.[17(pp515–519)]

The process of evaluative self-statements begins early in life. The child develops a self-directed verbal repertoire from the responses of others to the child's behavior and from observation of the self-administered praise and criticism of adults.[18] Self-administered praise can facilitate performance through enhancing feelings of esteem and perceived self-efficacy. Invariably self-criticism lowers perceptions of self-efficacy and inhibits effective behavior. The nurse should be aware of the fact that what sometimes appears to be a skill deficit in executing a new behavior may be self-inhibition of the appropriate response. This inhibition is the result of inappropriate self-statements.

Maladaptive emotions are often mediated by irrational self-statements that the client generates in specific situations. If negative emotions are aroused because individuals unthinkingly accept certain illogical premises or irrational ideas, there is good reason to believe that clients can be taught to think more logically and rationally and thereby create positive emotional states rather than negative ones, which in return change behavior and life experiences in positive directions.

Ellis and Grieger[15(pp8–9)] proposed the ABC framework for explaining the impact of self-generated thoughts or ideas on responses to specific environmental events:

- A—Activating experience or event
- B—One's beliefs about A (rational or irrational)
- C—Emotional–behavioral consequences

For effective cognitive restructuring to take place, self-generated thoughts (self-statements) must be accurately recalled and carefully analyzed. Irrational self-statements are often brought about by overgeneralization from past unpleasant experiences ("I'll never lose weight"), self-blame ("I don't have any willpower"), and negative self-attributions ("I'm weak and no good"). Irrational self-statements result in decreased self-esteem, depression, and lack of success in attempts at behavior change. Compare "I'll never be thin again!" (irrational belief) with "I have difficulty losing weight" (rational belief). Irrational beliefs contribute to feelings of powerlessness or lack of control, which can prevent clients from successfully managing health-related changes in their lives.[15(pp8–9)] Thus, skill and ability building accompanied by cognitive restructuring can be a highly effective approach for fostering constructive change.[19]

Nurses can assist clients in recognizing the irrationality of certain beliefs compared with actual reality, understanding that inability to initiate and sustain desired behaviors frequently results from irrational self-statements, and changing irrational self-statements to rational self-statements. Positive self-statements should be rehearsed by the client several times a day until he or she begins to replace irrational statements regarding adoption of a particular health behavior. The client must believe that he or she has the power to think positively and make desired lifestyle changes. The goal of cognitive restructuring is to teach clients to think more rationally, increase the incidence of positive emotions and positive self-appraisal, and thus augment perceptions of self-efficacy and control over their own lives and health.

Behavioral Processes

Reinforcement (Reward) Management

One of the most effective self-modification techniques available to clients is reinforcement management. This is a critical process during the preparation and action stages of behavior change.[12] It is based on the premise that all behaviors are determined by their consequences. If positive consequences result, the probability is high that the behavior will occur again. If negative consequences occur, the probability is low for the behavior's being repeated. When self-modification is the focus of nursing intervention, clients control the selection of behaviors to be changed and reinforcement contingencies to be used; that is, clients select what they will change, how they will change, and the rewards that they will receive for change. Positive reinforcement (reward) rather than negative reinforcement (removal of an aversive condition) or punishment (aversive experience) provide the most effective motivation for behavioral change. Behaviors that are to be reinforced must be clearly identified and a plan for managing reinforcements must be clearly delineated.

If a client wishes to increase the incidence of a specific health-promoting behavior or decrease the incidence of a health-damaging behavior, it is important that an initial frequency count of the target behavior (baseline data) be obtained so that extent of progress toward the desired change can be accurately assessed. The instrument or form on which behavior is to be recorded must be portable so that it is always available when the target behavior occurs. An example of a daily record of smoking behavior is presented in Figure 8–1. For many behaviors, times and situations are important because they represent the configuration of cues in which the behavior occurs. The period of baseline data collection can end when (1) the client has a good estimation of how often the target behavior occurs, or (2) when the client is confident that he or she understands the patterns of occurrence of the target behavior.[20] Although self-observation can be used to collect baseline data about the frequency with which health-related behaviors occur, studies of smoking cessation and other behavioral changes have failed to show sustained effects from self-observation or self-monitoring alone without use of other self-modification techniques.

Appropriate use of reinforcement is extremely important for self-directed behavior change. Reinforcers can be classified as tangible, social, or self-generated. Tangible reinforcers for desired behavior include objects or activities, such as purchasing a new magazine or going to a movie. Social reinforcers can include telephoning a friend or visiting with a neighbor. Both tangible and social reinforcers may be especially helpful during early efforts to adopt a healthy behavior or discontinue an unhealthy one. Self-generated

Behavior to Be Observed: Smoking

Observation Categories: Morning
Afternoon
Evening

Method of Coding Behavior:

E = Smoking after or during eating and drinking
S = Smoking while nervous in a social situation
D = Smoking while driving the car
O = Smoking at other times

Smoking Record

Date: Tuesday, August 26		
Morning	Afternoon	Evening
E E D O S S S E	O S S D S E E E	E O
Date: Wednesday, August 27		
Morning	Afternoon	Evening
E E E D D S S E E	S S S S D D E E E E	S E O

Figure 8–1. Self-observation sheet. (From Watson DL, Tharp RG,[20] with permission.)

reinforcers include self-praise, self-compliments, and other positive self-statements. The particular advantage of this type of reinforcement is that it is always available for administration and is under the client's control.

The time frame for application of reinforcement is critical. Immediate reinforcement is highly desirable, particularly in the early phases of self-change. Immediate reinforcement that is self-administered provides clients with moment-by-moment control over their own behavior. Initially, continuous reinforcement is also advisable. Continuous reinforcement promotes rapid learning of the desired behaviors. Intermittent reinforcement applied later stabilizes the behavior and makes it resistant to extinction. Over time, the nurse should decrease active participation in the reinforcement system of the client. Fading can occur in a number of ways. The nurse may move from tangible reinforcers to social reinforcers or from continuous reinforcement to intermittent reinforcement and then to complete fading.[21]

Many behaviors are too complex to be acquired all at once. Gradually shaping desired behaviors is an effective approach to making permanent changes in lifestyle. Shaping occurs when closer and closer approximations of the final behavior are rewarded. Reinforcement through the shaping process is contingent on increasingly higher levels of performance by the client. An example of shaping is the following:

- Brisk walk for 15 minutes 2 days of first week
- Brisk walk for 20 minutes 3 days of second and third week
- Brisk walk for 30 minutes 3 days of fourth and fifth week
- Brisk walk for 45 minutes 4 days of sixth and seventh week
- Brisk walk for 60 minutes 4 days of eighth and ninth week

Each step toward the final behavior should be mastered before the next step is attempted. The client can control the size of incremental steps to be rewarded and the rate at which the desired behavior is acquired. Problems that clients are likely to experience in the process of shaping behaviors include plateaus when progress seems impossible, cheating by reinforcing inadequate levels of performance, and problems in persistence. These problems should be anticipated and dealt with constructively, either through increased use of tangible reinforcers or through potent social reinforcers during plateau periods when persistence is waning.

Once the client starts engaging in a desired behavior, losing weight, feeling more relaxed, or feeling more energetic, these consequences of health behaviors have reinforcing properties. Deci and Ryan refer to use of these behavior-related sensations for reinforcement as intrinsic motivation. They have shown in some studies that when the behavior itself is self-rewarding, extrinsic rewards may actually interfere with level of intrinsic motivation to continue the behavior. When the behavior begins to offer its own reward, the nurse can counsel the client that other sources of reward may no longer be necessary.[22]

Modeling

Observation of models engaging in the desired behavior is important during the action phase to refine clients' performance capabilities and enhance self-efficacy. Modeling is especially helpful when clients are aware of their specific health goal but are uncertain about the exact behaviors that should be developed to move toward the goal. In early life, children learn a great deal through modeling. This form of learning is continued into adulthood. Individuals acquire social skills and learn how to relate with others through observing the interactions of persons whom they respect and admire.[17(pp 47–105)]

The following considerations are important in the effective use of modeling to facilitate behavior change:

- There must be models available with whom the client can identify (eg, gender-specific, age-specific, culture-specific).
- The client must take an active role in the selection of appropriate models.
- The learner must have an opportunity to actually observe the desired behaviors and must attend to important aspects of the behavior.
- The client must have the requisite knowledge and skills to reproduce the behavior.
- The client must have a sense of self-efficacy (confidence) that he or she has the personal competencies necessary to perform the behavior.
- The client must perceive incentives or rewards for imitating the target behaviors.
- The learner must have the opportunity for overt or covert rehearsal of the target behaviors.

By carefully choosing models that have achieved goals the client desires, opportunities can be provided to observe the model in events that contain the behaviors the client wishes to adopt. For example, how does an individual who is slim and trim eat? How much? Which foods? How long does eating take? What other behaviors does he or she engage in while eating? The client can acquire many useful ideas from models for modifying personal health behaviors.

Observation of others enriches the client's thinking regarding the range of behavioral options available. The success of many self-help groups can be partially explained through modeling techniques that generate new ideas for behavior or coping strategies for specific problems. The fact that health professionals are generally held in very high esteem by clients places the nurse in a strategic position to provide a model of healthful living that is attractive and consequently emulated by individuals to whom care is provided. Educational programs that prepare nurses to provide health-promotion and disease-prevention services to individuals and families are likely to be more effective if they initially focus on the health habits of the nurse and secondarily on various strategies for role-modeling healthy lifestyles to clients.[23] For example, health practitioners' personal physical fitness can have a great impact on their credibility when they are recommending increased exercise to clients. If health professionals smoke, are overweight, or do not exercise regularly, their credibility in the eyes of clients is diminished. A "do as I say, not as I do" approach to behavior change by health practitioners is detrimental to the success of any disease-prevention–health-promotion program. Those professionals involved in health fields must look closely at their own behavior before recommending lifestyle changes to others.[24]

Counterconditioning

Counterconditioning is a technique useful in the latter part of the action stage and in the maintenance stage of behavior change.[12(p99)] It is a classical conditioning procedure that is directed toward breaking an undesirable bond between a stimulus (conditioned stimulus) and a response (conditioned response). A conditioned response often represents an irrational or maladaptive response to one or more specific situations that has become automatic whenever the stimulus is presented. The goal of counterconditioning is to replace the undesirable stimulus–response bond with a more desirable one. For instance, anxiety may be replaced by relaxation in stressful situations, preventing the occurrence of the negative emotional response. Relaxation is actually incompatible with the previously conditioned response (anxiety).

The use of imagery for relaxation training (see Chapter 11) is an excellent illustration of a counterconditioning technique. When real-life situations for counterconditioning are not available, imagery provides a viable alternative. For example, when clients are being desensitized to stressful situations, they can be asked to imagine increasingly stressful events while they remain in a protected environment and progressively relax their muscles. Relaxation rather than tension in potentially stress-inducing situations is the stimulus–response bond that the nurse is helping the client to achieve. Once the client can relax during stressful imagery, relaxation techniques can be applied to stressful situations in real life to lower emotional and physiologic responses to stress, thus, decreasing "wear and tear" on the body.

Stimulus Control

By changing the antecedents of behavior, that is, the events that precede behavior, it is possible to decrease or eliminate undesired behavior and increase desired outcomes. The locus of attention in stimulus control is on the antecedents of a behavior, rather than on its consequences as in reinforcement management. To use stimulus control effectively, the client must have accurate information about when and where desirable behaviors could occur more frequently and under what conditions undesirable behaviors occur. The client must arrange for environmental cues to be encountered that promote only desired behaviors.

Stimulus control includes structuring cues that trigger the desired behavior in multiple environments. Multiple cues potentiate each other. Internal cues can be coupled with external cues, for example, "feeling good after brisk walking" coupled with "the invitation from spouse to take a walk." Table 8–2 presents an overview of possible cues (stimulus configurations) to health-protecting and -promoting behavior.

Individuals define for themselves the cues that are relevant based on past knowledge

TABLE 8–2. POSSIBLE CUES FOR HEALTH-PROTECTING AND HEALTH-PROMOTING ACTIONS

Internal Cues
Bodily states, eg, feeling good, feeling energetic, recognizing aging, fatigue, cyclical discomfort
Affective states, eg, enthusiasm, motivation for self-preservation, high level of self-esteem, happiness, concern
External Cues
Interactions with significant others, eg, family, friends, colleagues, nurse, and physician
Impact of communication media, eg, motivational messages from television, radio, newspapers, advertisements, and special mailings
Visual stimuli from the environment, eg, passing a diabetic screening clinic, billboards, attendance at a health fair, passing a gym or exercise center, or viewing others participating in target activity

and experience. For some clients, a postcard reminding them of an exercise class may be an adequate prompting for attendance, while for other clients a personal call from the nurse and several reminders from spouse may be needed to initiate action. The nurse must be aware of effective cues for specific clients in order to successfully prompt positive health behaviors. Dimensions of cues to be considered include relevance, strength (intensity), number, duration, and synergistic potential. Cues for behavior must be personally relevant, of varying intensity depending on the strength of intention to act, and extended or repeated across varying times and places to achieve maximal impact. Synergy of multiple stimuli or cues can be achieved by clustering environmental and interpersonal cues for healthy behavior. For example, to avoid eating foods high in fat, all such foods can be removed from the house, tasty low-fat foods can be stocked in cupboards, family members can eat healthy snacks, and individuals can focus only on healthy options when purchasing foods from vending machines (popcorn, cereal bars, fresh fruit, skim milk, etc).

The nurse, family, environment, or client may serve as the source of behavioral cues. Since the extent to which nurses can provide cues to action is limited, an important part of their professional role is to assist clients in (1) developing sensitivity to appropriate cues, (2) increasing chances for encountering appropriate cues, and (3) developing a system of internal cues that consistently trigger desired actions. It is important to remember that verbal and nonverbal cues, regardless of their source, must be consistent with each other. Any incongruity between cues can confuse and frustrate the client and inhibit action.

Antecedents of behavior need to be carefully analyzed in order to create a configuration of cues that will prompt specific health-protecting or -promoting behaviors. The client should describe the setting(s) in which the health-related behavior has occurred previously or could occur:

- *Physical setting:* Describe the setting(s) in which the behavior occurs. Describe when, where, and what is present.
- *Social setting:* Describe who is present when the behavior occurs and what they are doing.
- *Intrapersonal setting:* Describe what the client is thinking, feeling, or doing. What did the client say or think to him- or herself just before the behavior occurred?

Reconfiguring environmental stimuli can augment cues for desirable behaviors or decrease cues for undesirable behaviors. Specific approaches to stimulus refiguration or control include **cue restriction** or **elimination** and **cue expansion.**

In **cue elimination,** situational cues for undesired behaviors are decreased to zero. Although ideal, this may not represent reality. More frequently, cues cannot be totally eliminated but can be reduced or restricted. In **cue restriction,** for example, the cues to eating may be reduced to one room in the house, the kitchen or dining room. This is also called stimulus narrowing. A setting can also be selected that is incompatible with an undesirable response (cue elimination). Examples include sitting in no-smoking areas of restaurants or eating meals only with nonsmokers if cessation of smoking is the goal. Through stimulus restriction, the target behavior comes under the influence of only a few cues. By localizing the cues that activate behavior, arrangements can be made for limited encounter with these cues. In successful cue elimination, extinction of the behavior should result.

In **cue expansion,** the number of stimuli that prompt desired behaviors is increased. For instance, while personal preparation of food at home in one's own kitchen may prompt small servings of meats, fruits, and vegetables, the environment of a restaurant may prompt selection of rich entrees and desserts. An expanded configuration of cues can prompt health-promoting behavior in a variety of different settings. For instance, being given a menu at a restaurant can provide cues for looking at salad and vegetable options as opposed to less nutritious and higher-calorie offerings. By expanding the range of cues that elicit specific responses, desirable behaviors can occur more frequently and with greater regularity. Gaining conscious control over behavior rather than responding automatically will assist the client in acting more rationally and more in line with personal health goals.

Controlling antecedents of behavior through the restriction, elimination, or expansion of cues can assist clients in creating internal and external cue configurations supportive of positive health practices. Stimulus control is an important approach to successfully modifying behavior and lifestyle.

Dealing with Barriers to Change

Interference with action can arise from external barriers within the environment, such as lack of facilities, materials, or social support, or from internal barriers, such as lack of knowledge, skills, or appropriate affective or motivational orientation on the part of the client. The professional nurse facilitates the preparation, action, and maintenance stages of behavior change by assisting clients in minimizing or eliminating barriers to action. It is futile to encourage clients to take actions that are highly likely to be blocked or frustrated.

Internal barriers to self-modification toward more positive health practices can result from a variety of sources:

- Unclear short-term and long-term goals
- Insufficient skill to follow through with self-modification approach
- Perceptions of lack of control over environmental contingencies (cues, reinforcements, time) related to the target behavior
- Lack of motivation to pursue selected health actions

Barriers such as these often reflect insufficient attention to the preparation stage of behavior change.

Clients who find their course of action thwarted may reevaluate the decisions made regarding practice of specific health behaviors. They may seek more information to support change in behavior, discard the selected action in favor of another, rationalize the behavior as unnecessary, or deny the relevance of the selected health goal.

The interaction of level of readiness and barriers to action is depicted in Table 8–3. Consequences for the client and appropriate nursing actions are also presented. When clients evidence a high level of readiness to engage in health-protecting–promoting be-

TABLE 8–3. INTERRELATIONSHIPS AMONG LEVEL OF READINESS TO TAKE HEALTH ACTIONS, BARRIERS, CONSEQUENCES FOR CLIENTS, AND NURSING INTERVENTIONS

LEVEL OF READINESS	BARRIERS TO ACTION	CONSEQUENCES FOR CLIENT	NURSING INTERVENTIONS
High	Low	Action	Support and encouragement; provide low-intensity cue
High	High	Conflict	Assist client in lowering barriers to action
Low	Low	Conflict	Provide high-intensity cue
Low	High	No action	Assist client in lowering barriers to action and then provide high-intensity cue

haviors and barriers are low, only a low-intensity cue is needed to activate behavior. A high-intensity cue under these conditions may actually be aversive. When readiness is high and barriers to action are also formidable, barriers need to be reduced or eliminated. When both readiness and barriers are low, readiness to act should be increased in order to initiate action. When readiness is low and barriers high, both factors should be addressed, or behavior change is unlikely to occur.

Significant others can serve as barriers to health actions. One of the most important sources of information about the appropriateness of our own beliefs and actions are the attitudes and behaviors of others. When family members or other persons or groups disagree or are neutral or apathetic toward health behaviors, the extent of inhibition created for the client depends on the following factors:

- The relevance of disagreeing persons or groups
- Attractiveness to the client of disagreeing persons or groups
- Extent of disagreement of relevant persons or groups
- Number of persons relevant to the client who are in disagreement with behavior
- Extent to which client is self-directed rather than other-dependent

As the nurse listens to the client's account of efforts at implementation of health practices, he or she may well be able to provide insights concerning blocks to desired behavior. By analysis of the environment in which the behavior is to occur and preparation of the client with the appropriate knowledge and skills to deal constructively with potential or actual barriers to implementation, the nurse can facilitate accomplishment of personal health goals meaningful to the client.

• MAINTAINING BEHAVIOR CHANGE

The maintenance stage of health behavior raises special challenges for the client. Changes in behavior that are transient accomplish little in enhancing client health status. Not only must behavior be sustained in the environment in which it is learned, but the behavior must be generalized to other situations. Factors that affect continuation of positive health behaviors include:

- Extent of personal skill to carry out the behavior
- Number of personal beliefs and attitudes that support the target behavior, including beliefs about self-efficacy
- Extent of affective support (positive emotional response) and cognitive commitment (intention) to perform the behavior
- Ease of incorporating behavior into lifestyle
- Absence of environmental constraints to performing the behavior
- Extent to which the behavior is intrinsically rewarding
- Extent to which decision to take action has been communicated to others and there is social support for the behavior
- Consistency of behavior with self-image
- Personal attractiveness of incompatible actions

The maintenance phase is indeterminate in length, extending from beginning stabilization of the new behavior throughout the client's life span. Various strategies for maintenance include relapse prevention (see Chapter 2), booster sessions, iteration of the contemplation or preparation stages to reactivate the behavior, and habit formation.

Habits are behaviors that become automatic and are maintained on a stimulus–response level with little conscious effort. Habit formation results in stable patterns of behavior. The nurse can assist clients in habit formation by helping them plan for certain health-promoting behaviors to occur repeatedly in the same setting or context. For example, a client can exercise each noon in the company fitness center, 3 to 5 days a week. The client should head to the fitness center promptly at noon, allowing absolutely nothing else to interfere with the scheduled exercise activity. The decision to exercise or not exercise should not even be considered each day. The client should avoid any opportunity for choice once the initial commitment to exercise has been made. When the client arrives at the fitness center, the stimuli of the locker room, exercise equipment, and coworkers jogging or bicycling will prompt the client to get into proper attire, warm up, and start to exercise. After a period of time, if habituation has occurred, exercising at noon should become a habit just like brushing teeth or showering.[25]

ETHICS OF BEHAVIOR CHANGE

Within the nursing profession, the right of autonomy and self-determinism of the client is a major tenet of professional practice in situations in which autonomous behavior is not a threat to the health and welfare of other human beings. Thus, individuals and families should be allowed to select their behavioral patterns and lifestyle based on sound information from health professionals or other credible information sources. Not all members of society will choose the most healthful behaviors, and this is their right when their actions do not affect others.[26] As the nurse assists clients who have sought help in adopting health-promoting lifestyles, authoritarian and coercive strategies should be avoided. Allowing clients to assume leadership in modifying their lifestyles is an ethical, nonmanipulative approach to improving the health of individuals and families and other groups.

DIRECTIONS FOR RESEARCH IN BEHAVIOR CHANGE AND LIFESTYLE MODIFICATION

With escalating emphasis on modification of overall lifestyles to promote health and well-being, applications of theories of behavior change to health behaviors increasingly appear in the literature. Each theory has critical concepts, some with more empirical support than others. What is becoming evident is that a multitheory approach to intervention may be the most productive. Fitting the theory or constructs to the client in a culture-specific manner is an important area meriting further study. How to assess clients in order to select optimal behavior-change strategies and how to meaningfully combine change strategies in scientifically sound ways that are culturally relevant are not well understood. Further research in the following areas is warranted:

1. Developing and testing interventions that are based on a logical integration of multiple theories. Each extant behavioral theory does not alone seem powerful enough to predict health behavior.
2. Testing whether stages of behavior change actually represent extremely fluid and dynamic states of behavior that clients cycle in and out of, as opposed to an orderly progression of client states.
3. Determining the appropriate blend of intrinsic and extrinsic motivation to optimize probabilities of successful behavior change for individuals and families within their unique life circumstances
4. Determining developmental patterns in the importance of intrinsic versus extrinsic motivation for various health behaviors
5. Developing and testing the effectiveness of multisectoral interventions that focus on removal of environmental constraints and creation of environmental supports for behavior change at the community level
6. Developing and evaluating the outcomes of policy interventions that socially anchor change to facilitate the maintenance of health-protecting and health-promoting behavior over the life span
7. Evaluating the health-behavior change and health outcomes that result from implementation of theoretically based comprehensive primary health care models in diverse settings

This research will require the best thinking of scientists from numerous disciplines in collaboration with communities to develop and test the effectiveness of behavior-change intervention programs that are culture-sensitive and -specific rather than culture-stereotypic.

SUMMARY

A number of behavior-change strategies have been presented in this chapter. The *Handbook of Health Behavior Change*[27] as well as *Nursing Interventions Classification (NIC)*[11] provide additional valuable information on health behavior-change strategies.

The nurse, in assisting individuals and families to modify health behaviors, not only promotes desired changes but provides clients with skills for continuing self-change and self-actualization. Learning that has lifelong application can empower clients to engage in a wide array of behavior changes that will improve their health and well-being.

REFERENCES

1. Prochaska JO, DiClemente CC. *The Transtheoretical Approach: Crossing Traditional Boundaries of Change.* Homewood, Ill: Dow Jones-Irwin; 1984.
2. Prochaska JO, Velicer WF, Rossi JS, et al. Stages of change and decisional balance for 12 problem behaviors. *Health Psychol.* 1994;13(1):39–46.
3. Janis IL, Mann L. *Decision-Making: A Psychological Analysis of Conflict, Choice, and Commitment.* London, England: Cassell & Collier Macmillan; 1977.
4. Prochaska JO. Strong and weak principles for progressing from precontemplation to action on the basis of twelve problem behaviors. *Health Psychol.* 1994;13(1):47–51.
5. Velicer WF, DiClemente CC, Rossi JS, et al. Relapse situations and self-efficacy: an integrative model. *Addict Behav.* 1990;15:271–283.
6. Marcus BH, Selby VC, Niaura RS, et al. Self-efficacy and the stages of exercise behavior change. *Res Q Exerc Sport.* 1992;63(1):60–66.
7. Marcus BH, Banspach SW, Lefebvre RC, et al. Using the stages of change model to increase the adoption of physical activity among community participants. *Amer J Health Prom.* 1992;6:424–429.
8. Marcus BH, Owen N. Motivational readiness, self-efficacy and decision-making for exercise. *J Appl Soc Psychol.* 1992;22:3–16.
9. Marcus BH, Rakowski W, Rossi JS. Assessing motivational readiness and decision-making for exercise. *Health Psychol.* 1992;11:257–261.
10. Prochaska JO, Marcus BH. The transtheoretical model: application to exercise. In: Dishman RK, ed. *Advances in Exercise Adherence.* Champaign, Ill: Human Kinetics; 1994:161–180.
11. McCloskey JC, Bulechek GM. *Nursing Interventions Classification (NIC).* St Louis, Mo: Mosby Year Book; 1992.
12. Prochaska JO, DiClemente CC, Norcross JC. In search of the structure of change. In: Klar Y, Fisher JD, Chinsky JM, et al, eds. *Self-change: Social Psychological and Clinical Perspectives.* New York, NY: Springer-Verlag; 1992:87–114.
13. Fishbein M, Bandura A, Triandis HC, et al. Factors influencing behavior and behavior change: final report of theorist's workshop on AIDS-Related Behaviors National Institute of Mental Health, National Institutes of Health October 3-5, 1991; Washington, DC.
14. Rokeach M. *The Nature of Human Values.* New York, NY: Free Press; 1973.
15. Ellis A, Grieger R, eds. *Handbook of Rational-Emotive Therapy.* New York, NY: Springer; 1977.
16. Kendall PC, Turk DC. Cognitive-behavioral strategies and health enhancement. In: Matarazzo JD, Weiss SM, Herd JA, et al, eds. *Behavioral Health: A Handbook of Health Enhancement and Disease Prevention.* New York, NY: John Wiley & Sons; 1984:393–405.
17. Bandura A. *Social Foundations of Thought and Action: A Social Cognitive Theory.* Englewood Cliffs, NJ: Prentice-Hall Inc, 1986.
18. Kazdin AE. *Behavior Modification in Applied Settings.* 2nd ed. Homewood, Ill: Dorsey Press; 1980.

19. Martin RA, Poland EY. *Learning to Change: A Self-management Approach to Adjustment.* New York, NY: McGraw-Hill Inc, 1980:159–160.
20. Watson DL, Tharp RG. *Self-directed Behavior: Self-modification for Personal Adjustment.* Monterey, Calif: Brooks/Cole Publishing Co; 1972.
21. Berni R, Fordyce WE. *Behavior Modification and the Nursing Process.* St Louis, Mo: CV Mosby Co; 1977:68.
22. Deci EL, Ryan RM. *Intrinsic Motivation and Self-determination in Human Behavior.* New York, NY: Plenum Press; 1985:113–148.
23. Pender NJ, Sallis JF, Long BJ, et al. Health care provider counseling to promote physical activity. In: Dishman R, ed. *Advances in Exercise Adherence.* Champaign, Ill: Human Kinetics; 1994:215–216.
24. Sensenig PE, Cialdini RB. Social-psychological influences on the compliance process: implications for behavioral health. In: Matarazzo JD, Weiss SM, Herd JA, et al, eds. *Behavioral Health: A Handbook of Health Enhancement and Disease Prevention.* New York, NY: John Wiley & Sons; 1984:384–392.
25. Pender NJ. Self-modification. In: Bulechek GM, McCloskey JC, eds. *Nursing Interventions: Treatments for Nursing Diagnoses.* Philadelphia, Pa: WB Saunders Co; 1985:80–91.
26. O'Connell JK, Price JH. Ethical theories for promoting health through behavior change. *J School Health.* 1983;53:476–479.
27. Shumaker SA, Schron EB, Ockene JK, eds. *The Handbook of Health Behavior Change.* New York, NY: Springer; 1990.

9

Exercise and Health

Regular physical activity is essential for dynamic, energetic, and productive living. Physical activity is defined as any bodily movement produced by skeletal muscles that results in caloric expenditure.[1] Modern life with its automobiles, televisions, computers, video games, and high levels of inactivity in school and work environments necessitates the commitment of significant leisure time to physical activity in order to gain resultant health benefits. Furthermore, the competitive aspects of sports stressed in many school athletic programs results in few children and adolescents making a sustained commitment to systematic exercise as a lifelong activity and source of personal enjoyment. **Exercise** is generally defined as leisure-time physical activity.[2] However, another term has been coined recently, **lifestyle exercise.** Lifestyle exercise is characterized as integration of numerous short bouts of exercise into daily living.[3] Because of the centrality of both leisure time and lifestyle exercise to health, this chapter focuses on the benefits of exercise, the determinants of exercise for children and adults, the exercise process, interventions to promote exercise, and the importance of exercise counseling by health providers in primary care.

Healthy People 2000 has set goals for 20% of adults and 75% of children to engage in vigorous physical activity on 3 or more days per week for 20 or more minutes and at least 30% of people aged 6 and older to engage in light to moderate activity daily for at least 30 minutes. Attainment of these goals would significantly increase the level of activity of many children, adolescents, and adults.[4] Results from a review of physical activity patterns in North America suggest that the greatest decrease in physical activity across the life span occurs in adolescence.[5] Physical activity declines almost 50% throughout the childhood and adolescent years, with females becoming increasingly more sedentary than males.[6] There is a paucity of data describing developmental transitions in exercise attitudes and beliefs from childhood to adulthood that might explain different trends in exercise behavior. It does appear that sedentary patterns established in youth may persist into adulthood, leading to a life of inactivity and resultant low levels of fitness, poor body image, and actual physical deterioration. Without the cultivation of lifelong activity habits, adults find it much more difficult to develop regular exercise patterns and persist in such behavior over time. Thus, the challenge to health-behavior scientists is to understand the determinants of exercise behavior as a basis for intervention and counseling to influence exercise within various target groups, particularly youth. Although biologic differences between boys and girls are accelerated during puberty, with girls increasing in percentage of body fat compared with boys, it is likely that the observed gender and developmental differences in exercise result from the complex causal interplay of biologic, social, and environmental influences. Sherrill et al[7] found that highly fit boys in elementary school also had higher self-concepts than minimally fit boys. Interestingly, there was no difference in self-concept between highly fit and unfit girls. These findings suggest that exercise and fitness may not be integral to the female self-concept, an important issue to address if physical activity goals for women are to be achieved. Gender, developmental, and individual variations in attitudes and responses to exercise must be understood in order to design effective programs of exercise that persist across the life span.

Achieving the goal of regular exercise is largely dependent on sources of personal and social motivation within a person's day-to-day environment. Many individuals begin exercise programs on their own; some are able to continue them. Others rely on the school or work environments to create programs that help them achieve their exercise goals. With increasing emphasis on primary care, *Healthy People 2000* has set services objectives for health professionals to support the behavior-change goals for individuals. By 2000, the goal is to increase to at least 50% the proportion of primary care providers who routinely assess and counsel their patients regarding the frequency, duration, type, and intensity of physical activity practices. At present, it is estimated that less than one third of primary care practitioners offer physical activity counseling to their patients.[4(p105)] This is an important counseling opportunity that is missed, given that primary care providers have periodic contact with patients and thus the opportunity to positively impact health-related lifestyles. Physical activity counseling should be a team effort, at a minimum involving the physician and the nurse. Both **counseling** about exercise and **modeling** an active lifestyle are integral to effective physical activity promotion by health professionals.

BENEFITS OF EXERCISE

Habitual exercise contributes to physiologic stability and high-level functioning and assists individuals in actualizing their physical performance potential. There is also widespread agreement across a large number of research studies that exercise is beneficial to health. Indeed, millions of Americans are at risk for a wide range of chronic diseases that might well be prevented by active lifestyles. What is not clear is the extent of physical activity needed to influence health outcomes. For instance, is vigorous exercise and resultant physical fitness the key to the prevention of premature deaths from cardiovascular disease, or is moderate activity over time equally beneficial? To what extent does moderate versus vigorous activity prevent loss of bone mass, decrease in lean muscle mass, and decrease in basal metabolism rates? Should emphasis in exercise adoption programs at all ages be focused on the encouragement of regular moderate activity or on vigorous activity and resultant physical fitness to obtain important health benefits? These are critical questions yet unanswered. Furthermore, it is difficult to sort out the health benefits solely from exercise, because engaging in exercise may trigger other health behaviors such as changes in dietary and smoking habits and adoption of more effective methods of coping with stress. Despite the need for further research to understand the mechanisms connecting exercise and health, studies indicate a variety of beneficial effects from regular patterns of exercise that cannot be ignored.

Important benefits of exercise have been linked to many biologic responses and systems. For example, a meta-analytic review of laboratory studies on aerobic fitness and reactivity to psychosocial stressors among adults indicated that aerobically fit subjects had a reduced stress response. It is hypothesized that aerobic exercise may decrease sympathetically mediated cardiovascular responses to psychosocial stress through changes in core temperature, insulin, endogenous opiates, or renal function.[8] A prospective field study of adolescents yielded similar findings, with the negative impact of stressful life events on health declining as exercise levels increased.[9] Reducing the intensity and length of the stress response may reduce associated strain on a number of physiologic systems. Among 1057 adolescents from the 7th, 9th and 11th grades, higher levels of sports and nonteam physical exercise were associated with fewer physical symptoms, less depressed mood, higher self-esteem, and higher level of school achievement.[10] Among 1200 Icelandic adolescents, those who actively participated in sports reported fewer symptoms of anxiety and depression, rated their health more positively, and reported less involvement in other health-compromising behaviors such as smoking and drinking.[11]

Systolic and diastolic blood pressures tend to be reduced by regular exercise, possibly through a reduction in catecholamine levels. Thus, exercise may be an important component of nonpharmacologic management of essential hypertension. Active individuals also exhibit higher plasma concentrations of high-density lipoprotein (HDL) cholesterol and a higher ratio of HDL to low-density lipoprotein (LDL) cholesterol, both thought to lower the risk of cardiac events. Excess body fat is reduced through regular exercise. Acute bouts of activity in overweight individuals can lower insulin levels and improve glucose tolerance in the short term. Furthermore, exercise can improve pulmonary function in individuals, including those with impairment and disability.[2(p18–25)]

Epidemiologic evidence also suggests a lower risk of cancers of the breast and reproductive tract in women who exercise regularly. It is unclear what hormonal mechanisms may underlie this finding. Also, exercisers tend to increase their dietary intake, which may mean that they have a greater intake of nutrients and fiber than nonexercisers, which may contribute to the proposed effects of exercise, particularly on colon cancer, through mechanisms such as lowering intestinal transit time. An intriguing hypothesis is that exercise enhances immune function that may be protective against cancer by inhibiting tumor cell growth. Increased circulating leukocytes have been reported following bouts of exercise, but the exact mechanisms underlying this increase are yet to be determined. Further research is needed to determine the possible role of exercise in altering immunologic functioning and subsequently enhancing host defenses to carcinogens.[2(pp567–586)]

Proposed positive effects of regular exercise are summarized in Table 9–1. For a detailed discussion, see Bouchard et al.[2]

TABLE 9–1. PROPOSED POSITIVE EFFECTS OF PHYSICAL EXERCISE

Cardiopulmonary and Blood Chemistry Effects
Reduce systolic and diastolic blood pressure
Increase blood oxygen content
Decrease total cholesterol
Increase high-density lipoproteins
Reduce serum triglycerides
Increase peripheral blood circulation and return
Reduce resting heart rate by increasing stroke volume
Increase blood supply to heart and myocardial efficiency
Increase heart rate recovery after exercise
Immunologic/Oncologic Effects
Reduce incidence of selected types of cancer
Improve prognosis post-treatment for cancer
Increase circulating leukocytes
Endocrine and Metabolic Effects
Improve glucose tolerance
Decrease reactivity to psychosocial stressors
Decrease body fat
Increase endogenous opioid peptides, particularly beta-endorphins
Enhance oxidation of fatty acids
Increase metabolism rate
Musculoskeletal Effects
Increase lean muscle mass
Maintain bone mass
Prevent or ameliorate chronic back and joint pain
Increase muscle strength and endurance
Psychosocial Effects
Improve self-concept
Improve body image
Decrease anxiety and depression
Improve mental alertness
Enhance general mood and psychologic well-being

LIFE-SPAN PATTERNS OF EXERCISE

Studies indicate that most American adults are sedentary. For example, in a study of African-American young adults, the prevalence of very poor aerobic fitness was high for both men (71%) and women (82%). Only 4.5% of women and 6.4% of men reported regular participation in activities intensive enough to increase aerobic fitness. A similar profile is observed in other populations.[12] Folsom et al[13] further report that for both whites and blacks, leisure-time physical activity was higher in men than in women and decreased with age. Whites of both sexes compared to blacks had higher leisure-time energy expenditure. In contrast, blacks of both sexes compared to whites reported greater regular vigorous exercise at work.[16] Both racial groups need to make further progess in adopting active lifestyles that promote health and prevent the onset of chronic disease.

Interest in life-span patterns of exercise has been fueled by the realization that a number of risk factors including obesity, high blood pressure, and elevated cholesterol may be evident early in childhood and predispose to cardiovascular disease in adulthood. Early detection of risk factors that track into adulthood would promote a prospective approach to the promotion of health and prevention of chronic diseases—an approach that could begin in the infant and preschool years. Further, there is increasing evidence that habits of physical activity begun early in life may persist over time if they are tailored to the individual and less reliant on organized competitive sports than is currently the case in most physical activity programs in school settings.

Family influences during childhood may have a positive effect on the exercise patterns that children develop. For example, more active parents have been shown to have more active children of both genders.[14] In assessing the correlates of physical activity in a multiethnic sample of preschool children, family cardiovascular disease risk and father's body mass index (BMI) were negatively correlated with the preschoolers' level of physical activity, whereas the parents' reported level of vigorous activity was positively correlated with the preschoolers' level of physical activity.[15] Role modeling of active lifestyles, social support for exercise, and normative expectations that children will exercise are likely to have positive effects on the exercise patterns that children develop. Thus, the effects of early physical activity experiences of children with parents and siblings on lifetime physical activity patterns need to be further explored and cannot be dismissed lightly. In addition, active extended-family members, such as grandparents, can powerfully reinforce the message that exercise is for everyone and makes a difference in the quality of life and health well into the older adult years.

Understanding the determinants of exercise in various age groups is essential to effective intervention and counseling by health care providers to promote active lifestyles.

POTENTIAL DETERMINANTS OF EXERCISE IN CHILDREN AND ADOLESCENTS

Little is known about the determinants and health outcomes of exercise among school-age youth. This is surprising, considering the extensive exercise research conducted on middle-class, adult males. The dearth of research on physical activity in youth may reflect a commonly held misperception that children and adolescents are perpetually active and highly physically fit. Nothing could be further from the truth. Various studies indicate that greater than one third of youth have adopted sedentary lifestyles by 10 years of age. By age 18, less than 10% of the population report levels of physical activity that promote the development and maintenance of cardiopulmonary fitness.[4(p95)]

The long-term goal of exercise research among youth is to identify factors influencing exercise behavior as a basis for designing culturally appropriate interventions to increase exercise and improve exercise-related short- and long-term health outcomes. Of particular interest are the ways in which developmental and social transitions, which occur with great rapidity during late childhood and early adolescence, affect participatory patterns. Pubertal changes (onset of menarche, changing body fat distribution) and social transitions (moving from elementary school to junior high school and on to senior high school) undoubtedly exert important influences on sports participation, predisposition to exercise, and patterns of physical activity. Longitudinal studies are needed to identify changing activity patterns and probable influences on exercise across childhood and adolescence as most studies, to date, have been cross-sectional, identifying only correlates or potential influences on exercise behavior.

In their excellent paper summarizing the state of knowledge and identifying important gaps regarding determinants of physical activity and interventions for children, Sallis et al[16] propose that a variety of factors influence activity in children, with no one variable or category of variables expected to account for most of the variance in children's physical activity. In fact, what makes prediction of exercise behavior even more difficult is that variables may fluctuate in their predictive importance for different gender, race, or socioeconomic groups at different developmental time points. Thus it is important to clearly specify the group(s) being studied and their location within a developmental trajectory. In terms of determinants, Sallis and colleagues concluded that **exercise self-efficacy, intentions to exercise,** and perceived **barriers to exercise** are potent psychologic influences on exercise among youth. Interpersonal influences such as **parental role modeling of exercise** and **social support or encouragement of exercise** also appear to have considerable effect on children's and adolescents' exercise behavior.

Biddle and Armstong[17] identified interesting gender differences in psychologic correlates of physical activity. Among 11-to-12-year-old boys, activity was positively correlated with intrinsic motivation, that is, engaging in an activity for its own sake or for the sense of mastery and control. An opposite trend was found for the girls of the same age with extrinsic motivation of approval by their teacher being more motivating than the intrinsic challenge of the task. Garcia and colleagues, in applying the Health Promotion Model to exercise behavior in a racially diverse population, found definite gender differences between exercise-related beliefs and behaviors of fifth- and sixth-, as well as eighth-grade boys and girls. Compared to boys, girls reported less representation of self as athletic and lower levels of past and current exercise. Girls also reported lower levels of self-esteem and health status, which in part may be related to overweight or fatigue due to unfitness. The **benefits to barriers differential** (benefits-of-exercise score minus barriers-to-exercise score), **access to exercise facilities and programs,** and **gender** were significant predictors of exercise measured several weeks later. **Grade, health status, exercise efficacy, social support,** and **social norms** appeared to exert indirect effects on exercise mediated by the benefits to barriers differential, and **race** exerted indirect effects mediated by access to exercise facilities.[18]

Halfon and Bronner[19] found that seventh-grade boys had faster running times than girls. Furthermore, premenarchal girls ran faster than postmenarchal girls of the same age. Differentials in fat distribution may provide a partial explanation of longer running times postmenarche. Thus, biologic changes that occur in adolescence cannot be ignored as factors directly or indirectly influencing gender differences in exercise behavior and need further study.

In an effort to determine if there were differences in the factors distinguishing high fit versus low fit black adolescents compared to white adolescents, researchers studied the perceptions of exercise of a sample of 495 urban youth. The Health Belief Model variables explained a moderate 27% of variance in fitness of white youth and 14% variance in fitness of black youth. Beliefs about susceptibility to cardiovascular disease best differentiated high- and low-fitness white students, whereas beliefs about the severity of cardiovascular disease best differentiated high- and low-fitness black students. Current perceived fitness and intention to exercise in the future also predicted group membership for black adolescents. Social support, or having many friends who exercised, best predicted group membership for white adolescents. Further studies assessing the diversity of exercise perceptions among black and white youth are critical to developing effective exercise promotion strategies for particular child and adolescent populations.[20]

In terms of actual behavior, McKenzie et al[21] examined the activity patterns of 351 Anglo- and Mexican-American preschoolers at home and at recess. Ethnic differences were noted. Mexican-American children were less active than Anglo children at home and during recess. This may be related to environmental factors, as Mexican-American children spent more time in the presence of adults both at recess and at home and had access to fewer active toys.

Within various groups of youth, there is considerable variation in exercise attitudes and beliefs as well as in support for exercise in interpersonal and physical environments. Computerized methods for comprehensive assessment of exercise-related characteristics of individuals and of their environments need to be developed in order to "personally fit" exercise programs to youth, thus increasing their chances for success. For example, for a 12-year-old boy, cognitive evaluation theory[22] with its emphasis on intrinsic motivational orientation and enjoyment of exercise may be the most effective theoretical framework to use in encouraging physical activity. On the other hand, for a 12-year-old girl, social support theories may be more useful, as they emphasize the importance of receiving instrumental and social support from significant others to sustain physical activity. The appropriateness of different theories for promoting increased activity needs to be evaluated among youth with different belief constellations. Better approaches to assessment will facilitate decision making about use of specific theoretically based exercise promotion strategies and will avoid use of stereotypes as a basis for intervention.

Schools should play a major role in promoting involvement of children in sports and recreational activities as well as in nonsport exercise. By involving children on a daily basis in physical education, teaching the personal value of regular exercise, making sports and exercise enjoyable activities, and encouraging continuing involvement in moderate or vigorous activities in numerous settings, schools fulfill their responsibility for creating an active generation. Further, school-based programs should be supplemented by family-based programs, community-based programs, and exercise counseling programs in primary care services. Family-based programs encourage parents to be active with their children and design activities that make this an enjoyable, relationship-building experience. For example, weekend family bike outings and parent-child aerobic or recreational activities create opportunities for parents to be role models for active lifestyles. Community-based exercise programs that are widely publicized and well attended, such as community runs, community all-sports days, and neighborhood walking groups, establish norms of activity and participation across all age groups. Cultivating community-wide exercise habits can create an activated community and greater habituation to exercise for a larger segment of the population than an individualistic approach. Furthermore, exercise counseling programs offered by nurses and physicians in primary care can provide both the impetus and reinforcement for continuing participation of youth in physical activity. Efforts should be directed toward increasing current physical activity as well as the likelihood that children will continue to be active voluntarily and will develop into active adults. A cognitive–developmental approach to exercise promotion takes into consideration the increasing maturity of youth and changes in their decision-making patterns, perceptions of personal competence, and intrinsic and extrinsic motivation across time.[23]

In summary, coordinated school, family, community, and health professionals' efforts to promote exercise can be synergistic in positively influencing the level of physical activity among youth. Childhood and adolescence are ideal points in the life span to foster continuing exercise behavior that reaps rich health benefits throughout life.

POTENTIAL DETERMINANTS OF EXERCISE IN ADULTS

Increasing emphasis has been placed on carrying out the study of exercise determinants among adults using models and theories of human behavior. Most of the theories and models used in adult exercise studies to date have their origins in social psychology: social cognitive theory, theory of reasoned action, theory of planned behavior, Health Belief Model, protection-motivation theory, Health Promotion Model, and the Interaction Model of Client Health Behavior. The protection-motivation theory and the Health Belief Model postulate that exercise can be understood only in terms of prevention of disease; social cognitive theory and the theory of reasoned action propose that exercise behavior is comparable to other forms of behavior and can thus be understood in terms of its multiple cognitive and social dimensions.

Instead of testing a single theory, researchers have begun to contrast various theoretical models in terms of their ability to predict adult exercise behavior. For example, Dzewaltowski[24] contrasted Bandura's social cognitive theory and Fishbein and Ajzen's theory of reasoned action. Self-efficacy expectations (judgment concerning ability to execute a desired course of action) and outcome expectations (estimate that a given behavior will lead to certain outcomes) are central concepts in social cognitive theory. They have been shown in a number of studies to be predictive of adherence to an exercise program. According to the theory of reasoned action, behavioral intention is the direct determinant of behavior. In exercise research, it has predicted as little as 9% to as much as 67% of the variance in exercise behavior, leaving open to question the strength of intention as a predictor of exercise. In contrasting the two theories, the theory of reasoned action explained only 5% of the variance in exercise behavior whereas adding variables from social cognitive theory increased the amount of explained variance to 15%. Thus, social cognitive theory was more effective than the theory of reasoned action in predicting exercise behavior. Needless to say, much work must yet be done to develop models with greater predictive power for exercise behavior.

Godin and Shephard,[25] in a recent review article on use of attitude-behavior models in exercise promotion, point to the effectiveness of **past behavior, exercise self-efficacy, barriers to exercise, outcome expectancies** including **postive and negative health** and **nonhealth benefits,** and **intention** in predicting exercise. However, they concluded their review by pointing out that attitude-behavior models seldom explain more than 35% of the variance in exercise behavior. Models that sometimes explain more variance, do so inconsistently. They suggest that this may be due to the fact that the models used to study exercise behavior have focused on predisposing factors or those factors that result in the initiation of exercise. Other factors that need to be studied include facilitating factors, such as accessibility and availability of facilities, and reinforcing factors, such as rewards and incentives that accompany or follow exercise behavior and contribute to its persistence. The interaction of psychologic with environmental factors in the determination of exercise behavior requires further investigation.

In a study of 2020 adults, the determinants of exercise behavior were studied using the Health Promotion Model (HPM) as the framework. The sample consisted of subgroups of working adults, community-living older adults, cardiac rehabilitation patients, and ambulatory cancer patients. Perceiving many **benefits from exercise,** few **barriers to exercise** and good **perceived health status** predicted greater involvement in exercise behavior. In the two studies in which **exercise efficacy** was tested, higher perceived efficacy predicted greater involvement in exercise behavior. Among working adults, level of **prior exercise program participation** was highly predictive of continuing participation. Among older adults, **preference for a moderate to high level of physical exertion** and being high in **self-motivation,** factors not in the HPM, also contributed to the explanation of exercise frequency. The variance in exercise predicted across the four groups ranged from 23% to 59%.[26]

Using protection motivation theory, derived from the Health Belief Model, **perceived vulnerability to the aversive effects of a sedentary lifestyle** as well as **self-efficacy for increasing exercise** has been shown to affect young women's intentions to exercise. The effects of severity of potential cardiovascular problems and the efficacy of exercise in prevention of such problems were not significant predictors of intentions.[27]

A consistent finding is that after adoption, adults have difficulty maintaining regular exercise patterns, which results in a usual rate of dropout from organized programs of about 50% in the first 3 to 6 months. Further, those who might benefit most, such as overweight persons, are most susceptible to dropping out. Dishman and colleagues[28] summarized the potential determinants of continuation of adults in an exercise program as the personal determinants of **past program participation, being at high risk for coronary heart disease, perceiving health to be good, self-motivation,** and **having requisite behavioral skills.** Important environmental determinants were identified as **spouse sup-**

port, perceived available time, and **access to facilities.** Strong predictors of maintaining spontaneous exercise rather than exercise in an organized program were: **higher level of education, family support,** and **positive peer influences.**

Older adults merit special consideration in discussions of determinants of exercise. This group consists of the young old (aged 65 to 74 years), middle old (aged 75 to 84 years), and very old (aged over 85 years). Ability to exercise as well as determinants of exercise undoubtedly vary over the age spectrum. Almost all studies of exercise determinants in older adults have focused on the young old. Stephens and Craig,[29] in taking a longitudinal perspective, found that swimming and cycling decreased with age but walking and gardening increased with age. **Feeling better physically** and **improving fitness** were the most frequent reasons given for exercising. **Barriers to exercise,** an important consideration for the elderly, need further exploration because though work and family demands may lessen with age, convenience of facilities, cost, opportunities for exercising with others, fear of exercise-related illness or injury, disability, and sensory impairment become more salient with age. Concern about existing medical conditions can be a further deterrent to exercise. Shephard[30] suggests that focusing on personal beliefs rather than subjective norms (expectations of others) may be more effective. Further, assisting older adults to exercise should focus on providing transportation, facilitating companionship for exercise, building on prior activity habits, and tapping exercise skills that have developed over a lifetime. It is, indeed, possible for adults to be active into their very old years. However, in order to increase the frequency with which this happens, further studies of exercise capabilities and other determinants of exercise need to be conducted across the entire spectrum of older adulthood.

It is interesting to note that after consideration of the major behavior prediction and behavior-change theories, a group of prominent theorists concluded that none of their theories singly were sufficient to explain various health behaviors. Instead, they identified variables underlying behavioral performance that span a number of theories. They arrived as a set of eight variables that they believe account for the most variance in behavior: intention, environmental constraints (barriers), ability to perform the behavior, anticipated outcomes (benefits versus costs), social norms, self-standards for behavior, emotional reaction to behavior (positive or negative), and self-efficacy (perceived capabilities).[31] These variables are listed in Table 9–2. Of these variables, self-standards for behavior and emotional reaction to the behavior have received the least attention in the exercise research literature. Self-standards as determinants of behaviors refers to the degree to which performance of the behavior is consistent with one's self-image or self-schema. Although people may respond to social pressures, they do not constantly shift their behavior to conform to what others want. Rather, they adopt certain standards for their own behavior. These standards serve as positive or negative sanctions for behavior. The potential impact of self-standards on exercise behavior needs to be explored.

Affective evaluation of exercise (emotional response to exercise) is receiving increasing attention in adult exercise adherence literature as a potential determinant of exercise behavior. Godin[32] differentiated between an "enjoyment factor" and a "desirability factor." The enjoyment factor was proposed as a component of attitude representing af-

TABLE 9–2. MAJOR VARIABLES UNDERLYING EXPLANATION OF HEALTH BEHAVIORS AND RELATED EXERCISE-SPECIFIC TERMS*

Intention	Self-standards for behavior
Intent	Exercise Self-Image
Commitment	Exercise Self-Schema
Environmental constraints (external circumstances)	Exercise Goals
Barriers	Emotional reaction to the thought of the behavior
Ability to perform the behavior	Exercise-related affect
Exercise skills	Self-efficacy
Anticipated outcomes	Exercise self-efficacy
Benefits versus costs	
Positive outcomes versus negative outcomes	
Attitude	
Social norms	
Family expectations	
Peer expectations	
Health provider expectations	

*Major variables from Fishbein et al.[30].

fect toward the behavior itself, that is, the affect or emotion aroused by thinking about engaging in the behavior. Component adjectives of the enjoyment factor include: pleasant–unpleasant, interesting–boring, stimulating–dull. The desirability factor was viewed as more cognitive in nature, representing the benefits of performing a behavior such as healthy–unhealthy, good–bad, useful–useless. Interestingly, in a group of women who were expectant mothers, the enjoyment (emotional) factor was the predominant predictor of intention to exercise after birth of their child. This study suggested that a measure of affect, that is, perceived enjoyment or pleasure associated with exercising, is an important attitudinal dimension associated with intentions to exercise. In contrast, when Garcia and King[33] had a community-based sample of sedentary older men and women rate the exercise experience in terms of perceived exertion, enjoyment, and convenience, these measures obtained during the first 6 months of exercise were not predictive of exercise behavior measured during the subsequent 6 months. The authors acknowledged that more sensitive psychometric measures of enjoyment need to be developed to adequately capture the concept.

In subsequent psychometric work, Hardy and Rejeski[34] have differentiated between perceived exertion and the affect a person feels during exercise. They have proposed that rating of perceived exertion reflects a composite of physiologic, and cognitive input related to the stress and strain of physical work and thus may not measure precisely the affect a person feels during exercise. The differentiation between "what one feels" defined as perceived exertion and "how one feels" defined as affect was proposed. Gauvin and Rejeski[35] have developed the Exercise-Induced Feeling Inventory (EFI) to assess feeling states that occur in conjunction with acute bouts of exercise. The scale captures distinct feeling states of revitalization, tranquility, and positive engagement, as well as physical exertion. They propose that subjective states that occur during and following exercise are likely predictors of whether individuals are willing to adopt and maintain physically active lifestyles. McAuley and colleagues[36] have developed the Exercise-Induced Affect Scale (EIAS) to capture the affective responses during an exercise episode. The development of tools to measure preexercise, intraexercise and postexercise feelings states provide a basis for further research on affect as a potential determinant of exercise.

Many theories currently used to explain exercise behavior fall under the rubric of decision theory, for example, theory of reasoned action and social cognitive theory. Applying information processing theory to exercise behavior, Kendzierski and colleagues[37] have developed and tested an exercise self-schema measure. Schemata are cognitive structures that guide the processing (selecting, organizing, retrieving) of self-relevant information.[38] Kendzierski, in investigating the predictive value of exercise schemata, found that individuals with an exercise schema were more likely to initiate an exercise program.[39] Having an exercise schema was defined as: rating two of three exercise descriptors (someone who exercises regularly, someone who keeps in shape, physically active) as extremely self-descriptive and rating at least two of the three exercise descriptors as attributes that are extremely important to self-image. The relationship of self-schema to self-regulation of exercise behavior, exercise intentions, and actual exercise behavior merits further exploration.

Flexibility in using multiple theories may in the long-run be the best approach for assisting individuals of all ages to adopt a regular pattern of physical activity. Needed are intervention studies that clearly specify the theoretical dimensions of an intervention and evaluate outcomes. In the interim, programs and interventions to increase overall physical activity and exercise should be guided by what we know to date about the determinants of exercise, even though our knowledge is incomplete.

• THE EXERCISE PROCESS

Sonstroem[40] has recommended that the field of exercise research shift from primary reliance on predictive models to the use of process models that may aid in specifying the mechanisms underlying the adoption and maintenance of exercise behavior. Two process models are described below.

The stages of change as described by DiClemente et al[41] have been applied by Marcus and colleagues to exercise behavior.[42] The stages of change propose that individuals engaging in a new behavior move through a series of changes: precontemplation (not intending to make changes), contemplation (considering changes), planning or preparation (making minor changes), action (actively engaged in major behavior change), and maintenance (sustaining the behavior over time). The processes and strategies used to promote change are linked specifically to the stage of change of the client. That is, stage-specific interventions are proposed. The model of the stages and processes of change have been developed in the context of stopping addictive behaviors such as smoking, with to date few applications to starting positive health behaviors such as exercise. However, in testing the model on 1172 participants in a worksite health promotion project, Marcus and colleagues concluded that the constructs of the theory can be generalized to exercise behavior. Experiential processes suggested as useful in exercise promotion include: consciousness raising, dramatic relief, environmental reevaluation, self-reevaluation, and social liberation. Behavioral processes proposed as useful include: counterconditioning, helping relationships, reinforcement management, self-liberation, and stimulus control. Study participants used all 10 of the above processes. Precontemplators, as might be anticipated, used the 10 processes of change less than persons in other stages of change, and preparers tended to use behavioral processes more often than contemplators. Use of experiential processes did not differ between the precontemplation and preparation stages. Persons in the action stage used both experiential and behavioral processes more often than preparers, and there was a decrease in the use of experiential processes but not behavioral processes in the maintenance stage compared to the action stage.

After subjects were classified into the five stages of behavior change on the basis of responses to questionnaires, demographic differences were examined. Women were more likely than men to be in the contemplation or action stages and less likely to be in the maintenance stage. In another study, working women with young children in the home were more likely to be in the lower stages of exercise adoption than women without young children. Married women reported significantly fewer minutes of vigorous activity than unmarried women.[43] In a study of 286 women aged 50 to 64, precontemplators were significantly older, had lower exercise knowledge, perceived lower psychologic benefits from exercise, had lower family support for exercise, and did not perceive exercise as important compared to the action group. Both the precontemplation and the contemplation group perceived more barriers to exercise than did the action group.[44] Further, subjects who were less well-educated, had greater body mass index scores, or who scored higher on perceived stress were likely to be in the earlier stages of adoption. These findings suggest that certain groups may have unique issues to confront in developing habits of regular exercise. Special attention to the needs of these groups is required on the part of health care providers.

In examining the utility of self-efficacy theory and the decisional balance model within the stages of change model, Marcus and colleagues found that precontemplators scored the lowest on exercise self-efficacy, whereas those in maintenance scored the highest.[45] Persons in maintenance also scored the highest on the pro scale (benefits of exercise), the overall decisional balance index (pro scale minus con scale), and lowest on the con scale (costs of exercising) as predicted by the theories. Research focused on the changes in exercise self-efficacy and decisional balance (beliefs about the costs and benefits of exercise) throughout the stages of exercise behavior could provide important information for appropriately tailoring exercise interventions to groups at differing points in the change process.

Using a slightly different approach to exercise staging from DiClemente and colleagues, Sallis and Hovell[46] have identified the four phases of exercise adoption as sedentary, adoption, dropout or maintenance, and resumption. Three transitions between phases merit more attention by exercise researchers: the transition from being a nonexerciser to being an exerciser (Sedentary → Adoption), the transition after adoption of either dropping out or maintaining exercise (Adoption → Dropout or Maintenance), and the transition to resumption of exercise after dropping out (Dropout → Resumption). People vary widely in the amount of time that they spend in each phase and the number of times they cycle through the various phases.

INTERVENTIONS TO PROMOTE EXERCISE

Maintenance of the benefits of exercise requires commitment to an ongoing program of exercise throughout the life span. The optimum way to achieve maintenance is to promote behavioral carryover of regular exercise patterns from childhood into adulthood. To do this, health professionals must understand the complex motivation that underlies individual efforts to maintain physically active lifestyles from preschool through adulthood. Different motivational variables may be salient at different developmental points or for different individuals at the same developmental point. Thus, an analytical approach must be taken when applying general models of exercise motivation to specific clients.

Experimental studies in which manipulating certain variables increases adoption, maintenance, or resumption of exercise provides the most compelling evidence regarding the actual determinants of exercise. Behavioral strategies that have increased adherence to exercise among adults in experimental studies include: (a) establishing contracts with deposited valuables returned upon contract fulfillment, (b) maintaining self-monitoring diaries and periodic discussion with exercise coordinator, (c) training in relapse prevention, (d) providing personalized feedback and praise, (e) setting flexible goals, (f) using dissociative cognitive strategies that encourage attention to the environment and other pleasant distractions rather than the exercise-related sensations.[45(pp316–317)]

To date, most exercise studies have been conducted on white males, employed adults enrolled in corporate fitness programs, or college students. Thus, in some populations such as children, adolescents, older adults, and various racial and ethnic groups, descriptive work on the predictors of exercise and the process of exercise (stages of exercise behavior, stage transitions) is needed before sound experimental work informed by the most promising theoretical perspectives can proceed. A life-span developmental perspective should undergird these investigative efforts. "Fitting" an exercise-motivation approach to the individual on the basis of a comprehensive assessment of critical exercise-related parameters is particularly challenging.

It is quite clear that a one-time intervention without follow-up is unlikely to result in sustained activity for most individuals. Thus, tracking the impact of exercise-promotion interventions over a certain portion of the developmental trajectory (junior high into high school, college into career, employment into retirement) will provide valuable information about the intensity, repetitiveness, and timing of exercise-promotion interventions that are most effective in sustaining exercise across various life stages.

The efforts of DiClemente and colleagues to explicate a transtheoretical approach for understanding behavior change and to delineate stage-specific strategies for intervention offers one framework for structuring innovative intervention studies. For example, Marcus and colleagues[47] enrolled 610 adults 18 to 82 years old in a community-wide event directed at enhancing exercise behavior. The 6-week intervention consisted of providing written materials and an activity resource manual to increase physical activity.

Based on questionnaire responses regarding their exercise status, participants were divided into three stages of exercise adoption: contemplation, planning or preparation, and action. Print materials were created using the specific change processes matched with the different stages of behavior change. For example, persons in contemplation were sent a booklet entitled, "What's in it for You?" Persons in preparation received materials entitled, "Ready for Action." Examining representative samples from study participants in each stage, 31.4% of those in contemplation advanced to preparation and 30.2% advanced to action following the stage-matched intervention. For those in the preparation stage at baseline, 61.3% advanced to action. A major limitation of this study was lack of a control group. However, the study does suggest the potential effectiveness of a stages-of-change community intervention for increasing the adoption of physical activity. Known predictors of exercise should be analyzed for incorporation into staging studies.

Nurse scientists testing interventions to promote adoption and maintenance of exercise should proceed from a well-articulated theoretical framework. The limited number of intervention studies that do exist often have not been theoretically based. Considerable improvement has occurred in this area in recent years. Experimental interventions should focus on both individuals and aggregates. The ideal would likely be to have empirically tested interventions at individual, family, and community levels that are synergistic in effect, thus optimizing impact and ultimate effectiveness in achieving national physical-activity and physical-fitness goals.

• EXERCISE COUNSELING IN PRIMARY CARE

In Gordon's identification of functional health patterns, one that includes exercise is Activity–Exercise Pattern.[48] The focus is on describing patterns of exercise, activity, leisure, and recreation, including activities of daily living that require energy expenditure. The type, quantity, and quality of exercise is to be described as well as factors that interfere with activity. Diagnoses from the North American Nursing Diagnosis Association (NANDA) relevant to activity include: diversional activity deficit, activity intolerance, and high risk for activity intolerance. The reader is referred to the NANDA Taxonomy for further diagnostic information about definitions, defining characteristics, and etiologic or related factors.[49]

Physical activity counseling for persons of all ages in schools, worksites, and primary care settings is the responsibility of the professional nurse and the physician. When available, the exercise specialist, health educator, and sports or exercise psychologist may further augment the counseling team. The American Nurses' Association (ANA) as well as the American Academy of Family Physicians, American Academy of Pediatrics, American Medical Association, American College of Sports Medicine, and US Preventive Services Task Force provide guidelines for physical activity counseling by health professionals. In physical activity counseling for children, adolescents, and their parents, the ANA's *Clinician's Handbook of Preventive Services: Putting Prevention into Practice*[50(pp97–99)] recommends that every visit be seen as an opportunity to promote an active lifestyle consisting of at least 20 to 30 minutes of vigorous activity three times weekly. Assisting children and adolescents in the selection of appropriate activities should consider: enjoyment of the activity for its own sake rather than solely for competition, involvement in physical activities that can be enjoyed into adulthood, pursuit of activities that can be easily incorporated into a child's daily life and enjoyed all year around, engagement in activities that develop a range of physical activity skills, use of appropriate safety equipment, and avoidance of activities that would result in musculoskeletal injuries because of physical immaturity. Youth should be counseled to avoid use of any anabolic steroids.

Put Prevention into Practice guidelines for physical-activity counseling for adults indicate that all clients in primary care should be asked about their physical-activity habits during work and leisure to determine if these activities are of sufficient intensity to confer health benefits. Adults should be assisted in planning a program of physical activity that is medically safe, enjoyable, convenient, realistic, and structured to achieve patient-specified goals. Routine monitoring, follow-up, and booster sessions are essential to assist clients in maintaining their exercise programs.[49(pp311–314)] Home exercise programs may work for some adults, whereas for others structured programs may need to be offered at worksites or convenient community locations. Group activities may be particularly appealing to adults who prefer the social support and comradeship of group programs.

Nurses in primary care should be central figures in the development of exercise programs and in exercise counseling throughout the life span. This calls for enhancement of the theory-based counseling behaviors of nurses in primary care and other settings. Although few studies have been done of the physical-activity counseling practices of advanced practice nurses, Holcomb and Mullen[51] reported that certified nurse midwives were more likely to counsel their patients about smoking, weight, and alcohol intake than about their level of physical activity. Brown and Waybrant,[52] in examining the health promotion counseling practices of 110 nurse practitioners, found that 76% reported counseling at least one patient on the previous day about physical activity. The content of the counseling including the use of "state of the science" information about the determinants of exercise behavior was not ascertained. Specific protocols can be developed to guide content and process in counseling activities. For example, the Physician-based Assessment and Counseling for Exercise (PACE) program is an example of a theory-driven protocol developed for primary care providers' use in exercise-counseling activities. The protocol uses stages-of-change theory and stage-specific intervention strategies as the framework for recommended assessment and counseling activities.[53] Increasingly sophisticated guidelines and protocols for exercise counseling will need to be developed as knowledge concerning the motivational mechanisms underlying the adoption and maintenance of exercise behavior becomes available.

Barriers to physical-activity counseling sometimes cited by health professionals include: lack of time, lack of reimbursement, absence of theoretically sound protocols to guide counseling with diverse groups, lack of perceived effectiveness as a counselor, and lack of proper training to fulfill this role. If nurses are to provide quality counseling to clients regarding their physical activity, they must work to overcome these barriers. Providers who model active lifestyles themselves are likely to be much more effective counselors than their sedentary counterparts. According to social learning theory, observation of others is a powerful form for transmitting attitudes, beliefs, patterns of thought, and behaviors. Although few primary care clients may directly observe providers exercising, they are quick to recognize the extent to which their provider has actually experienced the challenges and the "ups and downs" of adopting and maintaining a regular program of leisure time physical activity. The physical appearance of health care providers also provides powerful cues to clients as to whether they actually "practice what they preach."

Intensity of Exercise

Vigorous exercise has been widely advocated with at least 20 minutes spent, three times per week at 60% or more of maximum heart rate. Recently, moderate exercise (less than 60% maximum heart rate) has been proposed as having some of the same health-protective benefits as vigorous exercise. Thus, the factors influencing both vigorous and moderate exercise should be studied, because the constellation of variables influencing each may be different. Furthermore, the factors influencing different types of exercise within a particular intensity classification may be different. Since some people dislike strenuous exercise, moderate activities may have fewer barriers to participation and therefore may be incorporated more easily into an individual's daily routine.[45(p311)] Blair et al[54] suggest that lifestyle exercise in which a person engages in numerous short bouts of physical activity throughout the day (stair climbing, walking to and from a distant parking place) resembles the physical activity measured in epidemiologic studies that have found cumulative energy expenditure to be inversely related to cardiac risk. Lifestyle exercise may be ideal for sedentary individuals not ready to undertake a more vigorous or formal exercise program. When sedentary individuals become accustomed to lifestyle exercise, they may be ready to begin a moderate program of exercise progressing to a vigorous one. Some combination of lifestyle exercise and somewhat vigorous leisure-time exercise is probably closer to the ideal for persons who can safely tolerate it.

Exercise Risks

An overly aggressive approach to exercise can exaggerate existing clinical conditions and put patients, particularly older adults, at risk for untoward effects. If an individual has an undiagnosed heart condition, strenuous exercise could create arrhythmias. Persons with cardiovascular disease or other chronic conditions should be cautioned to avoid exercising at levels that are physiologically untenable or result in untoward symptoms. Overstressing muscles and joints can result in muscle soreness and joint pain. Individuals over 50 years of age or with an existing chronic illness that may increase the risk of exercising should be evaluated medically before starting to exercise in order to determine any particular precautions required for structuring the exercise program. A program of gradually increasing exercise is recommended, with much more emphasis for older adults on moderate rather than vigorous exercise. Exercise prescriptions should result in an enjoyable exercise experience, optimizing the benefits of exercise while minimizing the risks.

• OPTIONS FOR EXERCISE PROGRAMS TO ENHANCE HEALTH

Individuals have a variety of options for integrating a greater level of physical activity into their lives. Two categories of exercise that should be considered for appropriateness in counseling any given client include: **lifestyle exercise** and **leisure-time exercise.**

Figure 9–1 illustrates the difference in patterns of energy expenditure over the course of the day for a person who is sedentary, engages in lifestyle exercise, and engages in vigorous leisure-time exercise. Although there is no confirmatory evidence to date, it is proposed by Blair and his colleagues that if the area under the dotted line (lifestyle exercise) is the same as under the dashed line (leisure-time exercise) the health effects will be comparable.[3(pp161–163)] One randomized clinical trial does suggest that three 10-minute periods of exercise spread throughout the day may produce essentially the same conditioning as one 30-minute session.[55]

Lifestyle Exercise

Lifestyle exercise, defined as physical activity that can be planned into activities of daily living, has been suggested as a new strategy for promoting physical activity in populations.[56] This approach to exercise may be an ideal way for persons who do not like to exercise or who have compromised capabilities for exercise to increase their daily energy expenditure. People should be encouraged by health providers to think about how they

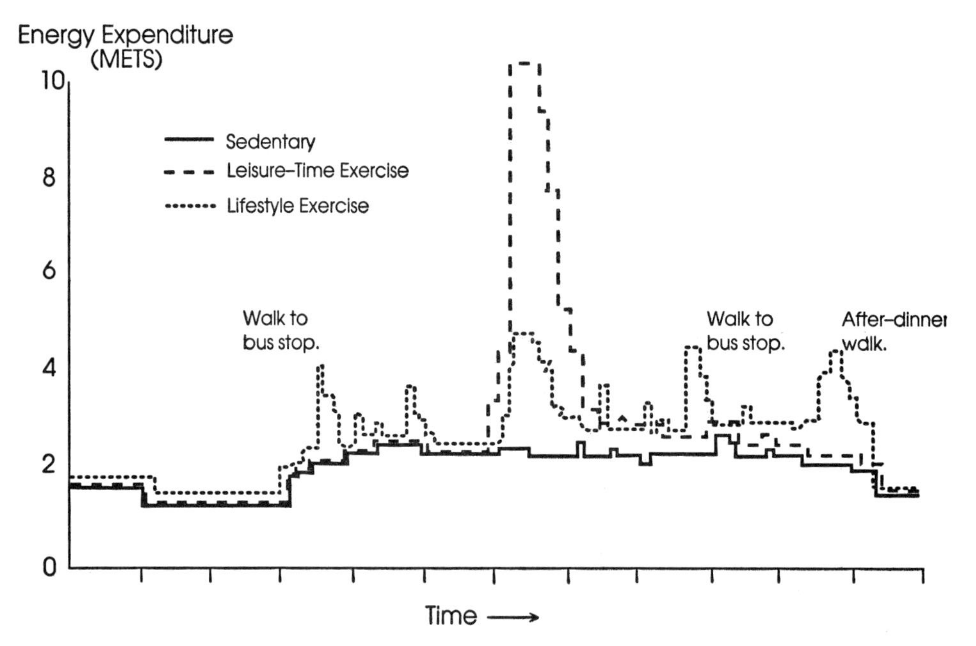

Figure 9-1. The solid line indicates the energy expenditure over the course of a day for a sedentary person. The dashed line represents the energy expenditure of an individual who engages in planned, vigorous exercise during leisure time (such as a jog at lunchtime) but is otherwise sedentary (that is, traditional exercise training). The dotted line illustrates energy expenditure for an individual with a sedentary job who seeks opportunities to integrate short bouts of physical activity (such as brisk walking, stair climbing, gardening, yard work, playing with children) into the daily routine (that is, lifestyle exercise). Comparable health effects are expected for both approaches if the total daily energy expenditure is the same. (From Blair SN, Kohl HW III, Gordon NF,[53] with permission.)

can spend less of their day being sedentary. To develop a plan by which this can happen gives clients a sense of control over their own lives and some concrete ideas to try out. Table 9–3 presents suggestions for substituting more active for less active approaches to work and home activities.

Leisure-Time Exercise

Exercise carried out in leisure time generally is of moderate or vigorous intensity. Activities may consist of walking, jogging, bicycling, swimming, or a myriad of other recreational and sports activities performed singly or in a group. Commonly referred to as endurance exercise, leisure-time physical activity generally should consist of three phases: warming-up, endurance exercise, and cooling down. Together they constitute a program of exercise that, sustained over time, will increase fitness and cardiorespiratory function.

Warming Up. Before extended exercise, warming up is important to increase blood flow to the heart and skeletal muscles, enhance oxygenation of tissues, and increase flexibility of muscles. The warming-up period allows the heart rate and body temperature to increase gradually and joints to become more flexible prior to exercise. A gradual increase in heart rate reduces chances of arrhythmias during exercise. An increase in body temperature may prevent muscle soreness and musculotendinous injuries. Increased blood flow to skeletal muscle aids in oxidative processes and the delivery of fuel substrates for energy. A low level aerobic activity is recommended. Only moderate stretching is recommended during warming up, as overstretching of muscles and joints may cause unnecessary soreness and possible injury. However, stretching does have a number of benefits including stimulating circulation, increasing flexibility, lengthening muscles, and preventing muscle strains during exercise. Warming up can include activities such as: walking briskly, arm circles, jumping jacks, leg exercises, or wall push-ups. The warming-up period need take no longer than 7 to 10 minutes and should be followed immediately by endurance exercise.

In physical activity counseling with clients of all ages, the importance of warming up before exercise should be stressed to avoid risk of injury and other untoward effects of exercise. In addition, endurance exercise may be more enjoyable if the body is readied for this challenge.

TABLE 9–3. SEDENTARY AND ACTIVE APPROACHES TO THE CONDUCT OF DAILY LIVING

SEDENTARY	ACTIVE
Take the elevator or escalator	Climb the stairs
Call on the telephone	Walk down the hall or walk next door
Drive to lunch	Walk to lunch
Sit in a chair throughout a meeting	Get up quietly and walk about the room
Park right next to your destination	Park some distance away from your destination
Remain sedentary at your desk	Take several minutes to do arm and leg exercises
Use the remote control for the TV	Get up and walk to the TV when you want to change the channel
Visit with your colleagues in the "break room"	Take a walking break and visit

Endurance Exercise. Aerobic exercise should be based on an appropriate exercise prescription that ultimately improves cardiopulmonary as well as muscular function at an incremental pace. Pacing should be based on age, fitness, health status, and activity preferences. The exercise prescription should identify the frequency, intensity, duration, and type(s) of exercise as well as the recommended pattern of progression. Endurance exercise should be planned as an integral part of lifestyle, since continued practice is essential for long-term health benefits. Children and adolescents may have different exercise preferences from adults but both should engage in their chosen activities three to five times per week. If the goal is weight reduction as well as conditioning, exercising five times a week is more likely to result in a weekly expenditure of 800 to 1200 calories. *Guidelines for Exercise Testing and Prescription* from the American College of Sports Medicine[57] or another reliable source should be used by qualified health professionals to determine appropriate exercise intensity. This determination is based on various formulas that take into consideration maximal and resting heart rate. It is recommended that the duration of an exercise episode be 15 to 60 minutes in length. Typical recommendations are 20 to 30 minutes at training heart rate. Lower-intensity activities for longer duration should be considered for individuals who are obese, elderly, or those with a chronic disease.

When the physiologic demands of endurance exercise are repeated on a regular basis, the body becomes more efficient in function and stronger. Appropriate activities include those that use large muscle groups and are performed in a continuous rhythmic manner such as walking, jogging, bicycling, cross-country skiing, swimming, and aerobics. Although endurance activities have a general effect of improving cardiorespiratory function, each type of exercise has specific benefits. For example, bicycling develops the quadricep muscles with little effect on upper extremities. It is important to assess the strengths and weaknesses of various endurance activities that are components of an exercise prescription.

Cooling Down. Taking time to cool down for a period of 5 to 10 minutes following endurance exercise is important because exercise raises heart rate, blood pressure, body temperature, and lactic acid within the muscles. Cooling down allows the heart rate to gradually decrease, minimizing the possibility of arrhythmias as well as preventing pooling of blood in muscles and resultant light-headedness. It helps eliminate lactic acid within muscles and maintains blood flow to and from the muscles. During the cooling down period, it is important to keep the lower extremities moving in activities such as slow walking, jogging, or cycling. At the end of the cooling-down period, the client's heart rate should be below 100.

• DIRECTIONS IN EXERCISE RESEARCH

This chapter has provided a research-based discussion of the benefits of exercise, factors influencing exercise behavior among youth and adults, the exercise process, exercise interventions, and the importance of physical fitness counseling. Research is still needed to develop valid tools for measurement of physical activity and exercise and to better understand how to tailor exercise programs to the needs of different populations. Although accumulating descriptive research has provided rich resources for experimental work, few theoretically based intervention studies have been conducted. Rigorous experimental studies will be critical to assisting nurses and other health professionals to increase the level of activity in the population through programs and primary care services proven to be effective. Particular focus should be placed on assisting children and adolescents to adopt exercise as an integral, enjoyable, and rewarding aspect of their lifestyle. King and colleagues[58] have made recommendations concerning directions for future research by interdisciplinary teams to better understand exercise phenomenon. Their recommendations have been incorporated into the following list:

1. Explore both the determinants and methods of changing individual patterns of physical activity.
2. Test the effectiveness of family interventions to increase physical activity and exercise.
3. Identify and examine the stages of physical-activity behavior including relapse and resumption.
4. Identify and describe the manner in which the important developmental milestones or life transitions influence the readiness and ability to be physically active.
5. Contrast the effectiveness of existing theoretical models of behavior change for structuring interventions to increase physical activity and identify the operative unique and common causal mechanisms among the models.
6. Design and evaluate physical-activity interventions as components of or adjuncts to other risk reduction-interventions and programs.
7. Evaluate programs for altering multiple health-related behaviors simultaneously or sequentially.
8. Evaluate methods of physical-activity assessment and interventions designed to increase individual adoption, maintenance, and relapse prevention of physical activity in the clinical setting, school setting, worksite setting, and various community settings.
9. Investigate the influence of the physical environment on the adoption and maintenance of physical activity.
10. Investigate the influence of social factors on the adoption and maintenance of physical activity (eg, family environment and structure, social support, societal norms, and role models).
11. Investigate the influence of biologic and affective factors that may influence the adoption and maintenance of physical activity and their relationship to other variables affecting physical activity.

• SUMMARY

Nurses, as key health professionals in the delivery of primary care, need to assume responsibility for using current and emerging knowledge to assist clients to develop lifelong exercise habits. Exercise must be an integral part of personal lifestyle if it is to have optimum effects on health. Maintaining physical fitness can be enjoyable and rewarding for persons of all ages and contribute significantly to extending longevity and improving the quality of life.

REFERENCES

1. Caspersen CJ, Powell KE, Christenson GM. Physical activity, exercise and physical fitness: definitions and distinctions for health-related research. *Pub Health Rep.* 1986;101:126–131.
2. Bouchard C, Shephard RJ, Stephens T, eds. *Exercise, Fitness and Health: A Consensus of Current Knowledge.* Champaign, Ill: Human Kinetics; 1990.
3. Gordon NF, Kohl HW III, Blair SN. Life style exercise: a new strategy to promote physical activity for adults. *J Cardiopulm Rehab.* 1993;13:161–163.
4. *Healthy People 2000: National Health Promotion and Disease Prevention Objectives.* Washington, DC: US Public Health Service; 1991. US Dept of Health and Human Services publication (PHS) 91-50212.
5. Stephens T, Jacobs DR, White CC. A descriptive epidemiology of leisure-time physical activity. *Public Health Rep.* 1985;100(2):147–158.
6. Rowland TW. *Exercise and Children's Health.* Champaign, Ill: Human Kinetics; 1990:1–7.
7. Sherrill C, Holguin O, Caywood A. Fitness, attitude toward physical education, and self-concept of elementary school children. *Percept Mot Skills.* 1989;69:411–414.
8. Crews D, Landers DM. A meta-analytic review of aerobic fitness and reactivity to psychosocial stressors. *Med Sci Sports Exerc.* 1987;19(suppl):S114–S120.
9. Brown JD, Siegel JM. Exercise as a buffer of life stress: a prospective study of adolescent health. *Health Psychol.* 1988;7(4):341–353.
10. Mechanic D, Hansell S. Adolescent competence, psychological well-being, and self-assessed physical health. *J Health Soc Behav.* 1987;28:364–374.
11. Thorlindsson T, Vilhjalmsson RT, Vilhjalmsson R, et al. Sport participation and perceived health status. *Soc Sci Med.* 1990;31(5):551–556.
12. Ainsworth BE, Berry CB, Schnyder VN, et al. Leisure-time physical activity and aerobic fitness in African-American young adults. *J Adolesc Health.* 1992;13:606–611.
13. Folsom AR, Cook TC, Pprafka JM, et al. Differences in leisure-time physical activity levels between blacks and whites in population-based samples: the Minnesota Heart Survey. *J Behav Med.* 1991;14(1):1–9.
14. Moore LL, Lombardi DA, White MJ, et al. Influence of parents' physical activity levels on activity levels of young children. *J Pediatr.* 1991;118:215–219.
15. Sallis JF, Patterson TL, McKenzie TL, et al. Family variables and physical activity in preschool children. *Dev Behav Pediatr.* 1988;9(2):57–61.
16. Sallis JF, Simons-Morton BG, Stone EJ, et al. Determinants of physical activity and interventions in youth. *Med Sci Sports Exerc.* 1992;24(6) (supp):S248–S257.
17. Biddle S, Armstrong N. Children's physical activity: an exploratory study of psychological correlates. *Soc Sci Med.* 1992;34(3):325–331.
18. Garcia AW, Norton MA, Frenn M, et al. Gender and developmental differences in exercise beliefs among youth and prediction of their exercise behavior. *J School Health.* 1995;65(6):213–219.
19. Halfon ST, Bronner S. Determinants of physical ability in seventh grade school children. *Eur J Epidemiol.* 1989;5(1):90–96.
20. Desmond SM, Price JH, Lock RS, et al. Urban black and white adolescents' physical fitness status and perceptions of exercise. *J School Health.* 1990;60:220–226.

21. McKenzie TL, Sallis JF, Nader PR, et al. Anglo- and Mexican-American preschoolers at home and recess: activity patterns and environmental influences. *Dev Behav Pediatr.* 1992;13(3):173–180.
22. Deci EL, Ryan RM. *Intrinsic Motivation and Self-determination in Human Behavior.* New York, NY: Plenum Press; 1985.
23. Fox K. Motivating children for physical activity: towards a healthier future. *J Phys Educ, Rec Dance.* 1991;62(7):34–38.
24. Dzewaltowski DA. Toward a model of exercise motivation. *J Sport ExercPsychol.*11:251–269.
25. Godin G, Shephard RJ. Use of attitude-behaviour models in exercise promotion. *Sports Med.* 1990;10(2):103–121.
26. Pender NJ, Walker SN, Sechrist KR, et al. *The Health Promotion Model: Refinement and Validation.* Final Report to the National Center for Nursing Research, National Institutes of Health (Grant no. NR 01121). DeKalb, Ill: Northern Illinois University Press, 1990.
27. Wurtele SK, Maddux JE. Relative contributions of protection motivation theory components in predicting exercise behavior. *Health Psychol.* 1987;6:453–466.
28. Dishman RK, Sallis JF, Orenstein DR. The determinants of physical activity and exercise. *Public Health Rep.* 1985;100:158–172.
29. Stephens T, Craig C. *The Wellbeing of Canadians.* Ottawa, Ont: Canadian Fitness and Lifestyle Research Institute; 1990.
30. Shephard RJ. Determinants of exercise in people aged 65 years and older. In: Dishman R, ed. *Advances in Exercise Adherence.* Champaign, Ill: Human Kinetics; 1994:343–360.
31. Fishbein M, Bandura A, Triandis HC, et al. *Factors Influencing Behavior and Behavior Change: Final Report of Theorists' Workshop on AIDs-related Behaviors*; October 3–5, 1991; Washington, DC: National Institute of Mental Health, National Institutes of Health.
32. Godin G. Importance of the emotional aspect of attitude to predict intention. *Psycholog Rep.* 1987;61:719–723.
33. Garcia AW, King AC. Predicting long-term adherence to aerobic exercise: a comparison of two models. *J Sport Exerc Psychol.* 1991;13:394–410.
34. Hardy CJ, Rejeski WJ. Not what, but how one feels: the measurement of affect during exercise. *J Sport Exerc Psychol.* 1989;11:304–317.
35. Gauvin L, Rejeski WJ. The exercise-induced feeling inventory: development and initial validation. *J Sport Exerc Psychol.* 1993;15:403–423.
36. McAuley E, Courneya KS. Self-efficacy relationships with affective and exertion responses to exercise. *J Appl Soc Psychol.* 1992;22:312–326.
37. Kendzierski D. Schema theory: an information processing focus. In: Dishman R, ed. *Advances in Exercise Adherence.* Champaign, Ill: Human Kinetics; 1994:137–159.
38. Markus H. Self-schemata and processing information about the self. *J Pers Soc Psychol.* 1977;35:63–78.
39. Kendzierski D. Exercise self-schemata: cognitive and behavioral correlates. *Health Psychol.* 1990;9:69–82.
40. Sonstroem RJ. Psychological models. In: Dishman R, ed. *Exercise Adherence: Its Impact on Public Health.* Champaign, Ill: Human Kinetics; 1988:125–154.
41. DiClemente CC, Prochaska JO, Fairhurst S, et al. The process of smoking cessation: an analysis of precontemplation, contemplation, and preparation stages of change. *J Consult Clin Psychol.* 1991;59:295–304.
42. Marcus BH, Rossi JS, Selby VC, et al. The stages and processes of exercise adoption and maintenance in a worksite sample. *Health Psychol.* 1992;11:386–395.
43. Marcus BH, Pinto BM, Simkin LR, et al. Application of theoretical models to exercise behavior among employed women. *Am J Health Prom.* 1994;9(1):49–55.

44. Lee C. Attitudes, knowledge and stages of change: a survey of exercise patterns in older Australian women. *Health Psychol.* 1993;12:476–480.
45. Marcus BH, Selby VC, Niaura RS. Self-efficacy and the stages of exercise behavior change. *Res Q Exerc Sport.* 1992;63(1):60–66.
46. Sallis JF, Hovell MF. Determinants of exercise behavior. In: Holloszy JO, Pandolf KB, eds. *Exercise and Sport Sciences Reviews.* Baltimore, Md: Williams & Wilkins; 1990:18:307–330.
47. Marcus BH, Banspach SW, Lefebvre RC, et al. Using the stages of change model to increase the adoption of physical activity among community participants. *Am J Health Prom.* 1992;6:424–429.
48. Gordon M. *Manual of Nursing Diagnosis, 1993-1994.* St Louis, Mo: Mosby Year Book; 1993:3, 159,161,185.
49. North American Nursing Diagnosis Association. *Nursing Diagnoses: Definitions and classification.* Philadelphia, Pa: NANDA, 1994.
50. American Nurses' Association. *Clinician's Handbook of Preventive Services: Put Prevention into Practice.* Waldorf, Md: American Nurses Publishing; 1994.
51. Holcomb JD, Mullen PD. Certified nurse-midwives and health promotion and disease prevention: results of a national survey. *J Nurse Midwifery.* 1986;31(3):141–148.
52. Brown MA, Waybrant KM. Health promotion, education, counseling and coordination in primary health care nursing. *Public Health Nurs.* 1988;5:16–23.
53. Pender NJ, Sallis JF, Long BJ, et al. Health-care provider counseling to promote physical activity. In: Dishman RK, ed. *Advances in Exercise Adherence.* Champaign, Ill: Human Kinetics; 1994:213–235.
54. Blair SN, Kohl HW III, Gordon NF. Physical activity and health: a lifestyle approach. *Med Exerc Nutr Health.* 1992;1:54–57.
55. DeBusk RF, Stenestrand U, Sheehan M, et al. Training effects of long versus short bouts of exercise in healthy subjects. *Am J Cardiol.* 1990;65:1010–1013.
56. Blair SN. *Living with Exercise.* Dallas, Tex: American Health Publishing; 1991:1–119.
57. American College of Sports Medicine. *Guidelines for Exercise Testing and Prescription.* 4th ed. Philadelphia, Pa: Lea & Febiger; 1991.
58. King AC, Blair SN, Bild DE, et al. Determinants of physical activity and intervention in adults. *Med Sci Sports Exerc.* 24(6)(suppl):S221–S236.

10

Nutrition and Health

Good nutrition is important to the nurturance of health. Accumulating evidence indicates that eating patterns play a major role in preventing disease and in creating the capacity for energetic and productive living. Although much is yet to be learned through nutrition research about mechanisms underlying the relationship between nutrition and health, community-based health education programs and national dietary and food production policies should be focused on promoting optimum nutrition among persons of all ages. In recognizing the importance of nutrition education, the *Healthy People 2000: National Health Promotion and Disease Prevention Objectives* identify the following nutritional service objectives to be achieved by the year 2000[1]:

- Increase to at least 75% the proportion of the nation's schools that provide nutrition education from preschool through 12th grade, preferably as part of quality school health education.
- Increase to at least 50% the proportion of worksites with 50 or more employees that offer nutrition education or weight management programs for employees.
- Increase to at least 75% the proportion of primary care providers who provide nutrition assessment and counseling or referral to qualified nutritionists or dietitians.

Since nurses are the health professionals most often in extended contact with clients, they are a valuable resource to individuals, families, and communities in providing information and assistance in regard to healthy nutrition. Dietary counseling and education should be an integral part of nursing practice in all settings. The professional nurse must be able to deal not only with therapeutic aspects of nutrition but also with nutrition as a critical element in prevention and health promotion. Nutritionists and psychologists are valuable colleagues of the nurse in planning sound nutrition education programs for individuals, families, or for entire populations.

• THE ROLE OF NUTRITION IN PREVENTION

Excess consumption of fats and highly refined carbohydrates is a major problem in the United States. Over 80% of children aged 2 through 5 years in the United States consume more total fat, saturated fat, and cholesterol than is recommended.[2] Furthermore, among boys there is a prepubertal increase in subcutaneous fat that is lost during adolescence, whereas prepubertal fat disposition in girls continues through puberty and into adulthood. A study comparing skin-fold data from three national surveys conducted between 1963 and 1980 found a 54% increase in obesity in children and a 39% increase in obesity in adolescents over the two decades.[3] It is estimated that 27% of children 6 to 11,[4] 15% of adolescents, and 24% of men and 27% of women aged 20 through 74 are overweight.[16(p114)]

The overconsumption of saturated fats, cholesterol, sugar, and salt has been linked to a number of chronic diseases that are the major causes of death and disability in the United States. The Committee on Diet and Health of the National Academy of Sciences, after a comprehensive review of epidemiologic, clinical, and laboratory evidence, concluded that diet influenced risk for several chronic diseases. The evidence was judged to be **strong** for a link between diet and atherosclerotic cardiovascular diseases and hypertension and **highly suggestive** for certain forms of cancer, especially those of the esophagus, stomach, large intestine, breast, lung, and prostate. Certain dietary patterns also appeared to predispose individuals to obesity, the risk of non–insulin-dependent diabetes mellitus, chronic liver disease, and possibly osteoporosis. Although these chronic diseases are complex, involving genetic and other environmental determinants, modifications in diet could play a significant role in reducing the risk of occurrence.[5]

For example, about 1,250,000 Americans suffer myocardial infarctions each year and many more have angina pectoris. Coronary heart disease (CHD) costs the US economy over $50 billion annually. A number of factors influence the development of cardiovascular disease. Factors that offer little possibility for control are genetic predisposition, gender, and advancing age. Factors over which individuals can have control include high blood cholesterol, cigarette smoking, high blood pressure, excessive body weight, and long-term physical inactivity. Addressing controllable risk factors can decrease deposits of cholesterol and other lipids, resultant cellular reactions, and the thickening of coronary artery walls and subsequent risk of myocardial infarction and sudden death.[6]

Accumulating evidence also indicates that dietary factors may be associated with both the occurrence of cancer and protection against cancer. Dietary constituents suspect in the occurrence of cancer include excessive intake of fat, kilocalories, nitrites, mutagens (contained in smoked, charbroiled, fried, or pickled meats), meats, and alcohol. Milk; fruits; vegetables; dietary fiber; vitamins A, C, and E; carotenoids; folate; and calcium have been suggested as protectants against cancer. Cox[7] compared the diets of 210 randomly selected low-income African-American and white women on intake of potentially cancer-promoting and cancer-protecting food components. For considerable numbers of the women in both groups, fat intakes were above the recommended 30%, fiber intakes were less than half the recommended amounts, and consumption of vitamins A,C,E; folate; calcium; fruits; vegetables; and milk were inadequate. Intake of meats and possible sources of nitrites were not excessive. Although the sample studied was relatively small, results of the study indicate the need for aggressive intervention programs to assist low-income populations to make healthy modifications in their dietary intake as a basis for possible protection against cancer.

TABLE 10–1. NUTRITION AND YOUR HEALTH: DIETARY GUIDELINES FOR AMERICANS

1. Eat a variety of foods.
2. Maintain a healthy weight.
3. Choose a diet low in fat, saturated fat, and cholesterol:
   - 30% or less of calories from fat;
   - less than 10% of calories from saturated fat.
4. Choose a diet with plenty of vegetables, fruits, and grain products:
   - 3 or more servings of vegetables daily;
   - 2 or more servings of fruit daily;
   - 6 or more servings of grain products daily.
5. Use sugars only in moderation.
6. Use salt and sodium only in moderation.
7. If you drink alcoholic beverages, do so in moderation:
   - 1 drink per day for women
   - 1 drink per day for men

From Nutrition and Your Health.[8]

The Dietary Guidelines for Americans, 1990[8] form the basis for a federal nutrition policy. In general these guidelines answer the question concerning how Americans over 2 years of age should eat for good health. Too many Americans eat too many calories, too much fat, cholesterol, and sodium and too few complex carbohydrates and not enough fiber, which may well contribute to the high rates of chronic disease in the United States. The dietary guidelines for the prevention of chronic diseases appear in Table 10-1. The *Food Guide Pyramid,*[9] consistent with these guidelines and published by the US Department of Agriculture, appears in Figure 10–1. The pyramid has replaced the Basic Four Food Groups and is useful for simple dietary screening and as a foundation for general nutrition education. Of calories consumed daily, 30% or less should be from fat (less than 10% saturated fatty acids, 10% polyunsaturated fatty acids, and 10% monounsaturated fatty acids). No more than 300 mg of dietary cholesterol should be consumed daily. Fat content of some commonly eaten foods appears in Table 10–2. Implementation of these recommendations would result in an approximate reduction of 10% or more in the average blood cholesterol level of the US population and lead to an approximate reduction of 20% or more in coronary heart disease, significantly improving the health and quality of life of the population. As fat in the diet is lowered, carbohydrate intake, primarily complex carbohydrates, should be increased to 50% to 60% of the diet, and protein should not exceed 10% to 20% of calories. Additional recommendations relevant to prevention of cancer include limiting intake of salt-cured, smoked, or nitrate-preserved foods.[10,11]

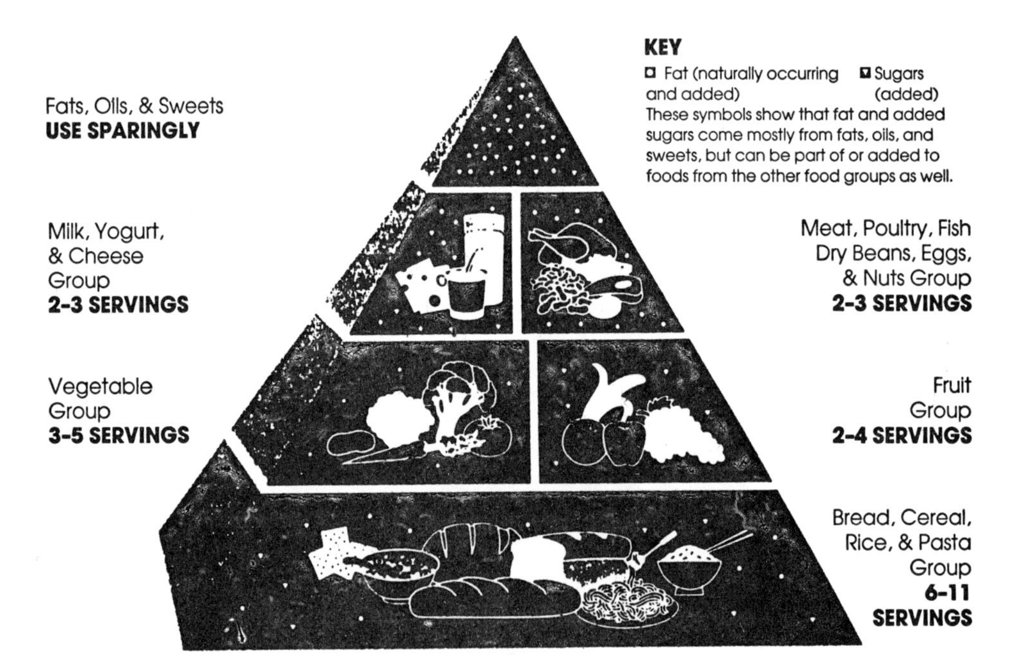

Figure 10–1. Food Guide Pyramid: A Guide to Daily Food Choices (Source: U.S. Department of Agriculture/U.S. Department of Health and Human Services)

TABLE 10–2. FAT CONTENT OF SOME FOODS

FOODS	FAT CONTENT (GRAMS)	TOTAL (KCAL*)
Milks and Yogurt	per c	per c
skim milk (milk solids added)	1	90
low-fat milk (1%)	3	100
low-fat milk (2%)	5	120
whole milk (3.3%)	8	150
low-fat yogurt, plain	4	145
low-fat yogurt , fruit-flavored	3	230
Table Fats	per tbsp	per tbsp
butter	12	100
margarine	12	100
whipped butter or margarine	8	65
mayonnaise	11	100
Creams	per tbsp	per tbsp
half-and-half	2	20
sour cream	3	30
nondairy whipped topping (frozen)	1	15
liquid nondairy coffee lightener	1	20
powdered nondairy coffee lightener	1 (per tsp)	10 (per tsp)
Desserts	per ½ c	per ½ c
ice cream (11% fat)	7	135
ice cream, soft serve	12	188
ice milk (4.3% fat)	3	93
sherbet	2	135
	per portion	per portion
apple pie, 1/4 of 9" pie	15	345
danish pastry, 4¼" diam × 1" deep	15	275
doughnut, glazed, 3¾" × 1¼" deep	11	205
Cheese	per 1 oz	per 1 oz
cheddar	9	115
American processed cheese	9	105
part-skim mozzarella	5	80
cottage cheese (4% fat)	5 (½ c)	118
cottage cheese (1% fat)	1 (½ c)	82
Meat, Fish, Poultry	per 3-oz serving	per 3-oz serving
ham, lean and fat	19	245
shrimp	1	100
rib roast, lean and fat	33	375
ground beef, 21% fat	17	235
ground beef, 10% fat	10	185
turkey, light meat	3	150

*Total kilocalories represent the kilocalories not only from fat but also from the protein and carbohydrate the food may contain.
Source: Nutritive Value of Foods, USDA Home and Garden Bulletin No. 72. Washington, DC: US Dept of Agriculture: 1981.

Undernutrition is also a problem in many segments of the population, resulting in retardation in linear growth of preschool children. Chronic iron deficiency in childhood may have adverse effects on growth and development. The prevalence of iron deficiency is higher in black children compared to white children and higher in children of families below the poverty level than in children of more affluent families. Inadequate calcium intake in youth may be related to failure to attain peak bone mass during the years of bone mineralization (up to age 20 years), possibly resulting in later predisposition to osteoporosis. Eating disorders resulting from undernutrition such as anorexia nervosa and bulimia are nutritional threats to the health of youth, particularly young women, that are not well understood.[1(pp112–123)] Further research is needed to explore mechanisms underlying these problems as a basis for effective interventions.

• FACTORS INFLUENCING EATING BEHAVIOR

A wide variety of factors influence overt eating behavior. These factors can be classified as biologic, psychologic, sociocultural, and environmental. The multicausal nature of eating behavior makes it highly complex and resistant to change. Eating behaviors are an integral part of individual and family lifestyle. Effective modification requires consideration of the factors that determine eating behavior and the use of appropriate change techniques.

Biologic Factors

Various neurotransmitters stimulate the process of eating behavior in animals, whereas other processes inhibit it. Norepinephrine, neuropeptide Y, and opioid peptides enhance eating behavior, whereas serotonin, epinephrine, calcitonin, and cholecystokinin inhibit it. It is proposed that norepinephrine, serotonin, and neuropeptide Y modulate the ingestion of carbohydrate-rich foods, whereas opiates regulate ingestion of high-fat foods. Some of the neurotransmitters, such as opiates, cholecystokinin, and substance P, may also play a role in taste. Biologic effects on eating behavior similar to those in animals are proposed for humans.[12]

The biologic changes of aging have a marked effect on eating behavior. A progressive loss of taste buds on the anterior tongue occurs with age, resulting in decreased sensitivity to sweet and salty tastes. In contrast, taste buds sensitive to bitter and sour increase with age. This taste distortion may result in decreased enjoyment of food and decreased intake of nutrients. Decreased gastric secretions can result in limited absorption of iron, calcium, and vitamin B_{12}. Decreased gastric motility augments the need for foods high in fiber (fresh fruits, raw vegetables, whole-grain breads, and cereals) and increases the importance of water consumption to promote regularity in bowel evacuation. A decrease in basal metabolic rate with aging has also been associated with a decrease in caloric intake. Many elderly people also suffer from isolation and depression. Altered hypothalamic-pituitary-adrenal–axis regulatory mechanisms have been noted in depression, including excessive cortisol secretion and an elevation in corticotropin releasing factor, a potent inhibitor of food intake.[13]

In regard to other physiologic influences, energy requirements also appear to be highly salient biologic determinants of eating behavior. Individuals exhibit awareness and sensitivity to low energy levels. Fatigue, listlessness, and apathy can indicate a caloric intake that is inadequate to meet energy needs. More studies are needed to document how various biologic factors affect eating behavior.

Psychologic Factors

Increasing knowledge of proper nutrition by itself does not necessarily improve eating habits. Although in a recent survey, 67% of 11th- and 12th-grade students reported that saturated fat and cholesterol should not be eaten in excess, this knowledge had only a slight influence on the consumption of foods high in these constituents.[14] Motivation and other psychologic factors must be addressed among persons of all ages if healthy nutritional practices are to become a reality for a larger portion of the population.

Psychologic factors can have positive or negative effects on eating behaviors. Perceiving many benefits from good dietary practices encourages individuals to select foods that are high in nutrients, low in fat and refined carbohydrates, high in fiber, and low in sodium and food additives. Health-conscious decisions about nutrition can be taught as early as preschool with systems such as "green" foods (foods high in nutrition), "red" foods (foods low in nutrition), and "yellow" foods (foods with limited but some nutritional value that are to be eaten sparingly). A positive self-concept also creates a psychologic climate that encourages persons of all ages to take care of themselves and watch what they eat because they place a high value on their own health and well-being.

Emotions, such as depression, and personal beliefs of low self-esteem and lack of personal control over one's life, particularly over eating behavior, can markedly impair nutritional practices. Negative emotions, such as anger, frustration, and insecurity, can lead to disturbances in eating behavior that lead to undernutrition (eg, anorexia nervosa, bulimia) or overnutrition (obesity). These problems frequently are indicative of a personal search for comfort, security, and nurturance through food intake. Focusing on enhancing or modifying self-concept and reducing depression may well be necessary before nutritional behaviors can be changed. Provision of nutritional guidance without attention to coexisting psychologic states may exaggerate rather than ameliorate nutritional problems.

Habits constitute another important determinant of eating behavior. A habit can be defined as a behavior that occurs often and is performed automatically or with little conscious awareness.[15] Habits are performed so frequently that many cues within the environment serve as signals for the behavior. They often result in a psychologic addiction to certain behaviors because they become a pervasive part of lifestyle. Such behaviors are known as consummatory because the response itself (eating) provides the reinforcement. People can also become psychologically addicted to the consequences of habitual behaviors such as the "energy spurt" experienced after the ingestion of highly refined sugars (doughnuts, sweet rolls, snack foods) or caffeine (sodas, coffee, chocolate). Habits can result in poor dietary practices because little or no conscious thought is given to eating behavior. Habits also depend on the availability of foodstuffs that can be readily consumed without preparation. Fast foods that are high in fats and refined carbohydrates and low in protein, minerals, and vitamins often meet this requirement.

Sociocultural Factors

The dietary habits of young children are profoundly impacted by family food preparation and eating behaviors. Numerous organizations have recommended that total fats and cholesterol be restricted in the diets of children over 2 years of age (saturated fats to 10% of calories, total fats to 30% of calories, and dietary cholesterol to less than 300 mg/d).

Black children and children from low-income families have diets least consistent with recommendations.[16,17] Parental beliefs about good nutrition for children may not match these recommendations and thus may actually contribute to an unhealthy diet. For example, in a study of 547 children between the ages of 2 and 5, the major food source of saturated fat for the total group was whole milk, which contributed 16.1% for white children, 18.5% for black children, and 26.9% for Hispanic children of saturated fat consumed. Many parents who drink reduced-fat or skim milk themselves will give their children whole milk in the belief that it is better for them. When the diets of black children were examined separately, their major sources of total dietary fat were franks, sausages, lunch meats, and bacon, with whole milk as a close second. This finding suggests cultural differences that may need to be considered in dietary counseling. Almost a third of total cholesterol consumed by children comes from eggs or egg products, with additional cholesterol added by whole milk, sweets, and beef. Children's diets could be considerably improved by changing the beliefs and practices of their care providers, including parents, other relatives, and day care or preschool personnel. Substituting 1% milk for all the whole milk consumed, part–skim-milk cheese for whole-milk cheese and skim milk for all the low-fat milks consumed would markedly decrease total fat intake. Not all children will find the substitutes acceptable and not all will use them all the time. However, moderate changes in food consumption patterns would result in favorable changes in dietary intake for most children.[2(pp800–802)]

Mass media are another aspect of an individual's sociocultural environment that exerts considerable influence over behavior, including health behaviors. Television and print media provide models of various behaviors that result in vicarious learning about the social desirability of behaviors and their positive and negative consequences. For example, in examining nutrition, dieting and fitness messages in a magazine widely read by adolescent women from 1970 to 1990, Guillen and Barr[18] report that both nutrition-related and fitness-related coverage emphasized weight loss and physical appearance. Less emphasis was placed on the role of good nutrition in improving health and well-being. The volume of content on nutrition and weight loss did not change over time but the hip : waist ratio of models decreased, becoming less curvaceous and more linear. This is a clear indication that the cultural norm expected of women, "thinness," is becoming **more** evident in media despite national concern about unhealthy nutrition practices among adolescent women that may lead to eating disorders. The peak onset of eating disorders occurs during adolescence. Ironically, in the same magazine, candy and snacks were the most frequently advertised food products. Rapid changes in body shape may make adolescents particularly vulnerable to these confusing messages. This is cause for concern, since early adolescence is a time of high nutritional demands because of high growth rates, energy demands, and calcium and iron requirements related to onset of puberty and menstruation.

Ethnic and cultural backgrounds serve as important influences on eating behavior. Ethnic foods are a source of pride and identity for many groups and may have deep emotional meanings for individuals because of their association with their country of origin or because of fond childhood memories of holidays on which particular foods were served. Food-consumption patterns of some ethnic groups provide good role models for other cultural groups within American society. For example, Choi and colleagues[19] found that when the nutrition and health status of elderly Chinese-Americans in Boston were analyzed, these elderly subjects consumed a high-carbohydrate and low-fat diet, were physically active, and were seldom obese. Compared with elderly whites, they had lower mean blood pressures and blood levels of total and low-density lipoprotein (LDL) cholesterol. Interestingly, high-density lipoprotein (HDL) cholesterol was also lower. Even more fascinating were the dietary attitudes and behaviors of Chinese-American middle school students when compared to Chinese middle-school students living in China. Chinese students living in China consumed less meat, dairy products, fats, sweets and snacks, and fast foods and consumed more fruits, vegetables, and starches.[20] Story and Harris[21] assessed the meals and snack patterns, food practices and beliefs, and food preferences of 207 Southeast Asian refugee high-school students to determine the extent to which they adhered to their traditional cultural diet rather than an American diet. Results of the study indicated that the youth maintained strong ties to their native foods and traditional meal patterns. Rice remained the staple food in their diet. Fruits, meats, and soft drinks, high-status foods in Southeast Asia, remained preferences. In terms of dairy products, white milk was positively viewed but cheese was disliked. Foods with little nutritional value such as candy bars, cakes, and potato chips were not consumed frequently. Overall, the Asian-Americans had much healthier nutritional practices than European-Americans. Thus, the nurse should be alert to cultural groups that can serve as positive role models for healthy eating behaviors to other Americans. Sharing health-promoting cultural practices with the larger society is an important asset of our increasing cultural diversity in North America.

Recognition of and respect for individual food preferences is important for professional nurses in dealing with adults from a wide variety of cultural backgrounds. Suggestions for health promotion in diverse cultural communities that can be extrapolated to the promotion of good nutrition in various ethnic groups include[22]:

- Understand cultural beliefs about the interrelationships between food and health.
- Recognize how food consumption practices contribute to cultural identity.
- Assess the extent to which acculturation to dominant-group nutritional behaviors has taken place.
- Consult with nutritionists or nurses of similar ethnic backgrounds to clients.
- Form a group of lay consultants on nutritional practices from the target ethnic community.
- Recognize nutritional attributes of ethnic foods.
- Reinforce ethnic nutritional practices that are positive.
- Make recommendations, when necessary, for changing ingredients to lower saturated fats, cholesterol, and sodium or increase fiber while still retaining taste.
- Provide information on nutrient values of ethnic foods to clients.
- Work with ethnic restaurants to offer healthy choices that are acceptable to target populations.
- Promote increased consumption of nutritious ethnic foods among the general population.
- Incorporate healthy ethnic food choices into worksite and school site cafeterias and vending machines.

The nurse should also be sensitive to the difficulties that ethnic groups may have in identifying the contents of foods packaged in the United States and in understanding nutrition labeling. Inability to obtain foods familiar to them and trying to eat foods that are unfamiliar can be a source of considerable frustration and distress. Lack of money, language barriers, day-to-day stresses of an unfamiliar environment, and confusing messages on mass media about nutritious foods often serve as barriers to good nutrition among members of varying ethnic groups.[23]

As part of their client's sociocultural milieu, health professionals serve as important role models in terms of healthy eating patterns. Thus, nurses and other health professionals should not only advocate healthy diets for others but put the dietary guidelines into practice as a part of their own lifestyles. Modeling recommended eating behaviors as well as struggling with the issues that surround maintenance of positive nutritional practices will indicate a sincerity and commitment to good health practices that speaks louder than words to the clients that they serve.

Environmental Factors

The American food environment is slowly changing to support healthier eating behavior on the part of all Americans. For example, new mandatory food labels on all packaged foods contain more complete, useful, and accurate nutrition information than ever before. Improved labeling can assist individuals and families in making healthier food choices. Parents should include children and adolescents in grocery shopping and make them a part of the search for healthy, appealing foods. Learning by active decision making about food selections is one way to increase the nutrition awareness of youth.

In 1994, nutrient content claims (eg, reduced fat) and health claims (eg, decreases cholesterol) on food-product labels became regulated to eliminate misleading statements. A section called Nutrition Facts on each packaged food product now provides per serving values of nutrient information. Daily value percentages of nutrients are derived from recommended daily allowances (RDAs) and are based on a 2000 calorie diet.[24] Legislation and regulation to achieve truth in advertising and open disclosure of information on food constituents is an important step toward facilitating consumers' awareness and use of knowledge to make nutritious point-of-choice decisions about food purchases.

Many environmental barriers to healthful eating still remain. The complexities of modern life make it difficult for many individuals to consistently maintain access to foods rich in important nutrients. For example, it has been estimated that 8 out of 10 American households report eating out regularly, with an average of 3.7 times per week per individual.[25] The major environmental factors influencing eating patterns appear to be accessibility, convenience, and cost. These factors can present barriers to positive nutritional practices during the action phase of health behavior. Seasonal variation in availability of foods such as raw vegetables and fresh fruits determines both accessibility and costs. Seasonal patterns in the types of fruits and vegetables used by clients need to be followed to maximize nutrient quality and minimize cost. Use of frozen fruits and vegetables in their natural juices rather than those canned during off-season is recommended to decrease the intake of sugar and salt. Home-frozen products can also be an important source of nutrients at reasonable cost.

Convenience foods constitute 60% of the American diet. Unfortunately, the nutrient quality of many fast foods is questionable. Such foods are frequently high in fat, salt, and refined carbohydrates and low in dietary fiber and important nutrients. Vending machines often have only foods high in fats and highly refined sugars. If access to more nutritious foods is inconvenient, individuals often select the easiest options. Ease of preparation also plays an important role in food selection. Quick and effortless preparation techniques appeal to many families because of busy work schedules. In addition, attractiveness of prepared foods is an important consideration. Assisting the client in selecting nutritious foods that are quickly prepared and esthetically appealing increases the likelihood of sustaining positive eating behavior. Cost of food is also a critical consideration for many families, given the increasing numbers of families living at or below the poverty level. Sources of complex carbohydrates (fruits, vegetables, and grains) may exceed the cost of highly refined sugar products. Proteins also vary greatly in per-unit cost. Assisting families in identifying low-cost, high-nutrition options within their "choice" environments is an important responsibility of the nurse providing nutritional guidance to diverse populations.

In modern society, food additives are used to retard spoilage and prevent deterioration of quality, improve nutritional value, enhance consumer acceptability, and facilitate preparation. Types of additives include preservatives, coloring agents, flavorings, bleaching and maturing agents, and nutrition supplements. By law, labels of many products must list the manufacturer, packer, and distributor, and the amount of each ingredient. Even when ingredients are listed, information on the products is often by itself insufficient to guide knowledgeable food selection. Not only are potentially carcinogenic additives used in preparation of foods (eg, nitrosamines in bacon and saccharin in low-caloric carbonated beverages), but unintentional food additives such as pesticides and other agricultural chemicals may appear in foods. A great deal of research must be done on the safety of large numbers of food additives. Unfortunately, some of the synergistic, cumulative, and long-term effects of many additives will only be determined after years of use and exposure within human populations.

• NUTRITIONAL NEEDS OF SPECIAL POPULATIONS

Infants and Children

The caloric and nutrient intake of children are critical for supporting growth and development. Infants whose diet is primarily mother's milk or infant formula consume 40% or more of their calories from fat, which is appropriate during infancy. When children reach 2 years of age, however, they should be encouraged to consume a diet lower in total fat, saturated fat, and cholesterol than the usual American diet (36% to 40%) as a basis for lowering risk for chronic diseases in later years.

Iron deficiency is also a problem for 21% of low-income children 1 to 2 years of age and for 10% of low-income children 3 to 4 years of age. Chronic iron deficiency may have adverse effects on both early and later growth and development. Anemia, an index of iron deficiency, can result in decreased physical ability, impaired body temperature regulation, lowered resistance to infection, and alterations in intellectual performance. A healthy start for infants means encouraging mothers to breast-feed or use iron-rich formulas for formula-fed infants. It is important that during pregnancy and lactation mothers maintain sufficient iron intake through iron-rich foods or supplements, as this increases the likelihood that their children will not be iron deficient during the early years of life.[1(p122)]

Infants and children in child-care facilities should be provided with adequate nutrition. Cost consciousness on the part of caretakers should not interfere with the provision of good nutrition. It is important that parents monitor the food provided to their children in care facilities until they are assured that healthy nutrition guidelines are followed.

Adolescents

Adolescence is a period of biologic and social change. Biologically, body size, composition, functions, and physical abilities are changing rapidly. Undernutrition slows height and weight growth and can delay puberty. Among adolescents, minimal dietary requirements are those that maintain an optimal rate of pubertal development and growth. Adolescents who are vigorously active also have increased energy needs. Thus, adolescents should consume diets providing more total nutrients than they consumed as young children. Moderation is a good rule as adolescents whose caloric intake is too high will gain weight, potentially leading to obesity. Those whose caloric intake is too low will experience loss of energy, weight loss, and in the extreme, eating disorders that can lead to health problems and even premature death. Adolescents with chronic diseases such as diabetes have special nutrition needs, since absorption, metabolism, or excretion of particular nutrients may change both as a result of adolescent biologic changes and as a result of their disease.[26]

In terms of fat intake, adolescents should be given dietary counseling on how to reduce total fat to less than 30% of calories per day and cholesterol to less than 300 miligrams per day to lower risk factors for chronic disease. Since adolescents consume many fast foods at lunchtime or during the evening hours, selecting low-fat fast foods can be a real challenge. As an example of high-fat, fast-food meals, a meal of double burger with sauce, milkshake, and french fries contains 46% of total calories from fat. Since the goal should be less than 30% calories from fats, it is easy to see why consumption of such meals day after day can create conditions of high risk for cardiovascular disease as early as adolescence. There is accumulating evidence that this "risk" carries over into adulthood.[26]

Adolescent girls in the United States typically begin menstruating at 12 1/2 years of age. Menstrual losses increase the need for iron, as does physical activity. Thus, particular attention should be given to adequate intake of this mineral in the diet for women in general, and in particular, for female athletes. The mineral calcium helps to build strong bones. It is also thought that adequate intake of calcium throughout childhood to age 25 will reduce the risk of osteoporosis in later life. Thus, girls should receive counseling on selecting diets that ensure adequate calcium and iron intake.[27]

Adolescents have special nutritional needs that require the attention of adolescents themselves as well as their families and primary-care health professionals. Nurses play a critical role in heightening awareness of the importance of good nutrition to overall adolescent health and performance. The challenge is to make nutritious food options appealing to adolescents who may eat primarily for taste rather than for nutritional or health reasons. Peer support for healthy eating practices is also critical, as the desire to be accepted by peers is extremely high during the adolescent years. Meal skipping contributes to poor nutrition and should be discouraged. Eating fast food but selecting lower-fat options creates opportunities for adolescents to be with their peers and yet limit fat intake. Pressure on fast food establishments to offer healthier options is also essential to creating a supportive environment for healthy nutritional practices among adolescents.

Schools have been increasingly used in the last few years by health professionals as a vehicle for early health-promotion and prevention activities. As of 1992, 9 states mandated nutrition education as a separate activity and another 21 included it as a required topic in mandated subjects such as health. The remaining states did not require it.[10(pp102–103)] Efforts on the part of major national health organizations should be directed toward ensuring that nutritional education is a part of all K-through-12 education programs. Efforts should also be made to integrate nutrition concepts throughout the entire curriculum including into courses where it is not traditionally taught, such as math, chemistry, and history.

Older Adults

Research on the nutritional needs of the elderly is expanding rapidly as the American population ages. Aging is thought to alter nutrient requirements for calories, protein, and other nutrients as a result of changes in lean body mass, physical activity, and intestinal absorption. Although many older Americans maintain healthy eating patterns, for some, changing nutritional needs may be accompanied by deterioration in diet quality and quantity, jeopardizing nutritional status, quality of life, and functional independence. Many elderly people skip meals and exclude whole categories of food from their diet because of reduced appetites, infrequent grocery shopping, lack of energy to cook, and difficulties in chewing and swallowing. For these individuals, supplementation may be required but should be initiated in consultation with health professionals. Too much self-medication can result in toxic levels of some vitamin and mineral supplements.[26(pp1–18)]

A word needs to be said about the interaction of foods and drugs. With polypharmacy common in older adults, some may take medications that interact with foods, decreasing nutrient absorption. Foods and drugs can interact, increasing the absorption of some foods and drugs and decreasing the absorption of others. The rate of absorption or the total level of absorption of drugs or nutrients may be affected. For example, crackers, dates, jelly, and other carbohydrates may slow down the rate of absorption of analgesics and limit their effectiveness in reducing pain. Milk, eggs, cereals, and dairy products can inhibit the absorption of iron. Antibiotics such as tetracycline are less readily absorbed when milk, dairy products, or iron supplements are taken. Prune juice, bran cereal, and high-fiber foods can increase intestinal emptying time to the point where some drugs cannot be adequately absorbed. There is a need for further exploration of food–drug interactions that commonly occur among the elderly.

For individuals over 65 years of age, recommended eating patterns lower in saturated fatty acids, total fat, and cholesterol help maintain desired body weight and lower the risk of CHD; generally these are nutritionally adequate. High-fat diets contribute to the overall risk of CHD. Risk factors are as follows: being male or a postmenopausal female, having a family history of premature CHD, cigarette smoking, hypertension, high

LDL cholesterol level, low HDL cholesterol concentration, diabetes mellitus, history of cerebrovascular or occlusive peripheral vascular disease, and severe obesity. All of these factors except cigarette smoking are influenced by diet in some way. Thus, there is international consensus among scientists that CHD is linked to nutritional pattern throughout life, with the ravages of risk manifest most frequently in middle-aged and older adults. Daily activity along with an adequate diet can prevent premature mortality from heart disease and maintain vigor into old age.[16(p23)]

The diets of older Americans generally would be healthier if they contained more complex carbohydrates and fiber. Many elderly people have tooth or mouth problems that make eating fruits and vegetables difficult. Average fiber intake among the elderly is less than half the recommended 20 to 35 grams. Health benefits attributed to fiber include proper bowel function, reduced risk of colon cancer, reduction of serum cholesterol, and improved glucose response. Six servings of whole grains are the recommended minimum for the elderly.

Energy requirements decline with reductions in body size, lean body mass, basal metabolism rate, and decreased physical activity. Because physical activity maintains muscle mass, it is highly desirable to keep physically active in later years. Diets of the elderly may also be deficient in protein along with calories as the result of inability to chew meat or the cost of protein-rich foods. Infections, trauma, and other metabolic stresses may increase protein needs. Protein-calorie malnutrition can lower resistance to disease and delay recovery from illness.[24(pp1–18)]

Older adults of limited economic means should be assisted in selecting low-cost foods that meet recommended nutritional requirements. They may need guidance on using label information to select foods and on how to prepare foods so that they are easier to chew and swallow. Nutrition is integral to quality of life for the elderly. Thus, it is a primary area for focus by nurses providing care to the elderly in primary care and long-term care settings.

• INTERVENTIONS TO CHANGE EATING BEHAVIORS

The functional health pattern inclusive of eating behaviors is the Nutritional-Metabolic Pattern. Gordon[28] describes this area of functional assessment as patterns of food and fluid consumption relative to metabolic need. Nursing diagnoses relevant to health promotion include: Altered nutrition: high risk for more than body requirements, Altered nutrition: more than body requirements, and Altered nutrition: less than body requirements. Diagnoses focus on the categories of obesity and undernutrition. An overview of definitions, defining characteristics, and etiologic or related factors can be found in Gordon's *Manual of Nursing Diagnosis: 1993–1994.*

Improving eating patterns involves changing knowledge, attitudes, and skills as well as the food consumption environment. Three key strategies recommended by the Food and Nutrition Board are to (1) enhance awareness, understanding, and acceptance of dietary recommendations for healthy eating; (2) create legislative, regulatory, commercial, and educational environments supportive of the recommendations; and (3) improve the availability of foods and meals that facilitate implementation of dietary recommendations.[29]

Altering nutrition education, the food acquisition environment, and food consumption patterns will all contribute to health. To alter nutrition education, there must be wide exposure of the general population at all ages to nutrition education through mass media, education at schools and worksites, do-it-yourself nutrition education packages, and nutrition counseling in primary health care services. New information technology must be used while at the same time making sure that nutrition education approaches are user-friendly. Interactive computer nutrition programs, nutrition videos, and integration of healthy nutrition messages into packaging are all important in broad-based nutrition education. The dietary advice offered needs to evolve as scientific discoveries about the contribution of diet to health take place.

The food acquisition environment still must undergo considerable change. It is affected by legislation and regulation regarding production of foodstuffs and by availability of food options. Many populations at schools and worksites are captive and rely primarily on others to provide and prepare their food for a considerable part of the day. The availability of healthy options within the environment, such as from cafeterias and vending machines, greatly affect nutrition behaviors. Furthermore, healthy food choices must have appeal in terms of taste and texture. Widespread research in the food production industry is creating more food options that are both consistent with dietary recommendations and acceptable to the public.

Food consumption patterns are not only affected by knowledge and availability but by the decision-making patterns of the individual or family. Kiosks at grocery stores and shopping malls to query about nutrients in specific foods as well as simple coding systems for fat, sodium, and fiber content all provide cues and easy assistance to consumers in making food selections.

The development of large-scale, low-cost strategies for changing eating behavior is an increasingly important goal for scientists in the fields of nutrition and behavior. Specific interventions to change eating behaviors of various groups are increasingly evaluated in the research literature. Several of these interventions are described below.

The San Diego Medicare Preventive Health Project

The San Diego Medicare Preventive Health Project[30] is one of five 6-year demonstration projects currently funded by the Health Care Financing Administration (HCFA) to examine the cost-effectiveness of adding selected preventive services, including nutrition education, to Medicare benefits. In a controlled clinical trial, 1800 members of a health maintenance organization were selected and randomly assigned to a preventive-care (intervention) group or a regular-care (control) group. The preventive-care intervention, implemented by students in the health sciences, was based primarily on Kanfer's model of self-control and self-regulation. Kanfer proposes that ability for self-change is a result of skill in (a) self-monitoring, (b) goal setting, (c) self-evaluation, and (d) self-reinforcement.[31] These processes comprised critical elements of the intervention. The preventive care group received counseling based on health-risk appraisal, assistance in goal setting, and a series of eight group health-promotion sessions. Nutrition information focused on drinking enough water; eating complex carbohydrates and fiber; eating enough protein; reducing fat, sugar, and sodium intake; and eating a variety of healthy foods. Of the subjects, 32% set a nutrition-related goal. In examining behavioral outcomes that the nutrition interventions sought to influence at 12-month follow-up it was found that intervention subjects decreased their fat intake (red meat, gravy, butter, fried foods) and caffeine consumption significantly more than control subjects. Surprisingly, control subjects showed a significantly greater increase in fiber intake relative to intervention subjects. Although a limitation of the study was self-reporting of nutrition intake, the noted changes in nutrition behaviors were encouraging. Further collection of data at 24, 36, and 48 months will determine if the changes were maintained or if additional booster sessions are necessary to alter eating and other health behaviors over the long term.

Point-of-Choice Intervention Programs

Mayer et al [25(pp31–43)] reviewed a number of research studies focused on the evaluation of interventions aimed at promoting healthy nutritional decisions at the "point of choice" in dining establishments and supermarkets. Of American families, 90% shop in supermarkets at least once every 2 weeks, and 8 out of 10 households report eating out regularly, with an average of 3.7 times per week per individual. Thus, the opportunity to reach a large number of people with point-of-choice nutrition interventions is high. Of the studies reviewed by Mayer and colleagues, six in supermarkets used brochures, shelf signs, posters, take-home fliers, and media to decrease fat, cholesterol, sugar, and total calories and increase the nutrient density of foods purchased. Only two studies showed changes in sales data of targeted items. In one study, a decrease in purchase of 3 of 5 targeted high-fat foods was noted. In the other study, sales of low-sugar cereals increased and high-sugar cereals decreased. Thus, much work yet remains to make point-of-choice nutrition interventions in supermarkets effective.

Eight studies reported interventions conducted in restaurants and cafeterias consisting of use of posters, labels, rebates, incentives, and nutrition games. The interventions focused on increasing the proportion of nutritious (eg, low-fat) foods purchased. All of the studies reported positive outcomes such as increased sales of low-calorie salads and vegetables, low-fat entrees, and skim milk and decreased purchase of desserts and breads. Incentives such as coupons, rebates, and specials on healthy foods tended to increase healthy choices in the studies in which they were used compared to provision of information (signs and labels) only. Further studies of the relative effectiveness of specific strategies and combinations of strategies in supermarkets, restaurants, and cafeterias to promote healthy nutrition are warranted. These studies are particularly important as they are contextually based in settings where a large number of individuals and families frequently make dietary decisions.

The San Diego Family Health Project

The San Diego Family Health Project[32] was a randomized controlled trial designed to test the effect of a family-based cardiovascular health intervention program. The behavioral goals to be achieved through the program were to increase the level of physical activity and decrease fat and sodium intake among family members. Families of fifth- and sixth-graders were recruited from 12 elementary schools. In half of the schools, Mexican-American families were recruited and in the other half, Anglo families were recruited. A total of 60 families (30 from each ethnic group) were recruited and randomly assigned to the intervention or control group. No significant differences were found at baseline between groups on dietary intake of fat, sodium, or total calories or on amount of exercise as measured by the Seven-Day Activity Recall. The 1-year intervention program was based on social learning theory and structured into 12 weeks of intensive intervention followed by six maintenance sessions distributed over 9 months at area schools. Each intervention session consisted of four parts: aerobic exercise, separate adult and child education segments, behavior management segment to set short-term goals, and heart-healthy snacks prepared by a different family each week. Session 1 provided training in self-monitoring, sessions 2 to 4 focused on physical activity, sessions 5 to 7 on sodium intake, sessions 8 to 10 on saturated and total fat intake, session 11 integrated all areas, and session 12 was a heart-healthy potluck dinner. Maintenance sessions covered behavior chaining, restaurants, grocery shopping, peer pressure, and planned and unplanned breaks in exercise and dietary routines. Five months after completion of the intervention, families were invited to the San Diego Zoo, where physical activities and eating behaviors could be monitored. During observation periods, observers noted which foods were purchased and which foods were consumed. Nutritional content for all food sold in concession stands in the zoo was provided. The amount of calories, fat, and sodium consumed was calculated for each subject. If the family had brought food with them, the mothers were interviewed as to what foods they had brought and nutritional content was subsequently calculated and divided by the number of persons in the family to estimate individual nutrient intake. Nutritional analysis of foods brought to the zoo indicated food brought by intervention families contained fewer calories and milligrams of sodium than control families' food. In foods eaten at the zoo, intervention group members ate fewer calories than control group members. Results indicate the effectiveness of such an intervention program that targets entire families rather than individuals and the feasibility of direct observation of dietary behaviors.

The Partners in Prevention Nutrition Program

This intervention[33] used a stage-of-change approach, based on the transtheoretical model developed by Prochaska et al,[34] to match tailored communications about dietary behavior to the needs of participants at different points in the change process. The 558 adult participants were recruited from four family practices in central North Carolina. The study sample was 73% female, 62.3% married, 19% minority (predominantly African-American) with a mean education level of 13.6 years, average age of 40.8 years, and median income level of $30,000 to $39,000. A randomized trial was used with pretest and posttest measures to determine the impact of tailored versus nontailored nutrition education materials on consumption of fat, fruit, and vegetables. Current dietary intake, stage of change in regard to dietary behavior, self-efficacy for dietary change, beliefs concerning perceived susceptibility to diet-related diseases, perceived benefits of dietary change to avoid health problems, and other psychosocial and physical variables were assessed at baseline. Participants were categorized at baseline as being in one of the following stages: precontemplation (not seriously thinking about change), contemplation (seriously thinking about change within the next 6 months), preparation (planning to change within the next 30 days), or action or maintenance (currently trying to change). Participants were randomly assigned to one of three groups: tailored nutrition messages, nontailored nutrition messages, or a control group that received no nutrition messages. Messages were mailed to participants 3 weeks after collection of baseline data. The tailored intervention consisted of a one-time, mailed nutrition information packet customized to participant's stage of change, dietary intake, and psychosocial information. For example, contemplators received information designed to decrease barriers to change and increase self-efficacy. Those individuals already trying to change received tailored recipes and messages aimed at preventing relapse. The nontailored messages provided standard risk information about the relation of diet to disease and gave dietary recommendations based on the *1990 Dietary Guidelines for Americans.*[8] The control group completed pretest and posttest surveys but received no nutrition information.

Members of the tailored message group, when surveyed approximately 6 months later, had significantly decreased total fat by 23% compared to 9% in the nontailored group and 3% in the control group. The tailored group reported decreased saturated fat by 26%, compared to 11% in the nontailored group and 3% in the control group. The tailored message did not affect reported intake of fruits and vegetables. Also, more individuals in the tailored message group, compared to the other groups, remembered receiving and reading the nutrition information packet. Thus, the stage-of-change approach to dietary modification looks promising. Further research is needed to determine whether interventions based on the transtheoretical model can be used to promote maintenance of dietary changes.

The Waianae Diet Program

The Waianae Diet Program[35] is an excellent example of a culturally sensitive program to change eating behaviors of the native Haiwaiian population, who have a disproportionately high rate of obesity. In 1993, the program received the Distinguished Community Health Promotion Program Award from the US Secretary for Health and Human Services. The primary intervention is a 3-week program of adhering to a strict, traditional Hawaiian diet with medical monitoring. Historical evidence suggests that prior to the adoption of western diets, Native Hawaiians had little cardiovascular disease or obesity.

The intervention includes a number of components. In the evenings, community participants come together to eat traditional foods such as taro (a starchy root similar to potato), poi (a mashed form of taro), sweet potatoes, yams, breadfruit, greens, fruit, seaweed, fish, and chicken. This diet approximates that of ancient Hawaiians, which was estimated to contain less than 10% fat, 12% to 15% protein, and 75% to 78% carbohydrates. Participants also attend educational sessions, which include cultural teachings, nutrition education, and motivational sessions. They are taught techniques for using the diet as a template for making food choices. A whole-person approach, with emphasis on spiritual aspects of living and group *ohana* (familylike) support, are additional features. Participants are particularly encouraged to act as role models for the modified eating behaviors they have learned. The program is viewed as a strategy for community empowerment, bringing community members together to address a problem they want to solve.

Early results suggest that the Waianae Diet Program has been successful. Weight, cholesterol, low-density lipoproteins (LDL), triglycerides, glucose, and systolic and diastolic blood pressures have decreased significantly in participants. Long-term evaluation is necessary to determine if modified eating behaviors and their health benefits can be sustained. The unique aspects of the program offer particular insight into how changes in dietary behavior can be integrated into the cultural, spiritual, recreational, and social aspects of participant's life perspective. This whole-person approach, espoused by nursing, may decrease the problems with compliance to new dietary behaviors evident in so many prior studies.

• MAINTAINING RECOMMENDED WEIGHT

Obesity is generally defined as being 20% or more overweight by standard height and weight tables. While the physical basis for excessive weight gain is relatively simple and straightforward (ie, the ingestion of more calories than needed for energy expenditure) the actual causes of being overweight are complex. They include:

1. Heredity
2. Cognitive factors (eg, unrealistic personal standards and expectations)
3. Affective factors (eg, emotional problems such as anxiety, boredom, and feelings of powerlessness)
4. Interpersonal factors (eg, family problems, difficulties with fellow workers or colleagues)
5. Sociocultural factors (food selection, food preparation, and food consumption practices)
6. Environmental factors (eg, salient cues for eating behavior and level of environmental sensitivity)

Although heredity plays a role in predisposition toward excessive weight gain, it is more important to focus on personal (cognitive, affective), interpersonal, sociocultural, and environmental influences.

The primary goal of interventions for weight loss is the permanent alteration of eating patterns and physical activity, rather than weight loss only. Actually, adopting more healthful eating behaviors is directed toward increasing rather than decreasing the pleasures derived from eating. New awareness of taste, texture, and form of foods allows the individual to participate to the fullest in the eating experience, totally involving gustatory, visual, olfactory, and tactile senses. Eating that promotes optimum health can be fulfilling, self-actualizing, and totally enjoyable.

The individual who maintains desired weight has taken a major step toward decreasing risk for many chronic health problems. Average recommended caloric intake for men and women of difference ages to maintain weight, assuming that they are moderately active, appears in Table 10–3. Not only does weight loss decrease the risk of chronic disease, it has been shown to increase self-esteem, perceptions of control, and feelings of social desirability and acceptance. Individuals of normal weight are more active than their overweight counterparts, and this further promotes health and decreases risk for health problems. On the other hand, frequent bouts of weight loss may be detrimental to health, as serum cholesterol is elevated during weight loss. Adipocytes are the fat cells within the body that increase in lipid content with weight gain. Weight reduction is achieved though decrease in size of cells. As increased by-products of fat metabolism enter systemic circulation, precautions must be taken to prevent their deposit in the lining of vessels and their detrimental effects to internal organs such as liver and kidneys. Stability of weight can prevent many of these potential hazards.

TABLE 10–3. AVERAGE RECOMMENDED CALORIC INTAKE FOR MEN AND WOMEN OF DIFFERENT AGES: MODERATE ACTIVITY (In kilocalories)

	MEN		WOMEN	
AGE	Mean	Range	Mean	Range
19–22	2900	2500–3000	2100	1700–2500
23–50	2700	2300–3100	2000	1600–2400
51–75	2400	2000–2800	1800	1400–2200
over 75	2050	1650–2450	1600	1200–2000

• INITIATING A WEIGHT-REDUCTION PROGRAM

The individual who desires to lose more than 20 pounds should obtain a medical history, physical examination, blood lipid and glucose analysis, and electrocardiogram before beginning a weight-loss program. Also, careful assessment of current dietary habits is essential in order to develop an individualized, effective program.

Other points to consider include the following:

- Is the person strongly motivated to change?
- Are there health conditions that make weight reduction a high priority?
- If change is desired, are expectations realistic?
- Does the person have a support system within or outside of the family to facilitate weight loss?
- Has the person had past successes in weight loss? If so, what worked? What did not work?

The best weight-loss program will be one that closely mirrors the *Dietary Guidelines* described earlier. Caloric reduction while maintaining adequate nutrient levels, adequate vitamins and minerals, and adequate fiber is the best way to achieve and maintain desired weight. Thus radical changes in food consumption patterns are not recommended as a means of weight loss.

A combination of dietary modifications that individuals find palatable and adequate exercise offer the best approach to achieving and maintaining recommended weight. Physical activity promotes expenditure of energy and can facilitate weight loss. Exercise is not only useful in burning excess calories; studies have suggested that it also prevents the loss of protein from muscle and minerals from bone that frequently occur when attempts at weight loss are accompanied by inactivity. Exercise in combination with restricted calories also assists in reducing undesirable lipoprotein lipids, increasing work capacity, lowering resting heart rate, and decreasing blood pressure. Increased physical activity generally decreases appetite and increases basal metabolism rate for several hours, offsetting the reduced metabolic rate that accompanies calorie restriction.[36] Further, positive changes in affect and mood that often accompany exercise can improve the long-term compliance with newly acquired eating behaviors. Both exercise during leisure time and lifestyle exercise should be increased as a complement to healthy nutritional practices. The reader is referred to Chapter 9 for discussion of further benefits of exercise and how to facilitate exercise adherence.

DIRECTIONS FOR NUTRITION RESEARCH

Further research is needed to understand the links between nutrition and health. Studies on the effects of fats, fiber, and sodium on the development of cardiovascular disorders and cancer are only a beginning. Further research is needed to explore the positive and negative effects of various food components on health as well as on specific disorders. A better understanding of factors related to undernutrition, particularly eating disorders in adolescents and young adults, and overnutrition is critically needed as a basis for effective nursing interventions.

To promote healthy eating habits across the life span, behavioral theories and models applicable to eating behavior should be tested predictively and, as warranted, incorporated into intervention studies. Existing theories in nursing, psychology, and public health can be used to design behavioral intervention evaluations that focus on the individual, the family, and the community. Studies should be conducted where assessments based on factors influencing eating behavior for a given individual allow determination of the most appropriate behavioral model to employ to augment positive eating behaviors. The availability of new technology provides the base for developing such powerful assessment tools to facilitate tailoring of nutrition interventions.

Nutrition is a powerful tool for positively influencing health. Further research will provide additional answers concerning the underlying mechanisms through which nutrition influences health and well-being.

SUMMARY

Professional support of the client by the nurse and suggestions for constructively dealing with barriers to changing eating behaviors will facilitate the client's efforts to eliminate or minimize obstacles that block attainment of desired nutritional goals. Promoting good nutrition is a critical concern in illness prevention and health promotion and an important dimension of competent self-care and dependent care. Cultural background is a major influence on eating behavior. The family and community should be considered as points for nutritional intervention that may, in the long run, be more productive than individual interventions. Since much is yet to be learned about nutrition and health, nurses and other health scientists should accept the challenge of exploring eating behavior as an important health-promotion activity.

REFERENCES

1. *Healthy People 2000: National Health Promotion and Disease Prevention Objectives.* Washington, DC: US Public Health Service; 1991. US Dept of Health and Human Services publication PHS 91-50212.
2. Thompson FE, Dennison BA. Dietary sources of fats and cholesterol in US children aged 2 through 5 years. *Am J Public Health.* 1994;84:799–806.
3. Gormaker SL, Dietz WH, Sobol AM, et al. Increasing pediatric obesity in the United States. *Am J Dis Child.* 1987;141:535–540.

4. Haddock CK, Shadish WR, Klesges RC, et al. Treatments for childhood and adolescent obesity. *Ann Behav Med.* 1994;16:235–244.
5. Committee on Diet and Health, Food and Nutrition Board, National Research Council. *Diet and Health: Implications for Reducing Chronic Disease Risk.* Washington, DC: National Academy Press; 1989.
6. National Cholesterol Education Program. *Report of the Expert Panel on Population Strategies for Blood Cholesterol Reduction: Executive Summary;* 1990. National Heart Lung & Blood Institute, National Institutes of Health publication NIH 90-3047.
7. Cox RH. Dietary cancer risks of low-income African-American and white women. *Fam Community Health.* 1994;17(3):49–59.
8. US Dept of Agriculture, US Dept of Health and Human Services. *Nutrition and Your Health: Dietary Guidelines for Americans.* 3rd ed. Washington, DC: US Government Printing Office; 1990. Publication USDA HG-232.
9. *Food Guide Pyramid.* Washington, DC: US Dept of Agriculture; 1992. Publication USDA HG-249.
10. Dwyer JT. Diet and nutritional strategies for cancer risk reduction: focus on the 21st century. *Cancer.* 1993;72(suppl):1024–1031.
11. Kritchevsky D. Dietary guidelines: the rationale for intervention. *Cancer.* 1993;72 (suppl):1011–1014.
12. Morley JE. Neuropeptide regulation of appetite and weight. *Endoc Rev.* 1987;8:256–287.
13. Morley JE, Mooradian AD, Silver AJ, et al. Nutrition in the elderly. *Ann Internal Med.* 1988;109:890–904.
14. Louis Harris Associates. *The Kellogg's Child Nutrition Survey.* New York, NY: Louis Harris and Associates; 1989.
15. Martin RA, Poland EY. *Learning to Change: A Self-Management Approach to Adjustment.* New York, NY: McGraw-Hill Inc; 1980:56.
16. National Cholesterol Education Program. *Report of the Expert Panel on Blood Cholesterol Levels in Children and Adolescents.* Bethesda, Md: US Dept. of Health and Human Services, 1991. US Dept of Health and Human Services publication NIH 91-2732.
17. American Academy of Pediatrics Committee on Nutrition. Statement on cholesterol. *Pediatrics.* 1992;90:469–473.
18. Guillen EO, Barr SI. Nutrition, dieting, and fitness messages in a magazine for adolescent women, 1970–1990. *J Adolesc Health.* 1994;15:464–472.
19. Choi ESK, McGandy RB, Dallal GE, et al. The prevalence of cardiovascular risk factors among elderly Chinese-Americans. *Arch Intern Med.* 1990;150:413–418.
20. Sun WY, Chen W. A preliminary study of potential dietary risk factors for coronary heart disease among Chinese-American adolescents. *J School Health.* 1994;64:368–371.
21. Story M, Harris LJ. Food preferences, beliefs, and practices of Southeast Asian refugee adolescents. *J School Health.* 1988;58:273–276.
22. Gonzalez VM, Gonzalez JT, Freeman V, et al. *Health Promotion in Diverse Cultural Communities.* Palo Alto, Calif: Health Promotion Resource Center, Stanford Center for Research in Health Promotion and Disease Prevention; 1991.
23. Gutierrez YM. *Nutrition in Health Maintenance and Health Promotion for Primary Care Providers.* San Francisco, Calif: School of Nursing, University of California, San Francisco; 1994.
24. Wellman NS. Dietary guidelines and nutrient requirements of the elderly. *Prim Care.* 1994;21(1):1–18.
25. Mayer JA, Dubbert PM, Elder JP. Promoting nutrition at the point of choice: a review. *Health Educ Q.* 1989;16(1):31–43.

26. US Congress, Office of Technology Assessment. *Adolescent Health Volume II: Background and the Effectiveness of Selected Prevention and Treatment Services.* Washington, DC: US Government Printing Office; 1991: II193–II228. Publication OTA-H-466.
27. National Academy of Sciences, National Research Council. *Diet and Health: Implications for Reducing Chronic Disease Risk.* Washington, DC: National Academy Press; 1989.
28. Gordon M. *Manual of Nursing Diagnosis. 1993–1994.* St Louis, Mo: Mosby Year Book; 1993.
29. Institute of Medicine, Committee on Dietary Guidelines Implementation. Improving America's diet and health: from recommendations to action. In: Lewis PR, ed. A Report of the Committee on Dietary Guidelines Implementation, Food and Nutrition Board, National Academy of Sciences. Washington, DC: National Academy Press; 1991.
30. Mayer JA, Jermanovich A, Wright BL, et al. Changes in health behaviors of older adults: the San Diego Medicare Preventive Health Project. *Prev Med.* 1994;23:127–133.
31. Kanfer FH. The many faces of self-control or behavior modification changes its focus. In: Stuart R, ed. *Behavioral Self-Management.* New York, NY: Brunner/Mazel Inc; 1977.
32. Patterson TL, Sallis JF, Nader PR, et al. Direct observation of physical activity and dietary behaviors in a structured environment: effects of a family-based health promotion program. *J Behav Med.* 1988;11:447–458.
33. Campbell MK, DeVellis BM, Strecher VJ, et al. Improving dietary behavior: the effectiveness of tailored messages in primary care settings. *Am J Public Health.* 1994;84:783–787.
34. Prochaska JA, DiClemente C, Norcross J. In search of how people change: applications to addictive behaviors. *Am Psychol.* 1992;47:1102–1114.
35. Shintani T, Beckham S, Kanawaliwali H, et al. The Waianae Diet Program: a culturally sensitive, community-based obesity and clinical intervention program for the native Hawaiian population. *Hawaii Med J.* 1994;53:136–147.
36. Bray GA. Exercise and obesity. In: Bouchard C, Shephard RJ, Stephens T, et al., eds. *Exercise, Fitness, and Health: A Consensus of Current Knowledge.* Champaign, Ill: Human Kinetics; 1990:497–510.

11

Stress Management

Stress is of both theoretical and practical interest to nurses. Nurse researchers have studied various aspects of stress in attempts to understand the stress–illness relationship as well as how to promote health through fostering stress resistance and overall resilience among individuals and families. It is estimated that 60% to 90% of visits to health care professionals are for stress-related disorders.[1] With this high an incidence of stress-related health problems, strategies for promoting stress reduction among clients are of critical importance to minimize insults to well-being and maximize positive challenge and realization of personal potential.

Stress is an inevitable human experience in any modern society characterized by rapid and accelerating change. Selye, a pioneer in stress research, defined stress as "the nonspecific response of the body to any demand made on it." Internal and external manifestations of stress are referred to by Selye as the General Adaptation Syndrome (GAS) or the "fight-or-flight" response. Specific physiologic or behavioral changes that occur in response to stressors include:

- Dilatation of pupils
- Increased respiratory rate
- Increased heart rate

- Peripheral vasoconstriction
- Increased perspiration
- Increased blood pressure
- Increased muscle tension
- Increased gastric motility
- Release of adrenalin
- Increased blood glucose level
- Raising of body hair
- Cold and clammy hands

The major sources of distress experienced by individuals in modern society originate in interpersonal relationships (communication) and performance demands (action) rather than from direct physical threat. Since communication and action represent two basic human processes, the potential for stress is always present.[2]

Stressors, the cause of stress, are defined by Lazarus and Folkman[3] as "environmental and internal demands and conflicts among them, which tax or exceed a person's resources." The body's response to stress involves the nervous, endocrine, and immunologic systems, which in turn affect all organ systems. Although all individuals experience stress, people interpret and react to it differently, resulting in differing vulnerabilities to the deleterious effects of stress. Some stressors are viewed as challenges, creating stimulation and excitement. Other stressors are viewed negatively, perhaps because they are considered undesirable, uncontrollable, or emotionally distressing. There is much scientific interest in the "resistance resources" that enable some individuals to successfully manage stressors and flourish while others find the same stressors debilitating.

Coping strategies assist individuals in dealing with stress and can be described as learned and purposeful cognitive, emotional, and behavioral responses to stressors used to adapt to the environment or to change it.[3] In the coping process, the ability to regulate emotions, behavior, and the environment are critical to successful adjustment. Cognitive appraisal and coping constitute the stress-coping process. Cognitive appraisal consists of two phases. In **primary appraisal,** the person evaluates whether he or she has anything at stake in the encounter. Is there potential harm or benefit to cherished commitments, values, goals, self-esteem, or the health and well-being of a significant other? In **secondary appraisal,** the person evaluates what if anything can be done to overcome or prevent harm or to improve the prospects of benefit. Various coping options are evaluated, such as altering the situation, accepting it, seeking more information, or holding back from acting in an impulsive way. Primary and secondary appraisals converge to determine if the person–environment transaction is primarily threatening or challenging.[4] Coping regulates stressful emotions (emotion-focused coping) and alters the person–environment relation that is causing the distress (problem-focused coping). Both forms of coping occur in stressful encounters. The success of problem-focused coping may in large part depend on the success of emotion-focused coping, since heightened emotions are likely to interfere with cognitive activity necessary to deal effectively with stressors. Problem-focused coping is likely to be dominant in encounters viewed as changeable, whereas emotion-focused coping often dominates in encounters viewed as unchangeable, with acceptance as the only recourse.[3(p294)] Encounters involving threat to self-esteem are often the most difficult to resolve. These threats include the possibility of losing the affection of someone one cares about, losing self-respect or the respect of others, and appearing to be unethical or incompetent.

It is estimated that disability, absenteeism, decreased productivity, and health-damaging effects of stress cost business and industry $150 billion annually. Thus, there are considerable financial incentives to businesses and health maintenance organizations to help individuals manage stress and avoid its costly, health-impairing effects.

The importance of developing healthy coping mechanisms is stressed in *Healthy People 2000* as critical to mental and emotional health. The following national goals have been identified[5]:

- Decrease to no more than 5% the proportion of people aged 18 and older who report experiencing significant levels of stress who do not take steps to reduce or control stress. (Baseline: 21% in 1985)
- Reduce to less than 35% the proportion of people aged 18 and older who experienced adverse health effects from stress within the past year. (Baseline: 42.6% in 1985)
- Increase to at least 40% the proportion of worksites employing 50 or more people that provide programs to reduce employee stress. (Baseline: 26.6% in 1985)

Although these goals focus on adults and the experience of debilitating stress, children and adolescents are also subject to numerous stressors in their daily lives. Thus, the stress-coping process throughout the life span and its importance to health and well-being are the focus of this chapter.

• STRESS AND HEALTH

Stress is linked to decreased life satisfaction, the development of mental disorders, the occurrence of stress-related illnesses (cardiovascular disease, gastrointestinal disorders, low back pain, headaches, etc), and decreased immunologic functioning, which has been implicated in cancer. In terms of heart disease, long-term stress is thought to sensitize arterioles to catecholamines, with even short-term stress responses causing overconstriction of the vessels and endothelial damage. Repetitive overconstriction can lead to hypertension, decreased myocardial perfusion, and arrhythmias.[6]

Social factors are considered to be intimately related to the experience of stress and subsequently to health and disease. In a review of a number of prospective studies, social isolation was found to increase morbidity and mortality, particularly among the elderly, poor, and black populations, even after controlling for possible confounding factors.[7] In other instances, the nature of interpersonal relationships may be detrimental to health. For example, the chronic stress of taking care of a family member with Alzheimer's disease has been associated with negative changes in immune function, particularly if the caregiver perceives little social support to be available.[8] Since both the absence of social relations and certain characteristics of social relations serve as stressors that can have an impact on health, understanding how social relationships affect the brain, physiologic processes, and health is of critical importance.[9]

Psychoneuroimmunology examines the effects of social and psychologic phenomena on the immune system as mediated by the nervous and endocrine systems. This arena of science is particularly important, since both acute and chronic infections as well as cancer have been linked to compromised immune functioning. In a series of studies, male undergraduate college students with high heart-rate reactivity to stressors (mental arithmetic test with noise superimposed) were compared to low heart-rate reactors on neuroendocrine and immune responses to stressors. High reactors compared to low showed higher stress-related levels of plasma cortisol and increased natural killer (NK) cell lysis. The finding that cortisol was elevated in high reactors is particularly interesting in view of the extensive literature linking cortisol with down-regulation of multiple aspects of cellular immune function. These findings suggest that interindividual variation in activation of the hypothalamic-pituitary-adrenocortical axis by brief psychologic stressors may explain why daily stressors have greater health consequences for some individuals than for others. Different mediating roles may be played by the hypothalamic-pituitary-adrenocortical axis and the sympathetic adrenomedullary systems. It appears that the immune system is influenced by central nervous system processes that are shaped by social psychologic factors.[9]

Although it has long been known that reduced cell-mediated immune function is found in depressed patients, Irwin and colleagues[10] compared 36 matched pairs of hospitalized depressed patients and nondepressed controls. Stressors were assessed in two categories in both groups: life events (discrete stressors) and difficulties (ongoing stressors in the individual's life). Both depressed patients and control subjects without signs of clinical depression but reporting high stress showed comparable reductions in NK cytotoxicity. Several biologic mechanisms common to states of depression and sustained high stress may mediate immunologic changes. Sleep disturbances and loss of slow-wave sleep may alter the secretory response of interleukin-1, important to the stimulation of NK cells. Furthermore, elevated concentrations of plasma catecholamines, often associated with depression, also have been correlated with suppression of NK activity. In yet another study, daily events were found to be associated with fluctuations in immune response. Immune response was measured by salivary immunoglobulin A (sIgA), a factor related to host defense. In a community-living sample of 96 men who completed daily event questionnaires, day-to-day reporting of more **desirable** events was related to more sIgA antibody. Reporting more **undesirable** events was related to less sIgA. **Positive affect** in relation to events was related to more sIgA and **negative affect** to less sIgA. Interestingly, desirable events were more strongly related to secretory immune response than undesirable events. These findings suggest that greater emphasis should be placed on the immune-enhancing capabilities of positive events. This area has been given little attention in previous research, compared to the extensive focus on the deleterious effects of undesirable events.[11]

A number of physiologic systems seem to be highly responsive to life experiences and the psychologic states that accompany them. Further studies of varying human responses to stress are important as a basis for: developing effective stress-management techniques, supporting healthy coping mechanisms, and restructuring faulty psychologic defenses.[12] A holistic approach that integrates the mind and body has long characterized nursing. Birney[13] emphasizes the importance of nurses understanding the relationships between stress and health as well as stress and illness as a basis for client assessment and provision of care. Nurses are in a key position to identify individuals and families who are coping ineffectively. The nurse should assess coping strategies for stress reduction; perceived controllability, intensity, and duration of stressors; emotional and behavioral regulation skills; and perceived availability of social support. This assessment can assist the nurse in structuring appropriate interventions or in making referrals to assist clients in dealing with stressors before they exert health-damaging effects.

• STRESS ACROSS THE LIFE SPAN

Children experience stress and develop coping patterns early in life. Nurses are concerned with children's stress-coping processes because of the hazards imposed by prolonged stress and because of the potential to increase children's well-being and health through constructive stress management. Environmental and social stressors that place children and adolescents at high risk for poor adjustment include prolonged poverty; physical handicap or chronic illness; early disruption of attachment relationships; parental dysfunction in the form of psychopathology or substance abuse; loss of a parent through divorce, imprisonment, or death; and living under conditions of continuing violence, disintegrated neighborhoods, or homelessness. Personal resilience and environmental protective factors that mediate the relationship between risk factors and healthy development need to be identified and incorporated into family, community, and school interventions.[14] Higher stress has been associated with a range of risk-taking behaviors such as smoking and alcohol use in early adolescence. On the other hand, use of behavioral coping (information gathering, decision making, problem solving), cognitive coping (minimizing distress, focusing on the positive), adult social support (talking with an adult), and relaxation were found to be inversely related to substance abuse.[15] Nurses and other health professionals may find that the best approach to avoidance of substance abuse and other risky behaviors is to assist children and adolescents in learning effective stress-coping processes to apply across a variety of life circumstances.

Most of the knowledge about stress has been gained from studies of adults. This information may or may not be directly applicable to children. Some factors that are known to be related to stress in children include: self-esteem, personality characteristics (type A behavior and temperament), gender, locus of control, social support, parental child-rearing behavior, and previous stressful experiences. The five most frequently occurring stressors identified by children themselves included: feeling sick, having nothing to do, not having enough money to spend, being pressured to get good grades, and feeling left out of the group. These differed from parents' perceptions of the most distressing events. Research is needed on sources of stress for children, developmental changes in stressors and coping strategies across childhood and adolescence, and how challenging rather than stressful environments can be created for youth. Wagner and Compas[16] found developmental differences in the stressors most strongly related to psychologic symptoms: family stressors in junior high, peer stressors in high school, and academic stressors in college. Particularly important are studies of the coping strategies used by resilient children who, despite high levels of stress, appear to cope well with adversity.[17] An excellent overview of instruments to measure stressors in children and physiologic and behavioral indicators of acute and chronic stress is provided by Grey and Hayman.[18]

The stresses often experienced in young and middle-aged adulthood relate to establishing oneself in a productive career, nourishing enduring relationships in a dyadic unit, child-bearing and child-rearing, and creating a sense of self-identity as an independent yet interdependent adult. Work is often cited as a source of stress, and worksite stress-management programs are increasingly offered by many employers. Sources of work stress include lack of control over job environment or production demands, being "caught in the middle" between supervisors and customers, being underprepared for the job, lack of clarity about job expectations, unexpected transfers across departments or company locations, feeling trapped in a particular job, and lack of positive relationships with coworkers. Stress often causes deterioration in performance, which can further escalate already-existing causes of stress and tension.

Support at home can buffer work-related stressors, or the existence of additional stressors at home can have a cumulative effect with those at work and further threaten health. The Double ABCX[19] model of family stress and adaptation describes how families manage stressful events over a period of time. The family demands or pile-up of stressors are referred to as the aA factor. Family changes and transitions as well as daily hassles among family members may cause stress. These demands on the family can produce internal tension that requires management. The bB factor represents all the assets and resources that a family can draw upon in a time of stress. These can include strengths of individual members, strengths of the family unit (open communication, cohesion), and strengths of the community (helpful agencies, supportive social networks). The third factor, cC, includes the family's definition and perception of all the demands, the family's stress-meeting resources, and actions that need to be taken to resolve the stress. The result of the interaction between a family's demands and capabilities is its state of adaptation, xX. This model has been useful to nurses in primary care settings in helping them to conceptualize the stressors and coping capabilities of families as a basis for assessment and intervention.

Constrained finances or arguments between spouses about how to spend limited income can markedly increase tension in the home. Single parents are particularly vulnerable to stress, as they may lack social support and also find that job demands leave them little time for parenting responsibilities. In the absence of authoritative parenting, children may get into difficulties that further stretch limited psychologic resources of parents. Stress-management programs that address changing work and home environments to minimize stress and developing effective coping strategies best meet the needs of young and middle-aged adults.

Although some sources of stress may abate in older adulthood, other stressors, particularly those resulting from loss, are more prevalent. The elderly are particularly vulnerable to negative life events such as death of a spouse, death of a close family member, personal injury or illness, health change of a family member, and retirement. Hassles of daily living may increase as a result of diminished sensory acuity, decreased dexterity and strength, loss of flexibility, and increased fatigue. The elderly may neglect health behaviors that augment their strength and resilience such as proper nutrition, adequate exercise, and proper rest and sleep. Cumulative stress along with depression can compromise immune function, leaving the elderly more vulnerable to acute and chronic infections and perhaps cancer.[20]

It is in old age when we begin to see the increased morbidity and mortality associated with years of daily hassles and cumulative major life events, particularly where coping strategies have been ineffective. Systemic effects on the cardiovascular, gastrointestinal, neurologic, endocrine, and immune systems may become increasingly apparent. Because of decreased resistance to disease, helping elderly adults to use existing coping techniques productively or learn new ones is of great importance. Nurses familiar with the problems of aging and the capabilities of older adults can equip them to manage the stressors that they encounter more effectively and efficiently, thus conserving valuable personal resources.

• APPROACHES TO STRESS MANAGEMENT

At any point in time, an individual or family may be subjected to many sources of potential stress. Multiple stressors can combine synergistically, resulting in cumulative stress. A number of nursing diagnoses specific to problems in stress management (defensive coping, ineffective family coping, etc) are described by Gordon in the functional health pattern category of Coping-Stress Tolerance Pattern. The reader is referred to the *Manual of Nursing Diagnosis: 1993–1994* for further diagnostic information.[21] The nurse and client together must assess the level of existing stress and the sources of stress and then determine the appropriate point(s) for intervention to achieve stress reduction.

The primary modes of intervention for stress management consist of the following:

- Minimizing the frequency of stress-inducing situations
- Increasing resistance to stress
- Counterconditioning to avoid physiologic arousal resulting from stress

In general, changing the environment to decrease the incidence of stressors should be the "first line of defense." When that is not possible, individual and family coping resources need to come into play to reinterpret stress as challenge, increase resilience against stress, or decrease the health-threatening effects of stressors.

Minimizing the Frequency of Stress-inducing Situations

In a technologic society, the need for adjustment to externally imposed change is continuous. Approaches to assisting clients in preventing stressful situations include (1) changing the environment, (2) avoiding excessive change, (3) time blocking, and (4) time management.

Changing the Environment

The environment in any society is shaped by its widely held values and beliefs. Changing the environment, when it is possible, is the most proactive approach to minimizing the frequency of stress-inducing situations. Major changes in societal beliefs, values, and actions are necessary if stress is to be reduced for some vulnerable populations. Sexism, racism, and ageism create stress for selected groups as a result of devaluation of their status and lack of acknowledgement of their contributions to society. Discrimination directed at any group can result in decreased educational and employment opportunities, poverty, and personal devaluation. Williams[22]argued that the primary causes of racial disparities in hypertension are rooted not in individual variation but in differences between races in exposure or vulnerability to pathogenic factors in the physical, social, economic, and cultural environment. For example, in the African-American population, darker skin color has been linked to higher blood pressure. When figures were adjusted for socioeconomic status (SES), this relationship disappeared. Recent work by Klag and colleagues [23] has shed new light on this relationship. They found that among urban blacks of low SES, blood pressure is higher among dark persons, whereas at higher levels of SES, skin color is unrelated to blood pressure. The researchers suggest that their findings are consistent with the conclusion that darker skin color creates an environment characterized by less access to economic and social resources, particularly among lower-SES persons. A related study documented that darker-skinned blacks in the United States are twice as likely to experience racial discrimination as their light-skinned peers.[24] Attempts to improve social environments for low-income black Americans must achieve changes in policies, values, and belief systems.

The work environment is frequently identified as a major source of stress. Changes in the work environment itself can reduce the incidence of stressful events. For example, instituting policies that provide flextime, job sharing, or child-care benefits or facilities can ease the stress on parents who must both maintain a job and care for young children. Protecting workers from job-related hazards, redesigning work assignments, creating pleasant work stations, instituting quality circles, or employing more participatory management styles also can foster lower levels of stress at work. Job-related stresses may also be avoided by becoming more aware of those persons or experiences that create personal stress and minimizing contact to the extent possible. Committee membership in groups that are stress-inducing might be better delegated to someone else who experiences less stress from the activity or who obtains actual enjoyment from participation.

If a job change is required by the client to decrease stress, new employment possibilities should be analyzed to make sure that stress phenomena similar to those already encountered are not an inherent part of the new employment setting.

Protective factors in the broader environment that can further decrease stress include: family characterized by warmth and cohesion, culture and ethnic events and customs that promote identity, supportive extrafamilial relationships, and involvement in community structures such as churches and neighborhood organizations that promote competence and support.[14(p483)]

Avoiding Excessive Change

When children as young as 8 to 12 years of age were asked to report the coping strategies that they used in anticipation of stressful events, they reported avoidance of change, or insulation from change or threat as the dominant strategies used.[25] Teaching children when and how to avoid excessive change is important, as coping strategies developed early in childhood often continue into adulthood and affect patterns of behavior throughout the life span.

During periods of high life change and resulting negative tension states, any unnecessary changes should be avoided. For example, if a family is experiencing the illness of one of its family members and a subsequent job loss, this may not be the time to consider geographic relocation, pregnancy, or any other change in lifestyle. Negative tension created by multiple changes is synergistic. Each time a distressing change occurs, the potency of previous changes for upsetting stability is increased. Deliberately postponing changes that result in negative tension assists clients in dealing more constructively with unavoidable change and prevents the need for multiple adjustments all at one point in time.

Any changes that are made in lifestyle during periods of high or moderate stress should be self-initiated and provide challenge to the client rather than threat. Increasing positive sources of tension that promote growth and self-actualization can offset the deleterious effects of negative tension. For instance, learning to play tennis, to swim, or to dance may provide an enjoyable challenge to counterbalance potentially debilitating stress.

Time Blocking

Girdano and Everly[26] have suggested a time-blocking technique that sets aside specific time for adaptation to various stressors. This block of time may be daily, weekly, or monthly. It offers clients time to focus on a specific change and develop strategies for adjustment. For instance, if a family member has just been diagnosed as diabetic, time must be set aside to meet the new needs of that individual and to learn more about the care and support that family members can provide. Acquisition of new information and thoughtful planning makes a specific change easier to adapt to and allows time for the expression of feelings and emotions that may hinder adjustment. Nurses, as health professionals, can be a rich resource of information and assistance as clients integrate unavoidable changes into their lifestyle. The major advantage of time blocking is that it ensures that important goals or concerns will be addressed and critical tasks accomplished. This can reduce the sense of urgency and lack of time, the level of anxiety, and associated feelings of frustration and failure.

Time Management

This approach to stress management actually refers to organizing oneself to accomplish those goals most important in life within the time available. Since lack of time is often given by individuals and families as a reason for not participating in health-promoting activities, assisting clients to manage time better can make a major contribution to their health and fitness. Time-pressured, type A clients with high risk for cardiovascular disease may be particularly in need of time-management skills.

Identifying values and goals and prioritizing goals can serve as a framework for time management. Identifying time wasted on activities unrelated to personal goals can permit the client to restructure how time is spent. Overcommitment to others or unrealistic expectations of oneself is a frequent source of stress. Time overload can be avoided by learning to say "no" to demands of others that are unrealistic or of low personal or family priority. Overload results in frustration and loss of satisfaction from the work accomplished, since one can seldom expend one's best efforts under strain and pressure.

An important approach to time management is the reduction of a task into smaller parts. A task as a whole may appear as an overload; however, if the task is broken down into smaller segments, accomplishment becomes feasible. An example of this for a client may be learning several effective conditioning exercises before learning a complete conditioning routine, or developing skill with a conditioning routine before beginning a walk-jog activity. To take the whole health-promoting behavior as one task may be overwhelming. Breaking it down into component parts allows mastery and feelings of competence.

Avoiding overload by delegating responsibilities to others and enlisting their assistance is also important. Making use of the skills of others and recognizing their ability to perform assigned tasks provides freedom from the expectation of having to be "all things to all people."

Another important aspect of time management is to reduce the perception of time pressure and urgency. Not all perceptions of time urgency are warranted; some are needlessly self-imposed. The client should differentiate between time urgencies that are valid and others that are needlessly created. Time urgency can also be minimized by avoiding procrastination. Leaving tasks that need to be completed until the last minute can result in needless pressure and stress.[27]

Increasing Resistance to Stress

Resistance to stress is achieved through either physical or psychologic conditioning. Physical conditioning for stress resistance focuses on exercise. Psychologic conditioning to increase resistance resources focuses on (1) enhancing self-esteem, (2) enhancing self-efficacy, (3) increasing assertiveness, (4) developing goal alternatives, and (5) building coping resources.

Promoting Exercise

Exercise is discussed at length in Chapter 9. However, the relationship between exercise and stress is addressed here briefly. Norris and colleagues[28] investigated the effects of exercise on psychologic stress in a group of 80 adolescents. Four groups of approximately 20 students each were formed: high-intensity exercise (70% to 75% maximum heart rate) group, moderate-intensity exercise (50% to 60% maximum heart rate) group, flexibility training group, and control group. The exercise and flexibility groups met twice a week for 25 to 30 minutes. The control group did not formally meet. Following the intervention, the high-intensity exercise group had significantly lower heart rates following the step test, lower diastolic blood pressure, and lower perceived stress scores. These data suggest that among adolescents, aerobic training may offer some stress-resistance benefits.

In another study, 48 (24 white, 24 black) 25- to 40-year-old women participated in two counterbalanced experimental conditions: an attention control with no aerobic activity and a 40-minute bout of aerobic exercise at 70% heart-rate reserve. Each condition was followed by 30 minutes of rest, exposure to mental and interpersonal threat, and 5 minutes of recovery. Blood pressure, heart rate, and self-reported distress were monitored at intervals throughout the study. Compared to the other groups, the exercise group had lower blood pressure reactivity and reduced frequency and intensity of anxiety-related thoughts in anticipation of interpersonal threat.[29]

Three processes have been suggested in accounting for the positive effects of exercise on responses to mental stress. The first is that psychologic changes are the by-products of improvement in cardiorespiratory fitness. However, this explanation is weakened by the fact that psychologic responses and fitness are frequently uncorrelated. A second possibility is that changes in exercise-related self-efficacy and mastery generalize to other situations, resulting in improvements in self-concept and coping ability. A third process that may underlie decreased stress responses following bouts of exercise is a blunting of psychophysiologic responsiveness to stressors.[30] Further research is needed to validate if and under what conditions exercise can actually enhance stress-resistance.

Enhancing Self-Esteem

Self-esteem is the value attributed to self. This valuation is based on a person's concept of his or her desirable and undesirable attributes, strengths and weaknesses, achievements, and success in interpersonal relationships. Thomas and colleagues[31] found in a study of 323 high school freshmen that females were more concerned with self-concept and self-esteem issues than were males. These issues were particularly related to dissatisfaction and distress over personal appearance. Nurse practitioners and school nurses have excellent opportunities to promote positive self-concepts and healthy levels of self-esteem in female adolescents as a basis for healthy functioning throughout life.

Although self-esteem is developed over time, studies have shown that the level of self-esteem can be changed. One approach is positive verbalization. In using this technique, clients identify positive aspects of self or personal characteristics that they value highly. They should also ask significant others to comment on their positive attributes. Each characteristic, one per day, is placed on a 3×5 index card, and the cards placed in a conspicuous place. Each card should be read several times a day. This technique helps clients to spend more time thinking positively about themselves and decreases the amount of time spent in self-devaluation. Increased self-awareness of positive characteristics and their presence in conscious thought will result in more frequent behavior that reflects these attributes and more positive responses from significant others.

Enhancing Self-Efficacy

Mastery experiences also appear to positively build a sense of competence to perform effectively and overcome obstacles. Experiencing successful performance of a particular, valued behavior provides positive messages concerning personal skills and abilities. Counseling clients to undertake tasks that are challenging but from which they can experience success rather than failure can build a sense of efficacy in a particular domain. Self-beliefs about personal efficacy have wide-ranging ramifications affecting level of motivation, affect, thought, and action. Perceiving oneself to be efficacious has been shown to predict performance better than actual ability. In other words, if people's beliefs in their efficacy are strengthened, they approach situations more assuredly and make better use of the skills that they have.[32(p4)]

Persons with high levels of efficacy, compared to low levels, mentally rehearse success rather than failure at a task, set high goals and make a firm commitment to attain them, perceive more control over personal threats, and are less anxious in the face of day-to-day challenges. Highly efficacious persons also tend to be more assertive in accessing the support that they need to optimize their chances of success.[32(pp10–32)] The nurse can help clients to identify areas of skill most important to them and then help them plan to augment their efficacy in these highly valued areas.

Increasing Assertiveness

Substituting positive, assertive behaviors for negative, passive ones can increase personal capacity for psychologic resistance to stress. Assertiveness is the appropriate expression of oneself, one's thoughts, and one's feelings and can result in greater personal satisfaction in living. Assertiveness is more constructive than aggression and deals more effectively than aggression with most problems encountered in the course of living. Many books and articles have been written on assertiveness training. Assertiveness allows individuals to share their perceptions and feelings with others in a way that facilitates rather than inhibits personal or group productivity. Several suggestions for becoming more assertive that clients ought to be encouraged to use include the following:

- Making a deliberate effort to greet others and call them by name
- Maintaining eye contact during conversations
- Commenting on the positive characteristics of others
- Initiating conversation
- Expressing opinions
- Expressing feelings
- Disagreeing with others when holding opposing viewpoints
- Taking initiative to engage in a new behavior or learn a new activity

The webs and constraints that entangle human beings are frequently self-constructed and disappear easily when efforts are made to become more open, assertive, and self-fulfilling. While it is possible for clients through use of simple techniques to become more assertive, very passive and reserved clients might well benefit from more comprehensive assertiveness training by a competent instructor or counselor. The nurse can assist clients in locating such resources for personal development.

Developing Goal Alternatives.[26(pp129–133)]

Clients must be aware not only of the goals that they have set but of why accomplishment of those goals is rewarding. Similar sources of reward or reinforcement may be possible through accomplishment of alternative goals. For example, a client's wished-for advancement within his or her current work situation may not materialize. If the primary reasons for wanting advancement are recognition and increased income, these rewards may be achieved by accomplishing similar goals. Recognition can come through community or organizational involvement and additional monies may be generated through wise investments. Flexibility on the part of the client permits achievement of desired outcomes through several approaches. As a result, lack of success in initial attempts to reach goals becomes much less ominous because of the probability of success in achieving alternative goals that bring similar rewards.

Building Coping Resources

Stress results when there is an imbalance between appraised demands and appraised coping capabilities.[33] Hobfall[34] has suggested that more attention be directed to the resource side of the equation rather than the demand side. He maintains that coping resources are more predictive of reactions to stressors than the actual demands. General coping resources that have been identified for development to enhance stress resistance include:

- Self-disclosure: Predisposition to share one's feelings, troubles, thoughts, and opinions with others
- Self-directedness: Degree to which a person respects his or her own judgment for decision making and, therefore, demonstrates assertiveness in interpersonal relationships
- Confidence: Ability to gain mastery over one's environment and to control one's emotions in the interest of reaching personal goals
- Acceptance: Degree to which persons accept their shortcomings and imperfections and maintain a positive and tolerant attitude toward others and the world at large
- Social support: Availability and use of network of caring others
- Financial freedom: Extent to which persons are free of financial constraints on their lifestyles
- Physical health: Overall health condition including absence of chronic disease and disabilities
- Physical fitness: Conditioning resulting from personal exercise practices
- Stress monitoring: Awareness of tension build-up and situations that are likely to prove stressful
- Tension control: Ability to lower arousal through relaxation and thought control
- Structuring: Ability to organize and manage resources such as time and energy
- Problem solving: Ability to resolve personal problems

These resources can be assessed by use of the Coping Resources Inventory for Stress. This is a promising research and clinical instrument to identify stress coping resources of individuals.[35] After assessing the extent to which the various coping resources are present, nurses should assist clients in maximizing existing strengths and in developing additional resistance resources.

Counterconditioning to Avoid Physiologic Arousal

Research findings have substantiated the ability of individuals to intentionally control autonomic nervous system functions such as respiratory rate, heart rate, heart rhythm, blood pressure, and temperature in the extremities, functions previously thought to be under unconscious control. Training aimed at assisting clients to attain volitional control of physiologic responses to stressful events provides an important set of strategies for the management of stress. The goal of counterconditioning is to replace muscle tension and heightened sympathetic nervous system activity produced by stress with muscle relaxation and increased parasympathetic functioning. The three interventions most frequently used to assist the client in accomplishing this are relaxation training, biofeedback, and imagery.

Progressive Relaxation Through Tension-Relaxation Techniques

Edmund Jacobson, who began his work on relaxation as early as 1908 at Harvard University, proposed that relaxation decreases voluntary muscle activity and activity within the sympathetic nervous system while increasing parasympathetic functioning.[36] There has been increasing accumulation of evidence in the scientific literature that supports Jacobson's findings that tension levels can be reduced through use of relaxation skills. Relaxation appears to be a way of turning off the body's response to the sympathetic nervous system and of actually decreasing neurohormonal changes that take place in reaction to the experience of negative tension states.[37]

Relaxation is thought to result in the following changes:

- Decrease in the body's oxygen consumption
- Lowered metabolism
- Decreased respiration rate
- Decreased heart rate
- Decreased muscle tension
- Decreased premature ventricular contractions
- Decreased systolic and diastolic blood pressures
- Increased alpha brain waves
- Enhanced immune function

Green and colleagues[38] found that a 3-week period of daily bouts of relaxation affected the concentrations of the serum immunoglobulins. Subjects reporting greater practice of relaxation had higher levels of sIgA, IgA, IgG, and IgM. These findings suggest that relaxation may enhance humoral immunity.

A very pleasant, quiet, soundproofed room where lighting can be dimmed, with reclining lawn or lounge chairs for clients, provides an optimum setting for relaxation training. Tight clothing should be loosened, glasses removed, shoes removed, and a comfortable position assumed in the chair. Relaxation should never be taught with clients lying flat. Although this is a common position assumed for rest and sleep, it often results in muscle strain in upper back and neck along with drowsiness, which interferes with training. A reclining position or sitting position is most appropriate.

At the beginning of each session, clients should be encouraged to focus on their own breathing as the air moves gently in and out. The purpose of this focusing activity is to increase awareness of self and the often imperceptible functions of the human body. Following the focusing activity, clients are moved slowly through tension and relaxation cycles for each of the major muscle groups listed in Table 11–1, maintaining tension for 8 to 10 seconds and releasing tension instantaneously on cue. The entire tension–relaxation cycle should be repeated twice during the first session to increase clients' awareness of the differences in body sensations during tensed and relaxed periods. The tension–relaxation instructions should be given very slowly, allowing clients to enjoy the feelings of relaxation they are experiencing. The guidance provided by the nurse is critical for successful relaxation.

TABLE 11–1. FIFTEEN-MUSCLE GROUP SEQUENCE FOR TENSION–RELAXATION CYCLE

MUSCLE GROUP	ABBREVIATED INSTRUCTIONS
1. Right hand and forearm	Make a fist.
2. Right upper arm	Pull elbow tightly into side.
3. Left hand and forearm	Make a fist.
4. Left upper arm	Pull elbow tightly into side.
5. Forehead	Wrinkle brow.
6. Upper cheeks and nose	Squint eyes and wrinkle nose.
7. Lower cheeks and jaws	Place teeth together and make a "forced" smile.
8. Neck and throat	Pull chin toward chest.
9. Chest, shoulders, and upper back	Take a deep breath. Push shoulder blades toward each other.
10. Upper abdomen	Pull stomach in and hold.
11. Lower abdomen	Bear down against the seat of the chair.
12. Right upper leg	Push down against the foot of the chair.
13. Right lower leg and foot	Point toes toward head and body.
14. Left upper leg	Push down against the foot of the chair.
15. Left lower leg and foot	Point toes toward head and body.

Training tapes can be used by clients at home to facilitate daily practice of relaxation techniques. Clients should keep a schedule of the frequency and length of time that relaxation is practiced. Clients are encouraged to "think through" the relaxation procedure and do their own coaching. A "prompt sheet" on the sequence of the muscle groups should be sent home with them for easy reference. This is intended to move clients toward independent practice of relaxation rather than encouraging reliance on the nurse or the coaching tape as a means of providing relaxation cues.

Some common problems that clients report include:

- Overly rapid self-pacing through the relaxation sequence
- Distraction by environmental noise
- Difficulty keeping attention on own monologue
- Interruption of distracting thoughts during relaxation
- Residual tension in some muscles after tension–relaxation

The problem of overly rapid self-pacing can usually be solved by encouraging clients to slow down internal speech or coaching pace. Autogenic phrases like "I feel calm," "I feel very relaxed," and "my arms and legs feel heavy" can be interspersed throughout self-instruction. Encouraging family members to join in the relaxation practice sessions can foster stress-management skills among the entire family unit.

Progressive Relaxation Without Tension

While tension–relaxation techniques result in high levels of voluntary muscle relaxation, clients can be taught how to relax without first tensing muscles. Relaxation through counting down and relaxation through imagery are strategies frequently used. The major advantage of these techniques is that tension is no longer required. This is particularly important for clients with hypertension or coronary heart disease, since elevations in blood pressure caused by prolonged or extensive muscle tensing may be contraindicated.

Deep relaxation without tension is the goal. Phrases that might be repeated to facilitate relaxation include:

- I feel quiet.
- I am beginning to feel quite relaxed.
- My feet feel heavy and relaxed.
- My ankles, my knees, and my hips feel heavy.
- My solar plexus and the whole central portion of my body feel relaxed and quiet.
- My hands, my arms, and my shoulders feel heavy, relaxed, and comfortable.
- My neck, my jaws, and my forehead feel relaxed. They feel comfortable and smooth.
- My whole body feels quite heavy, comfortable, and relaxed.
- I am quite relaxed.
- My arms and hands are heavy and warm.
- I feel quite quiet.
- My whole body is relaxed and my hands are warm—relaxed and warm.
- My hands are warm.
- Warmth is flowing into my hands. They are warm, warm.
- I can feel the warmth flowing down my arms into my hands.
- My hands are warm, relaxed, and warm.
- My whole body feels quiet, comfortable, and relaxed.
- My mind is quiet.
- I withdraw my thoughts from the surroundings and I feel serene and still.
- My thoughts are turned inward and I am at ease.
- Deep within my mind, I can visualize and experience myself as relaxed, comfortable, and still.
- I am alert, but in an easy, quiet, inward-turned way.
- My mind is calm and quiet.
- I feel an inward quietness.

These phrases have been suggested by Elmer and Alyce Green as a result of work in biofeedback at the Menninger Foundation. Such phrases result in physiologic imagery that can decrease both sympathetic nervous system activity and tension in voluntary muscles.

Relaxation through the countdown procedure initially focuses on each of the muscle groups used previously. The client is encouraged to relax each muscle group progressively as the count proceeds from 10 down to 1. When the client has practiced and becomes skilled with this procedure, total body countdown can be used: relaxing the entire body while silently counting down from 10 to 1. This is a particularly useful procedure for the office or when facing stressful social situations. In 2 to 3 minutes, the skilled client can achieve total body relaxation while in a sitting position with eyes open and focused on a specific object. This is one of the shortest procedures through which relaxation can be accomplished. Mini-relaxation sessions several times throughout the day can promote generalization of relaxation training to everyday life.

Relaxation Through Imagery

Using imagery to relax requires that the client passively concentrate on pleasant scenes or experiences from the past to facilitate relaxation. Recalling the warmth of the sun, the feeling of warm sand, the sensations of a gentle breeze, the vision of palm trees swaying, or sounds of ocean waves may be comfortable and pleasant for clients. Such recall can promote muscle relaxation.

Each client will vary in those scenes or images that result in actual changes in muscle tension. For some clients, visualizing specific colors, shapes, or patterns will be as effective as visualizing landscapes or scenes. If clients initially have difficulty in using imagery or visualization for relaxation, the nurse may use one of the following techniques:

- Have the client, with eyes closed, visualize a particular room of his or her house (living room, bedroom, kitchen), focusing on colors, shapes, and specific objects. The client's mind should wander about the room, with the client describing verbally what is seen in as much detail as possible
- Have the client focus on a particular piece of clothing that is a personal favorite. The client should describe the color, texture, design, and trim of the clothing and how it feels when worn (eg, soft, loose, fitted, light, warm)

As individuals become more vivid in descriptions of concrete objects, their ability to use less concrete imagery for purposes of relaxation increases. Imagery is a highly useful relaxation technique in many settings in which muscle tension or biofeedback equipment would be obtrusive.

Relaxation Through Biofeedback

Clients can be assisted in acquiring greater skill in relaxation through providing biofeedback regarding level of muscle tension and skin temperature. Biofeedback has in recent years offered the possibility for awareness and control of processes previously thought to be under unconscious rather than conscious control. Biofeedback can be defined as a process in which a person learns reliably to influence physiologic responses that are not ordinarily under voluntary control. The four basic operations in biofeedback are[39]:

1. Detection and amplification of bioelectric potentials
2. Conversion of bioelectric signals to easy-to-process information
3. Feedback of information to the client
4. Voluntary control of target response through learning based on feedback

The foundations of biofeedback hinge on a very simple idea: Clients need to be provided with information about what is going on inside their bodies, since bodily functions cannot be controlled unless information about them is available to the controller.[40] A wide range of autonomic processes can be controlled through response to feedback. Some of the physiologic parameters that have been controlled or modified through feedback include the following:

- Heart rate: Acceleration and deceleration
- Heart rhythm: Occurrences of premature ventricular contractions
- Blood pressure: Systolic and diastolic

- Peripheral vascular responses: Skin surface temperature
- Muscle tension: Muscle contractility
- Alpha wave activity: Brain wave patterns
- Galvanic skin response: Resistance of skin to passage of electrical current

Biofeedback is an important modality for facilitating stress management. The ultimate goal is establishing self-regulation that allows the client to control one or more of the autonomic responses identified above. A permanent change in the target response following training is desired. While biofeedback instrumentation facilitates learning during the training period, the client must learn to read and interpret body signals without the aid of equipment and to function effectively in modifying responses.

DIRECTIONS FOR RESEARCH ON STRESS MANAGEMENT

The ability to regulate processes previously considered to be under autonomic rather than voluntary control has been one of the most exciting research discoveries during the last several decades. In addition, major advances toward understanding the effects of stressors on the neuroendocrine and immune systems has offered new possibilities for managing the brain–body interface to promote health. A number of coping strategies have been tested. More research is needed concerning the profile of stressors most likely to occur at different developmental stages and the best way to match stressors with targeted coping processes. A very exciting research challenge is discovering how to build coping resources, resilience, and personal competence in the early childhood years so that patterns of successfully coping manifest themselves throughout adolescence and adulthood.

Most of all, research that suggests how to decrease environmental and family stressors for vulnerable populations is needed. Human tolerance for stress is finite—with the best of coping strategies, people can only stand so much. What are the changes in social policies, social structures, and relationships across cultures that need to be addressed to get at the root of the problem: the social injustice, discrimination, and inequity that is the unfortunate experience of many? Through the efforts of scientists from multiple disciplines, the phenomenon of stress pervasive in our society can be addressed. Results of the research can be applied to create a better world for all.

SUMMARY

Research on relaxation techniques indicates the usefulness of such approaches in the prevention and treatment of a variety of stress-related diseases. Relaxation also has been shown to increase feelings of energy, vitality, and self-control. However, like any other skill, continued use and practice of approaches to relaxation is essential if clients are to experience maximal prevention and health-promotion benefits from their use.

A number of different approaches for assisting individuals and families in managing stress have been presented in order to familiarize the reader with the range of strategies available. Some approaches suggested are relatively unstructured, while others are more formally defined and require instrumentation. The decision regarding which strategies to use must be made collaboratively by the client and the nurse. This decision should be based on the characteristics of the client, sources of stress experienced by the client, and general patterns of response to stressful events. The reader is encouraged to consult several references at the end of this chapter for further information on use of stress management strategies as nursing interventions.[20,41–43]

REFERENCES

1. Pelletier KR, Lutz R. Healthy people—healthy business: a critical review of stress management programs in the workplace. *Am J Health Prom.* 1988;5:12,19.
2. Seelye H. Introduction. In: Wheatley D, ed. *Stress and the Heart.* New York, NY: Raven Press; 1977.
3. Lazarus RS, Folkman S. *Stress, Appraisal and Coping.* New York, NY: Springer; 1984:293.
4. Folkman S, Lazarus RS, Dunkel-Schetter C, et al. Dynamics of a stressful encounter: cognitive appraisal, coping, and encounter outcomes. *J Pers Soc Psychol.* 1986;50:992–1003.
5. US Public Health Service. *Healthy People 2000: National Health Promotion and Disease Prevention Objectives.* Washington, DC: US Public Health Service; 1991:214–218. US Department of Health and Human Services Publication, PHS 91-50212.
6. Eliot SR. Stress and the heart: mechanisms, measurement, and management. *Postgrad Med* 1992;92(5):237–248.
7. House JS, Landis KR, Umberson D. Social relationships and health. *Science.* 1988;241: 540–545.
8. Kiecolt-Glaser JK, Dura JR, Speicher CE, et al. Spousal caregivers of dementia victims: longitudinal changes in immunity and health. *Psychosom Med.* 1991;53:345–362.
9. Cacioppo JT. Social neuroscience: autonomic, neuroendocrine, and immune response to stress. *Psychophysiology.* 1994;31:113–128.
10. Irwin M, Patterson T, Smith TL, Caldwell C, et al. Reduction of immune function in life stress and depression. *Biologic Psychiatry.* 1990;27:22–30.
11. Stone AA, Neale JM, Cox DS, et al. Daily events are associated with a secretory immune response to an oral antigen in men. *Health Psychol.* 1994;13:440–446.
12. Houldin AD, Lev E, Prystowsky MB, et al. Psychoneuroimmunology: a review of literature. *Holistic Nurs Pract.* 1991;5(4):10–21.
13. Birney MH. Psychoneuroimmunology: a holistic framework for the study of stress and illness. *Holistic Nurs Pract.* 1991;5(4):32–38.
14. Barbarin OA. Coping and resilience: exploring the inner lives of African American children. *J Black Psychol.* 1993;19(4):478–492.
15. Wills TA. Stress and coping in early adolescence: relationships to substance use in urban school samples. *Health Psychol.* 1986;5(6):503–529.
16. Wagner BM, Compas BE. Gender, instrumentality, and expressivity: moderators of the relation between stress and psychological symptoms during adolescence. *Am J Community Psychol.* 1990;18:383–406.
17. Ryan NM. The stress-coping process in school-age children: gaps in the knowledge needed for health promotion. *Adv Nurs Sci.* 1988;11(1):1–12.

18. Grey M, Hayman LL. Assessing stress in children: research and clinical implications. *J Pediat Nurs.* 1987;2(5):316–327.
19. Mays RM. Family stress and adaptation. *Nurse Pract.* 1988;13(8):52–56.
20. Weinberger R. Teaching the elderly stress reduction. *J Gerontol Nurs.* 1991;17(10):23–27.
21. Gordon M. *Manual of Nursing Diagnosis, 1993–1994.* St Louis, Mo: Mosby Year Book; 1993:249–339, 353–377.
22. Williams DR. Black-White differences in blood pressure: the role of social factors. *Ethn Dis.* 1992;2:126–141.
23. Klag MH, Whelton PK, Coresh J, et al. The association of skin color with blood pressure in US blacks with low socioeconomic status. *JAMA.* 1991;265:599–602.
24. Keith VM, Herring C. Skin tone and stratification in the black community. *Am J Soc.* 1991;97:760–778.
25. Ryan NM. Stress-coping strategies identified from school-age children's perspective. *Res Nurs Health.* 1989;12(2):111–122.
26. Girdano D, Everly G. *Controlling Stress and Tension.* Englewood Cliffs, NJ: Prentice-Hall Inc; 1979.
27. Everly GS. Time management: a behavioral strategy for disease prevention and health enhancement. In: Matazzo JD, Weiss SM, Herd JA, et al, eds. *Behavioral Health: A Handbook of Health Enhancement and Disease Prevention.* New York, NY: John Wiley & Sons; 1984:363–370.
28. Norris R, Carroll D, Cochrane R. The effects of physical activity and exercise training on psychological stress and well-being in an adolescent population. *J Psychosom Res.* 1992;36: 55–65.
29. Rejeski WJ, Thompson A, Brubaker PH, et al. Acute exercise: buffering psychosocial stress responses in women. *Health Psychol.* 1992;11(6):355–362.
30. Roy M, Steptoe A. The inhibition of cardiovascular responses to mental stress following aerobic exercise. *Psychophysiology.* 1991;*28*:689–700.
31. Thomas S, Shoffner DH, Groer MW. Adolescent stress factors: implications for the nurse practitioner. *Nurs Pract.* 1988;13(6):20–29.
32. Bandura A. Exercise of personal agency through the self-efficacy mechanism. In: Schwarzer R, ed. *Self-Efficacy: Thought Control of Action.* Washington, DC: Hemisphere Publishing Corp; 1992.
33. Coyne JC, Lazarus RS. Cognitive style, stress perception and coping. In: Kutash IL, Schlesinger LB, eds. *Handbook on Stress and Anxiety: Contemporary Knowledge, Theory and Treatment.* San Francisco, Calif: Jossey-Bass Inc Publishers; 1980:144–158.
34. Hobfoll SE. *The Etiology of Stress.* Washington, DC: Hemisphere Publishing Corp; 1988.
35. Matheny KB, Aycock DW, Curlette WL, et al. The coping resource inventory for stress: a measure of perceived resourcefulness. *J Clin Psychol.* 1993;49(6):815–829.
36. Bernstein DA, Borkovec TD. *Progressive relaxation training: a manual for the helping professions.* Champaign, Ill: Research Press; 1973.
37. Cautela JR, Groden J. *Relaxation: a comprehensive manual for adults, children, and children with special needs.* Champaign, Ill: Research Press; 1978.
38. Green ML, Green RG, Santoro W. Daily relaxation modifies serum and salivary immunoglobulins and psychophysiologic symptom severity. *Biofeedback Self-Regul.* 1988;13(3):187–198.
39. Blanchard EB, Epstein LH. *A Biofeedback Primer.* Reading, Mass: Addison-Wesley Publishing Co Inc; 1978.
40. Gaarder KR, Montgomery PS. *Clinical Biofeedback: A Procedural Manual.* Baltimore, Md: Williams & Wilkins; 1977.

41. Snyder M. Relaxation. In: Fitzpatrick JJ, Taunton RL, Benoliel JQ, eds. *Annual Review of Nursing Research.* New York, NY: Springer; 1988;6:111–128.
42. Peddicord K. Strategies for promoting stress reduction and relaxation. *Nurs Clin North Am.* 1991;26:867–874.
43. Pender NJ. The pursuit of happiness: stress and health. In: Wold S, ed. *Community Health Nursing: Issues and Topics.* Englewood Cliffs, NJ: Prentice-Hall Inc; 1989:145–175.

12

Social Support and Health

In the course of human interaction, individuals and groups both give and receive social support. It is a reciprocal process and an interactive resource that provides comfort, assistance, encouragement, and information. Social support fosters successful coping and promotes satisfying and effective living. Individuals and aggregates differ in the amount of social support that they give and that they provide. Further, the amount and type(s) of social support needed fluctuates across the life span and across varying situations. Individuals and families often call on internal resources first for coping with unanticipated, difficult, or threatening circumstances. Contacts with social support may then be initiated only when self-reliance fails. All individuals need a system of sustaining support to realize their full potential. Given that social support is a basic human need, researchers have explored its dimensions, defined it operationally in various ways, and studied the relationship between social support and health. Social support is considered to be person–environment interactions that decrease the occurrence of stressors, buffer the impact of stress, and decrease physiologic reactivity to stress.

Much of our understanding of the effects of social support on health has come from the field of mental health. From this literature, the empirical generalization can be made that social support is related to decreased stress during times of life crisis. Advances in our understanding of how social support actually affects mental and physical health are essential to the design of interventions to promote mental, social and physical well-being.[1] Relationships among social support, health behaviors, and health are addressed in this chapter. In addition, the role of the nurse in assisting clients to assess, modify, and develop effective social support systems that meet their needs will be explored.

• SOCIAL NETWORKS

A social network is the set of people with whom one maintains social contact and has some form of social bond.[2] Norbeck[3] emphasizes that the concepts of social network and social support are not interchangeable. A **social network** is made up of persons that an individual or family knows and interacts with. These interactions may occur frequently or infrequently and may include a large number of individuals. **Social support** refers to the subset of social interactions that are supportive. The social support system for any given individual or family is usually much smaller than the social network as identified by an array of contacts. Focusing on the individual for purposes of illustration, each individual is a node in the social network and each exchange is a link. An individual influences the environment at any point in time through network links, and links provide pathways through which the environment influences the individual. Networks can be defined in the following terms:

- Size (number of individuals)
- Composition (eg, friends or relatives)
- Geographic dispersion (distances separating network members)
- Homogeneity (common characteristics shared by network members)
- Strength of ties (extent of bonding)
- Density or integration (number of relationships among members of the network)

Low-density networks with few relationships among members are less likely to include strong ties than high-density networks.[4] Networks can be preorganized to a large part for the individual (fellow employees, clubs, schools) or determined by personal choice (friends, neighbors).

Kahn and Antonucci[5] proposed the convoy model for social networks. The convoy is depicted by three progressively enlarging concentric circles around an inner circle designating the individual. Each concentric circle depicts a layer of the person's social network. The inner circle consists of close, intimate relationships such as family and long-time friends. Individuals in the middle layer may be relatives, friends, and neighbors. The outer circle reflects contacts as a result of social roles, such as coworkers. This convoy or set of relationships moves about with the individual throughout life. Middle and outer layers are more likely to change; the inner layer is likely to be more stable. Inner circle members are difficult to replace and when they are no longer available, there is a sense of grief and loss.

Networks are important to individuals and families to the extent that they fulfill members' needs. Network contacts shape social identity, provide for reflective appraisal, provide information, and serve as avenues for new social contacts.

• SOCIAL SUPPORT

Social support, rather than social networks, are considered to be more directly related to health and well-being. Social support can be defined as the subjective feeling of belonging, of being accepted, loved, esteemed, valued, and needed for oneself, not for what one can do for others.[6] Important dimensions of social support to consider when assessing a client are the source, the function it serves, and the intimacy characteristic of the relationship. Throughout the social support literature, the following types of support are proposed: emotional support, instrumental aid, informational support, and affirmation. The type of support that is beneficial at any given time may differ, depending on the nature and stage of the confronting situation. Emotional support (encouragement, empathy) may help in depressing circumstances, whereas informational support may be more useful in assisting an individual to understand how to relate effectively with his or her peers. Instrumental aid provides assistance with specific tasks, such as the preparation of nutritious meals or the transport of children to recreational activities. Affirmation helps individuals to realize their own strengths and potential.

Ethnic and racial differences in social support transactions, an area of increasing interest to researchers and health practitioners alike, were studied by Silverstein.[7] Using data from the 1987–88 National Survey of Families and Households, differences among middle-aged to older Euro-Americans and African-Americans in providing and receiving instrumental and emotional support were examined for both men and women. Overall, both racial groups were equally likely to provide and receive the two types of support. When gender subgroups were looked at, African-American women reported less provision of instrumental support to others compared to Euro-American women. However, in old age, this pattern changed. African-American women were as likely as Euro-American women to provide instrumental support and more likely to receive it. Although more definitive research is needed in this area, the study results do indicate that the effects of race on social support should be examined for differing patterns across genders and stages of life.

Several social support systems relevant to health have been identified and described in the literature: natural support systems, peer support systems, organized religious support systems, organized support systems of care-giving or helping professionals, and organized support groups not directed by health professionals. In most instances, the family (natural support system) constitutes the primary support group. Families, in order to provide appropriate support, must be sensitive to the needs of family members, establish effective communication, respect the unique needs of members, and establish expectations of mutual help and assistance.

Peer support systems consist of people who function informally in meeting the needs of others. These individuals make contacts easily and enjoy being involved with other people. They maintain a reputation of helpfulness because of support provided to others. Many of these individuals have encountered an experience of major impact in their own life and achieved successful adjustment and growth. Because of personal insight, their advice is sought primarily in relation to resolving a problem of immediate concern with which they are familiar. Examples include the avid runner, the health-food enthusiast, the widow, or the parents of a retarded child. Successful coping is the primary credential of an individual credible as a source of peer support.

Organized religious support systems such as churches or other religious meeting places constitute a support system for individuals because the congregation share a common value system, a common set of beliefs about the purpose of life, traditions of worship, and a set of guidelines for living. Even highly mobile individuals may find a ready support system in the local church or synagogue. The church takes particular responsibility for support directed toward enhancing the spiritual dimension of health, which Chapman[8] defined as the ability to develop our spiritual nature to its fullest potential. This includes the ability to discover and articulate one's basic purpose in life, learn how to experience love, joy, peace and fulfillment and how to help ourselves and others achieve full personal potential.

A third type of support system is composed of care-giving or helping professionals with a specific set of skills and services to offer clients. The professional support system is seldom the first source of help for an individual. Family and close friends or peers are sought out initially for advice and support. It is often only when this source of help is unavailable, interrupted, or exhausted that health professionals enter the support scene. Norbeck reported that according to research data, clients rarely consider health professionals as a part of their social network, even though they describe supportive relationships that are helpful and important to them. Reasons for this may be that the relationship between client and provider is seldom reciprocal, assistance flows only in the direction from the professional to the client, the relationship is limited to only one sphere of the client's life, health care, and most care episodes do not result in an intensive, ongoing relationship with a care provider over time.[3(p9)]

Organized support systems not directed by health professionals include voluntary service groups and mutual help groups. Voluntary service groups provide assistance to individuals who are in need or for some reason are unable to provide services for themselves. Mutual help groups (Alcoholics Anonymous, Take Off Pounds Sensibly (TOPS), Recovery, Inc.) attempt to effect change in behavior of members or promote adaptation to a life change such as chronic health problem, terminal illness, or a disabled family member. The number of self-help groups has grown into a major movement in the United States within the last several decades. Some have sprung up because of disenchantment with the health establishment. Others have emerged as a result of attempts to deal with problems uncommon in the general society. Service groups and mutual help groups have played a significant role in social support relevant to health.

All support systems of a given individual or family are synergistic. In combination, they represent the social resources available to the client to facilitate stability and actualization. Various systems will attain dominance at different points in the life cycle, depending on stage of development and the stressors or challenges at hand.

Functions of Social Support Groups

The functions of social support groups in promoting and protecting health can be conceptualized in four ways, as depicted in Figure 12–1. Social groups can contribute to health by (1) creating a growth-promoting environment supportive of health-promoting behaviors, self-esteem, and high-level wellness, (2) decreasing the likelihood of stressful life events, (3) providing feedback or confirmation that actions are leading to anticipated and socially desirable consequences, and (4) buffering the negative effects of stressful events through influencing interpretation of events and emotional responses to them, thus decreasing their illness-producing potential.

The primary functions of social support groups are to augment personal strengths of members and promote achievement of life goals. Persons with undifferentiated or minimal social support systems exhibit poorer coping behavior and less emotional stability than do those with well-developed, mutually supportive relations.

Within a support aggregate, the persons are dealt with as unique individuals. There is heightened sensitivity to needs, and they are deemed worthy of respect and satisfaction. Support groups can be characterized as: sharing common social concerns, providing intimacy, preventing isolation, respecting mutual competencies, offering dependable assistance in crises, serving as a referral agent, and providing mutual challenge.

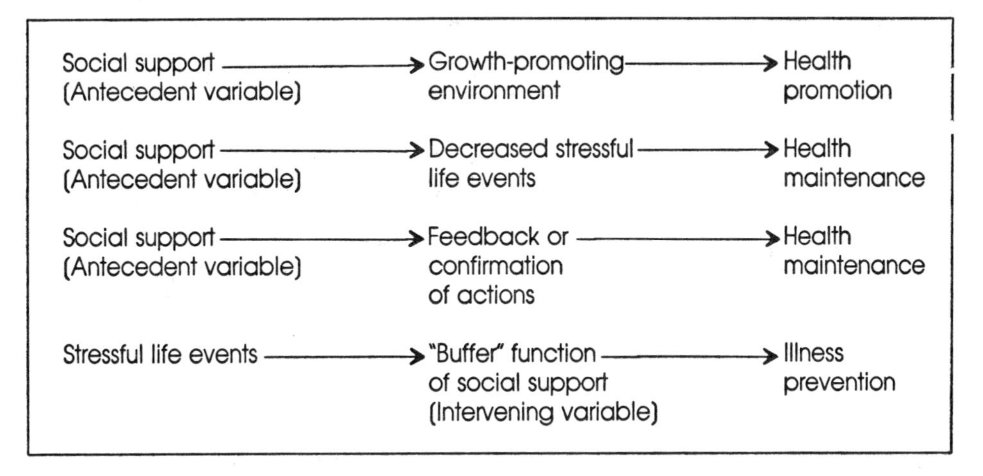

Figure 12–1. Possible impact of social support on health status.

Family as the Primary Support Group

The family is the primary context for learning about giving and receiving social support. The critical role of the family in social support is apparent from the dominant place given to family-related items in many instruments measuring social support.[9] In studying factors that create resilience in children in adverse settings and circumstances, Garmezy[10,11] found that critical protection was offered by family support through warmth, cohesion, family harmony, or by the presence of a caring adult, such as a grandparent, when absence or marital discord of parents made them unavailable to their children. External support in the form of a maternal substitute (neighbor, teacher, parents of a peer) when the child's mother was unresponsive also enhanced resilience. In a longitudinal study of children of Kauai raised in adverse conditions (poverty, perinatal stress, a disorganized caretaking environment), competent parenting styles that were supportive and enhanced self-esteem fostered resilience. Interestingly, high-risk youth who grew into resilient adults reported a period of required support or helpfulness that they had to provide to others in order to minimize the recipients' (often family members) stress or discomfort.[12] It is important to note that early experiences of **giving** social support as well as receiving it appeared critical to later adjustment. This finding, if replicated, has implications for structuring effective resiliency-enhancing interventions. Overall, sources of resilience or the means for fostering it seem to reside in the social context, with nuclear or extended family support playing a critical role.[13,14]

Family social support exerts complex effects on the physical and mental health of its members. For men, being married is related to lower mortality than is being single.[15] However, the mechanisms underlying this relationship are not well understood. Depressive symptoms have been associated with an adverse family environment that offers low levels of social support.[16] Studies that have compared the influence of family and other sources of support on depressive symptoms and health behaviors have shown the family to be important in fostering mental health[17] and increasing health-enhancing behaviors.[18] In studying 249 adult family practice patients, Parkerson and colleagues[19] found family support to be positively associated with emotional health status but not with physical or social health or symptom status. The interplay between family stressors and family support is depicted in Figure 12–2.

Within families, both positive and negative interactions occur. Negative interactions can be viewed as stressors, whereas positive, helpful interactions constitute support. A family's ability to foster positive interactive styles among its members may also relate to the extent to which the family has its own social network of long-term supportive relationships and the extent to which the family is accorded respect within the community. Positive emotional bonds of the family with its social network appear to buttress the family's competence and effective functioning. Families that are reciprocal in their network relationships and open to constructive feedback augment their versatility and resourcefulness for providing social support to family members.[20]

Community Organizations as Support Groups

The characteristics of a community and its organizations have a direct bearing on the level of well-being of individuals and families that reside in it. The quality of social inter-

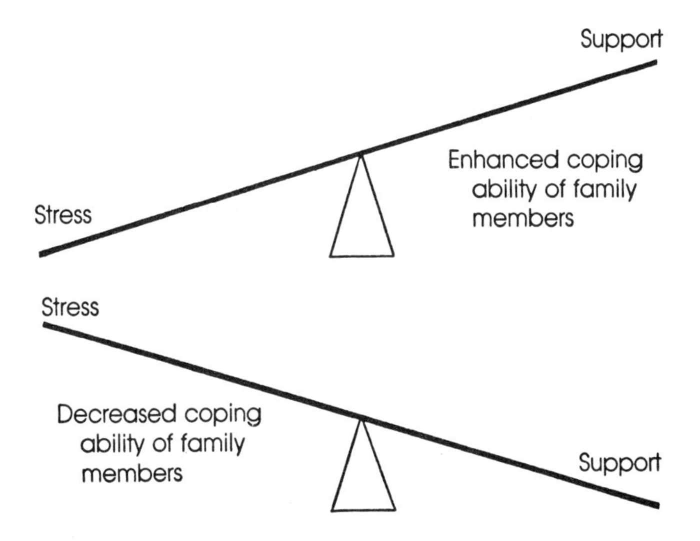

Figure 12–2. Family as a source of support or stress.

action and the life experiences of residents can contribute positively to health or negatively to social disorganization and overt illness. Stability within a community tends to promote close-knit ties among residents that mitigate the effects of crises on community members. Stable communities are characterized by value similarity, mutual assistance, mutual trust, and concern for members.

Organizations, particularly churches, are viewed as a source of support in the community. This is especially true for African-Americans. Walls and Zarit[21] found that perceptions of support from a church network contributed to feelings of well-being among elderly black women. Davis and colleagues[22] examined the efficacy of a church-based model of social influence and support to improve participation of underserved minority women in a cervical cancer control program. Thirty lay workers served as messengers, recruiters, and organizers for their own church congregations. Social support structures such as child care, meals, or transportation were organized. Over 1000 women attended the educational sessions. Postintervention data indicated that black women were 6.6 times more likely than Hispanics to have been screened for cervical cancer during the past 2 years. The community support program expanded the number of women reached with this critical preventive service.

Another example of community organizations as support groups is the De Madres a Madres community partnership for health. To increase the number of Hispanic women beginning early prenatal care, a community health nurse trained 14 volunteer mothers living in the targeted communities to identify women at high risk for not beginning early prenatal care and to provide social support and community support that was culturally appropriate. Within the first year of the project, over 2000 women at risk for not starting early prenatal care had been contacted. This community support program augmented the number of women initiating appropriate and timely prenatal care.[23]

Self-Help Groups

This chapter would not be complete in exploring sources of social support if self-help groups were not included in the discussion. While family and friends generally serve as primary sources of support, self-help groups are an important source of assistance within most communities. Examples of self-help groups include Mended Hearts, Compassionate Friends, Weight Watchers, and physical fitness clubs. Characteristics of self-help groups include a critical mass sufficient to form a group, a form of publicity or recruitment to attract appropriate members, and a central goal or activity that gives the group purpose and sustains the psychologic investment of its members. The question has been raised as to why individuals use self-help groups rather than other resources, such as professional services. Two hypotheses have been offered: (1) self-help groups arise in society to fulfill a need for services not being offered, or (2) self-help groups arise because of disappointment with the inadequate assistance or lack of meaningful resources within the community.

Self-help groups have been found to share the following common characteristics[24]:

- Membership consists of those who share a common condition, situation, heritage, symptom, or life experience.
- The group is self-regulating and self-governing, emphasizing peer solidarity rather than hierarchical governance.
- Members advocate self-reliance and require intensive commitment and responsibility.
- The group has a code of precepts, beliefs, and practices.
- Members maintain a face-to-face or phone-to-phone support network.
- The more experienced members provide anticipatory guidance.
- Members provide empathy for one another.
- The group provides specific guidance in dealing with a dilemma or life problem.
- Members can suggest practical ways for handling day-to-day problems.

Levy[25] identified the following four types of self-help groups by purpose: behavioral control or conduct reorganization, stress coping and support, survival orientation, and personal growth or self-actualization. The process operating within the groups appeared to be behaviorally and cognitively oriented.

Behaviorally oriented processes included:

- Direct and vicarious social reinforcement for the development of desirable behaviors and the elimination of troublesome behaviors
- Training, indoctrination, and support in the use of various kinds of self-control behaviors
- Modeling of methods of coping with stresses and changing behaviors
- Providing members with agenda of actions they can engage in to change the social environment

Cognitively oriented processes were the following:

- Removal of members' mystification over their experience
- Provision of normative and instrumental information and advice

- Expansion of the range of alternative perceptions of members' problems and circumstances and of the actions they might take to cope with their problems
- Support for change in attitudes toward self, one's own behavior, and society
- Social comparison and consensual validation leading to reduction or elimination of members' uncertainty and sense of isolation or uniqueness regarding their problems and experiences
- The emergence of an alternative or substitute culture within which members can develop new definitions of their personal identity and new norms upon which they can base their self esteem

Self-help groups are a valuable source of support within many communities. Their records of success in assisting millions of individuals in coping with a variety of different life experiences attest to their continuing viability as an integral part of community health resources.

• REVIEWING SOCIAL SUPPORT SYSTEMS

It is important for clients to be aware of sources of social support available to them. Approaches for reviewing the social support networks of clients are suggested below.

List those individuals below who provide financial, emotional, or instrumental support (assistance with tasks) to you. Indicate the type of support provided by placing the appropriate letter next to each name. *F* = financial support, *E* = emotional support, and *I* = instrumental support. Any individual may provide more than one type of support. Next, indicate whether the supportive other is a family member (*FM*), fellow worker (*FW*), or social acquaintance (*A*). Finally, after each person who has been a source of support for 5 years or more, place the number *5*.

John	*F, E, I, FM (husband), 5*	*Nancy*	*E, A*
Peter	*E, FM (son), 5*	*Larry*	*E, I, A*
Carmen	*E, FM (daughter), 5*	*Arlene*	*E, I, A*
Helen	*E, FM (mother), 5*	*Duane*	*I, A, 5*
Ted	*E, FM (father), 5*	*Elaine*	*I, A, 5*
Audrey	*E, FM (cousin), 5*	*Margaret*	*E, I, FW*
Andrew	*E, I, FM (cousin), 5*	*Marlene*	*E, I, FW*
Jane	*E, I, A*	*Frances*	*I, FW*
David	*E, I, A*	*Rose*	*I, FW*
Tom	*I, A, 5*	*Karen*	*I, FW*
Elsa	*E, I, A, 5*	*Theresa*	*I, FW*
Jack	*E, A*	*Diane*	*I, FW*

Figure 12–3. Support systems review.

The individuals identified on the previous page should be grouped in the following way:

Sources of Emotional Support

FAMILY	WORK	SOCIAL GROUP
John	*Margaret*	*Jane*
Peter	*Marlene*	*David*
Carmen		*Elsa*
Helen		*Jack*
Ted		*Nancy*
Audrey		*Larry*
Andrew		*Arlene*

Sources of Instrumental Support

FAMILY	WORK	SOCIAL GROUP
John	*Margaret*	*Jane*
Audrey	*Marlene*	*David*
Andrew	*Frances*	*Tom*
	Rose	*Elsa*
	Karen	*Larry*
	Theresa	*Arlene*
	Diane	*Duane*
		Elaine

Sources of Financial Support

FAMILY	WORK	SOCIAL GROUP
John		

Sources of Support for More than 5 Years

FAMILY	WORK	SOCIAL GROUP
John		*Tom*
Peter		*Elsa*
Carmen		*Duane*
Helen		*Elaine*
Ted		
Audrey		
Andrew		

Figure 12–3. (continued)

These approaches can be useful in giving both client and nurse increased insight into existing support resources.

Support Systems Review

Glaser and Kirschenbaum[26] have suggested a straightforward approach to be used in reviewing sources of social support for clients. In the support systems review the client is asked to list those individuals that provide personal support (financial, emotional, or instrumental). The client is then asked to indicate whether the supportive others are family members, fellow workers, or social acquaintances. By next identifying those individuals that have been sources of support for 5 years or more, the client gains increased awareness of the stability of personal support systems. After examining current sources of support, the client and the nurse can mutually determine the adequacy of support. If it is inadequate, decisions should be made concerning what can be done to enhance existing social support networks. Figure 12–3 provides a sample support system review for a hypothetical client. Following review of the client's social support systems, the following additional questions can be explored:

- In what areas do you need more support: financial, emotional, instrumental?
- Who within your present support system might provide the support but is not already providing it?
- What other individuals could become a part of your support system?
- What could you do specifically to add the people whom you believe you need in your support system?

Answers to these questions suggest actions that the client could take to expand sources of personal support.

Emotional Support Diagram

Sources of emotional support can also be diagrammed in such a way that strength of support is readily apparent. Figure 12–4 presents a sample emotional support diagram that is coded to indicate strong, moderate, and weak sources of support, as well as current conflicts with supportive individuals. The length of each line can be used to indicate geographical proximity to the client. This approach is particularly appropriate for clients who need a more visual presentation of their emotional support system in order to take action effectively to sustain or enhance emotionally satisfying relationships.

Review of social support systems is an integral part of the decision-making phase of health behavior. Through review, the client is assisted in recognizing current sources of support and in identifying barriers in social relationships that may thwart desirable health actions. The nurse must always be alert to client situations where social support is minimal or nonexistent. Extensive review of support systems may cause anxiety and depression for the client. In this case, a more informal, nonthreatening approach should be used.

• SOCIAL SUPPORT AND HEALTH

During the past decade, numerous studies have demonstrated the importance of social support to mental and physical health. In fact, between 1984 and 1991, 4247 papers on

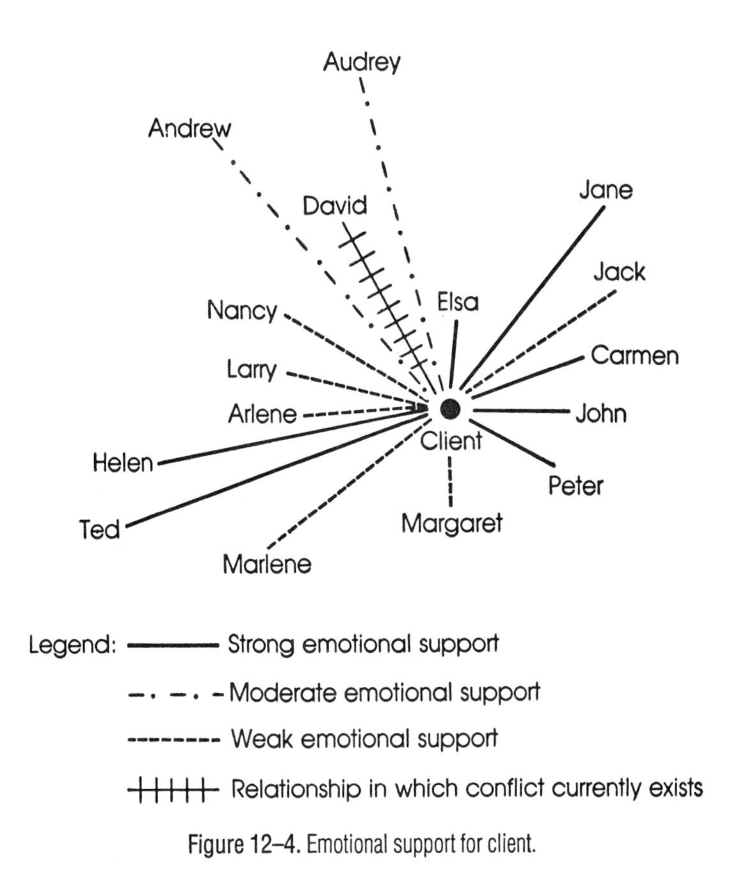

Figure 12–4. Emotional support for client.

social support were published in the medical, nursing, psychology, and sociology journals.[27] Lower levels of support appear consistently linked to higher rates of morbidity and mortality. House and colleagues have proposed that insufficient social support be considered a "risk factor" for mortality from a number of acute and chronic diseases.[28]

The actual mechanisms linking social support to health are not well understood. Several differing mechanisms have been proposed. Social support may directly link to health by promoting healthy or unhealthy behaviors, by providing information, or by providing tangible resources (child care, opportunities for work). Psychologically, social support may provide a sense of meaning to life or be associated with more positive affective states, such as improved sense of self-worth and increased sense of control. In a positive mood, individuals may appraise events as less threatening resulting in less physiologic arousal. Biologically, social support may enhance positive neuroendocrine and immunologic responses despite the presence of stressors.[29] All of these possible mechanisms present challenging questions for social support research.

The question has been raised as to whether gender differences exist in the dynamics of social support. In exploring gender differences, the relationship between social support and physical health may be weaker and more complex for women than for men, whereas the relationship between social support and mental health may be stronger for women than for men.[28(pp542–544)] Interestingly, women appear to be less biologically reactive to stressors than men.[30] Therefore, it is logical to ask if there are gender differences in the mechanisms linking social support and health, in socialization into use of social support as a coping strategy, or in learned behaviors of care and support to dependent others. Research has substantiated that women are more likely than men to be both social support providers and social support recipients. Married men rely heavily on their wives for social support, so a viable marriage is related to their satisfaction with support. Women rely on a balance of familial and nonfamilial support relationships, as some married women do not obtain personal social support from their spouse so turn to friends as confidants.[31] Women are primarily responsible for maintaining social networks that both men and women use. Thus, networks demanding high energy for maintenance can be a source of strain as well as potential support for women.[32] Interestingly, some studies have found higher mortality rates in women with high levels of social support.[33] This is a result that needs further exploration in diverse female populations.

Early adolescence is a period of high life stress when social support is critically needed. Cauce et al[34] examined the relationships among negative life events, locus of control, social support, and psychologic adjustment among 120 sixth- and eighth-graders. Students were predominantly white and middle class. Three sources of social support were evaluated: family support, peer support, and school support. Family support was correlated positively with perceived general, peer, and physical competence. Higher scores on locus of control for success were related to more positive adjustment, whereas locus of control for failures was unrelated to all measures of adjustment. School support was positively related to school competence; peer support was negatively related to school competence. Understanding these differing patterns of support is critical to the well-being of children, as impaired school performance is often the first sign of maladjustment. Yarcheski and colleagues[35] conducted an interesting study of the mediating role of hopefulness in the relationship between social support and general well-being among midadolescents. Hopefulness was defined as the degree to which an adolescent possesses a comforting belief that a personal, positive future exists. Study results indicated considerable mediation of the social support and general well-being relationship by hopefulness.

Thompson and Peebles-Wilkins[36] explored the impact of formal and informal social support networks on the psychologic well-being of black adolescent mothers. Survey data indicated that both lay and professional social support were important to the young mothers' well-being. Psychologic stress and depression were decreased by support from a male partner, caseworker contact, and membership in a support group. Support from a male partner also enhanced psychologic well-being. Interestingly, support from friends increased psychologic distress. The support for young black adolescent mothers needs to be explored in order to creatively combine the best components of lay and professional support to optimize the well-being of the mother as well as the infant. For a review of social support theories and instruments used in adolescent mothering research, the reader is referred to the work of Secco and Moffatt.[37]

The positive effects of providing support to others is a relatively new area of social support research. Most studies have focused on the positive effects of receiving support. Giving help may have positive effects on well-being for at least three different reasons:

the realization that one has helped an individual in need is a self-validating experience that can bolster feelings of psychologic well-being; giving aid to others fosters intimacy and trust, thereby strengthening existing social bonds, and giving support to significant others increases the probability that one's own need for assistance will be met in the future. An analysis of data from a national sample of persons 65 years of age and over revealed that as the level of education increased, individuals gave more informal and formal support to others. Informal support provided to others increased perceptions of personal control. Furthermore, as feelings of personal control increased, affective and somatic depressive symptoms decreased and perceptions of well-being increased. Helping others informally had a greater impact on well-being than helping others through formal organizational structures.[38] This contrast between providing informal and formal support and its relationship to health needs further exploration.

Social Networks and Social Support and Use of Prevention Services

The role of social networks and social support in promoting use of prevention services has been demonstrated by the findings of a number of studies. It is widely accepted that social networks function as conduits for information and as links to broader societal contacts. These social network functions may account for the finding by Kang and colleagues[39] that African-American women with larger social networks compared to smaller ones showed increased use of mammography screening. Interestingly, the amount of instrumental and social support that these women reported had no effects on use of preventive screening. Further study of cancer screening practices of older African Americans indicated that use of occult blood stool examination to detect colo-rectal cancer was highest among those who reported larger social networks.

Among low-income Mexican-American women, a group with the lowest rate of cancer screening in the United States, Suarez and colleagues[40] studied the extent to which differences in social networks accounted for differences in breast and cervical cancer screening. Women were grouped into three strata of social networks, low, medium, and high. The 2-year reported prevalence of Pap smear and mammography use increased with social network scores. Of the six social network components measured, the number of close friends was the most important predictor of use of mammography and Pap smear screening.

The mechanisms linking social support and use of preventive services need to be better understood. Particularly important is understanding how beliefs about personal vulnerability to disease or illness interact with the level and type of social support experienced to motivate use of screening services for early detection.

Social Support and Health Behavior

Research to date indicates that social networks, particularly persons in the network who provide social support, affect observed health behavior. It is well known that significant others function as an important lay referral system for individuals making decisions to seek professional care for health promotion, illness prevention, or care in illness. The resultant effects can be negative or positive. When a client is a member of a culture that differs markedly from that of health professionals, an extended lay-consultant structure may be available, which delays seeking professional care. For example, cultural rituals without therapeutic value may be applied before health professionals are consulted. In contrast, where the culture is similar to that of health professionals, the lay system may be bypassed and contact with health providers made early in the course of a problem or concern. Individuals use their lay referral system not only during the decision phase, concerning whether to seek care, but also during the action phase to make decisions about adherence. Diagnostic decisions, prescriptions for medication, and life changes recommended by health professionals frequently are discussed with significant others who constitute the individual's lay referral system. Concurrence by the lay referral system often determines the extent to which advice from health professionals is actually followed.

In the classic Alemeda County studies, which focused on the relationship between health behaviors and well-being, researchers found a positive association between social support from friends, relatives, and church groups and preventive behavior.[41] This finding has been confirmed in the National Survey of Personal Health Practices and Consequences. Results indicated that persons who visited friends and relatives more frequently, were married, or participated in various social groups were more likely to engage in physical activity, have positive nutrition habits, and discontinue smoking.[42] Zimmerman and Connor have offered a number of suggestions as to ways in which significant others can influence health behaviors[18(pp57–75)]:

1. Other asking person to change behavior because it is disturbing to them
2. Perceiving that other desires a change in one's habits
3. Other approval of persons making similar changes
4. Other having control over one's behavior (food preparation)
5. Concern of other for one's health elicits self-care behaviors
6. Participating with other in a health-promotion program and learning skills for change
7. Other modeling healthy behaviors

Maintenance of health-behavior change over time is difficult unless the behavior is encouraged through social support from significant others. This conclusion is supported by a number of studies. Zimmerman and Connor[18(pp57–75)] found among 84 adults, primarily women, that social support and extent of social network together added to explanations of health-behavior change. Families were more influential on health-behavior change than friends or coworkers. Supportiveness and encouragement by others to sustain the new behaviors were more explanatory of maintenance than other's actual health behavior change or modeling. Aaronson[43] in studying a group of pregnant women found that perceived behavior-specific support (encouragement to not drink, not smoke, and not use caffeine) was predictive of women's health behavior, whereas general support was not. In contrast to the findings of Zimmerman and Connor, received support (family behavior congruent with health recommendations for pregnant woman) was related to health behaviors. That is, persons who lived with individuals who abstained from alcoholic or caffeine drinks and therefore modeled these behaviors, were less likely to drink these beverages themselves. Both perceived and received support for healthy behaviors from significant others increased the incidence of these behaviors in the pregnant women.

While many retrospective studies have been done to determine the impact of social support on health behavior, prospective studies are needed in which networks of social support are identified and differences between health-promotion and illness-prevention behaviors are observed. The results from studies to date appear promising, but additional research is needed to delineate in detail the impact of social support on health behaviors.

• IDENTIFYING SOCIAL SUPPORT STRENGTHS AND NEEDS

Functional health patterns relevant to the area of social support include: self-perception–self-concept pattern, role–relationship pattern, and coping–stress tolerance pattern. Each functional health pattern contains a number of diagnoses relevant to social support problems or needs such as altered family processes, hopelessness, self-esteem disturbance, and chronic low self-esteem.[44] The diagnostic taxonomy, while facilitating problem identification, does not allow clear specification of social support assets and resources. Houldin et al[45] have attempted to address this gap by proposing nursing diagnosis for wellness as a basis for clearly identifying and supporting client strength. Inclusion of assets and strengths of clients as phenomena relevant to nursing care is extremely important if nurses are to provide leadership in developing positive strategies for enhancing the health of populations.

• ENHANCING SOCIAL SUPPORT SYSTEMS

Support-enhancing strategies have three goals: assisting individuals and families to strengthen existing supportive relationships, helping individuals and families to establish satisfying interpersonal ties, and preventing disruption of ties from evolving into or contributing to mental or physical illness.

Facilitating Social Bonding

Social skills training represents one approach to changing the characteristics of clients to enable them to develop supportive interpersonal relationships with others. Training can be carried out with individual clients or with groups of people who have similar skills deficits, such as dysfunctional families.[46] Social skills training is based on the belief that socially competent responses can be learned just like other behaviors. Initially, training is directed toward assessing and modifying perceptions of appropriate behavior in social situations. In addition, persons are taught to reevaluate their thoughts about themselves in a more positive manner. Attempts are made to improve social interaction patterns through modeling, role playing, performance feedback (eg, videotapes), coaching, and homework assignments. Skills to be taught can include initiating conversations, giving and receiving compliments, handling periods of silence, enhancing physical attractiveness, nonverbal methods of communication, approaches to physical intimacy, and dealing with criticism and conflict. Within the school setting, training in social skills and problem solving can be provided in the classroom as an approach to preventing the acquisition of socially alienating behaviors. To complement such work, the broader aspects of the school environment should be assessed to determine the extent to which they facilitate or inhibit students' opportunities for and skills in developing social ties.[47]

Enhancing Coping

Preventing the lack of social ties from resulting in serious psychologic and physical problems is particularly important during developmental or situational transition periods. Seminars or groups for widows, children of separated or divorced parents, parents who have lost a child, or relatives of persons imprisoned can assist such persons in coping with life stress. Benefits from such programs include help in understanding puzzling and disturbing emotional reactions, reducing feelings of alienation, and assisting people to cope with the crisis and move ahead into the future. It is important that programs be tailored to the unique needs of the populations served in terms of content and composition.[48]

Persons who have experienced recent loss may or may not have the skills necessary to spend time alone in productive and satisfying activities. Thus, assisting such persons to develop hobbies or skills that can be carried out alone may increase feelings of self-sufficiency and self-confidence. Such activities may be particularly useful to persons who are geographically isolated or who are disabled and cannot participate in formal or informal group activities.

Preventing Loss of Support and Loneliness

Preventing loneliness is a more desirable approach than treatment of loneliness and isolation after it has occurred. Two approaches to prevention include the identification of high-risk groups and educational interventions for persons of all ages focused on developing social support ties.[48] Young, unmarried, unemployed, and low-income persons appear particularly vulnerable to lack of support and loneliness. Obstacles to social participation, such as lack of transportation for the elderly or constant caretaking responsibilities for middle-aged women with elderly parents, can create high-risk populations. When such groups are identified, programs can be planned to decrease aloneness and isolation. Possible programs include transportation vehicles manned by volunteers for those in need, respite programs to provide relief for caretakers, community support groups for families with disabled or impaired members, and teleconference or computer-mediated support groups that can be accessed at home. Modern information technology offers many avenues for person-to-person linking not previously available. Nurses should be in the forefront in applying new and emerging technologies to augment social support.

Educational approaches to prevention of loss of social support and subsequent loneliness include classroom experiences for school children that help them gain experience in making friends, working cooperatively with others, and resolving differences or conflict. Over the past 30 years there is a growing body of evidence that poor social functioning of children often leads to serious personal adjustment problems in later life. Most experts would agree that children require the security of positive reciprocal relationships with their peers, parents, and teachers for maximum growth and development.[46]

For older adults, public service announcements concerning the importance of building sound relationships with relatives and friends may be the cues needed to initiate support-enhancing behavior. In addition, pamphlets, community programs, and neighborhood activities can be geared to helping persons build their own relationships or to reaching out to others in need of friendship and companionship.

Other general suggestions for enhancing social support include:

- Mutual goal setting with significant others to achieve common directions in actions and efforts

- Providing additional encouragement, personal warmth, and love to significant others
- Dealing constructively with conflict between oneself and support group members
- Offering assistance more frequently to individuals within personal social network to show concern and promote trust
- Seeking counseling, if needed, to enhance marital adjustment
- Making use of the nurse and other health professionals as community support resources
- Capitalizing on ties to a number of social groups in order to expand horizons for new growth opportunities

In attempting to enhance personal support networks, clients should be encouraged to identify specific goals to be achieved. By focusing on one or two changes at a time relevant to goals of highest priority, clients can often markedly alter the breadth and depth of social support available to them.

DIRECTIONS FOR RESEARCH IN SOCIAL SUPPORT

A convincing number of studies have demonstrated the importance of social support to health. Discovery of this link raises many additional research questions that to date remain unanswered. Current areas for fruitful research include[49,50]:

1. Distinguish empirically separable dimensions of social support.
2. Develop valid and reliable measures of social support as a multidimensional construct.
3. Determine the causal pathways between social support and physical and mental health.
4. Further clarify relationships between emotional state and the status of the immune system.
5. Determine if social support improves health outcomes independent of stressors or acts to decrease susceptibility to poor health only in the presence of increased stress.
6. Identify the mechanisms through which social support creates or activates resilience in children living in adverse conditions.
7. Differentiate between the constructs of social networks and social support and develop valid, reliable, and culturally sensitive measures of both including their component dimensions.

SUMMARY

With the important role that social support appears to play in the health and well-being of clients, the nurse cannot provide comprehensive health-protective and health-promotive care without considering the social context of the client, be it individual or family. Social support groups appear to be instrumental in assisting clients to cope with everyday hassles and major stressful life experiences and in enhancing emotional and physical well-being. The extent to which stressful events threaten health may well depend on the support available from core (family) or extended (community and professional) social networks. The design and evaluation of nursing interventions to enhance social support is critical. These studies will contribute to the development of scientifically sound nursing care interventions directed toward enhancing the quality of human social transactions across the life span.

REFERENCES

1. Bloom JR. The relationship of social support and health. *Soc Sci Med.* 1990;30:635–637.
2. Tolsdorf C. Social networks, support and coping: an exploratory study. *Fam Process.* 1976;15:407–417.
3. Norbeck JS. Challenges in social support research. The 8th Helen Nahm Research Lecture. San Francisco, CA: School of Nursing, University of California, 1988, p. 9.
4. Bowling A, Browne PD. Social networks, health, and emotional well-being among the oldest old in London. *J Gerontol.* 1991;(suppl. to No. 1)46(1):S20–S32.
5. Kahn RL, Antonucci TC. Convoys over the life course: attachment, roles and social support. In: Baltes PT, Brim O, eds. *Lifespan development and behavior.* New York, NY: Academic Press; 1980;3:253–286.
6. Moss GE. *Immunity and Social Interaction.* New York, NY: John Wiley and Sons; 1973.
7. Silverstein M, Waite LJ. Are blacks more likely than whites to receive and provide social support in middle and old age? Yes, no and maybe so. *J Gerontol.* 1993;48(4):S212–S222.
8. Chapman LS. Developing a useful perspective on spiritual health: love, joy, peace and fulfillment. *Am J Health Prom.* 1987;2:12–17.
9. Franks P, Campbell TL, Shields CG. Social relationships and health: the relative roles of family functioning and social support. *Soc Sci Med.* 1992;34:779–788.
10. Garmezy N. Resiliency and vulnerability to adverse developmental outcomes associated with poverty. *Am Behav Scientist.* 1991;34:416–430.
11. Garmezy N. Children in poverty: resilience despite risk. *Psychiatry.* 1993; 56:127–136.
12. Werner EE. The children of Kauai: resiliency and recovery in adolescence and adulthood. *J Adolesc Health.* 1992;13:262–268.
13. Rutter M. Resilience: some conceptual considerations. *J Adolesc Health.* 1993;14:626–631.
14. Fonagy P, Steele M, Steele H, et al. The Emanuel Miller Memorial Lecture 1992: the theory and practice of resilience. *J Child Psychol Psychiatry.* 1994;35(2):231–257.
15. Schoenbach VJ, Kaplan BH, Fredman L, et al. Social ties and mortality in Evans County, Georgia. *Am J Epidemiol.* 1986;123(4):577–591.
16. Keitner GI, Miller IW. Family functioning and major depression: an overview. *Am J Psychiatry.* 1990;147(9):1128–1137.
17. Schuster TL, Kessler RC, Aseltine RH. Supportive interactions, negative interactions, and depressed mood. *Am J Community Psychol.* 1990;18(3):423–438 .
18. Zimmerman RS, Connor C. Health promotion in context: the effects of significant others on health behavior change. *Health Educ Q.* 1989;16(1):57–75.
19. Parkerson GR, Michener JL, Wu RL, et al. Associations among family support, family stress, and personal functional health status. *J Clin Epidemiol.* 1989;42(3):217–229.
20. Kane CF. Family social support: toward a conceptual model. Adv Nurs Sci. 1988;10(2):18–25.

21. Walls CT, Zarit SH. Informal support from black churches and the well-being of elderly blacks. *Gerontologist.* 1991;31(4):490–495.
22. Davis DT, Bustamante A, Brown CP, et al. The urban church and cancer control: a source of social influence in minority communities. *Public Health Rep.* 1994;109(4):500–506.
23. Mahon J, McFarlane J, Golden K. De Madres a Madres: a community partnership for health. *Public Health Nurs.* 1991;8(1):15–19.
24. Lieberman MA, Borman LD. (eds). *Self-help Groups for Coping with Crisis.* San Francisco, Calif: Jossey-Bass Inc Publishers; 1979.
25. Levy L. Processes and activities in groups. In: Leiberman MA, Borman LD, eds. *Self-help Groups for Coping with Crisis,* San Francisco, Calif: Jossey-Bass Inc Publishers; 1979. pp 234–271.
26. Glaser B, Kirschenbaum H. Using values clarification in a counseling setting. *Personnel and Guidance Journal,* 1980;59:569–575.
27. Callaghan P, Morissey J. Social support and health: a review. *J Adv Nurs.* 1993;18:203–210.
28. House JS, Landis KR, Umberson D. Social relationships and health. *Science.* 1988;241: 540–544.
29. Shumaker SA, Hill SA. Gender differences in social support and physical health. *Health Psychol.* 1991;10(2):102–111.
30. Manuck SB, Polefrone JM. Psychophysiologic reactivity in women. In: Eaker ED, Packard B, Wenger B, et al, eds. *Coronary Heart Disease in Women.* New York, NY: Haymarket Doyma; 1987:164–171.
31. Antonucci TC, Akiyama H. An examination of sex differences in social support in mid and later life. *Sex Roles.* 1987;17:737–749.
32. Rook KS. The negative side of social interaction: impact on psychological well-being. *J Pers Soc Psychol.* 1984;46:1097–1108.
33. Orth-Gomer K, Johnson JV. Social network interaction and mortality: a six year follow-up study of a random sample of the Swedish population. *J Chronic Dis.* 1987;24:83–94.
34. Cauce AM, Hannan K, Sargeant M. Life stress, social support, and locus of control during early adolescence: interactive effects. *Am J Community Psychol.* 1992;20(6):787–798.
35. Yarcheski A, Scoloveno MA, Mahon NE. Social support and well-being in adolescents: the mediating role of hopefulness. *Nurs Res.* 1994;43(5):288–292.
36. Thompson MS, Peebles-Wilkins W. The impact of formal, informal, and societal support networks on the psychological well-being of black adolescent mothers. *Soc Work.* 1992;37(4):322–328.
37. Secco ML, Moffatt MEK. A review of social support theories and instruments used in adolescent mothering research. *J Adolesc Health.* 1994;15:517–527.
38. Krause N, Herzog AR, Baker E. Providing support to others and well-being in later life. *J Gerontol.* 1992;47(5):300–311.
39. Kang SH, Bloom JR, Romano PS. Cancer screening among African-American women: their use of tests and social support. *Am J Public Health.* 1994;84(1):101–103.
40. Suarez L, Lloyd L, Weiss N, et al. Effect of social networks on cancer-screening behavior of older Mexican-American women. *J Natl Cancer Inst.* 1994;86(10):775–779.
41. Wingard D, Berkman LF. A multivariate analysis of health practices and social networks. In: Cohen S, Syme L, eds. *Social Support and Health.* New York, NY: Academic Press; 1985:161–175.
42. Gottlieb NH, Green LW. Life events, social networks, life-style and health: An analysis of the 1979 National Study of Personal Health Practices and Consequences. *Health Education Quarterly,* 1979;14:91–105.
43. Aaronson LS. Perceived and received support: effects on health behavior during pregnancy. *Nurs Res.* 1989;38(1):4–9.

44. Gordon M. *Manual of Nursing Diagnosis, 1993–1994.* St Louis, Mo: Mosby Year Book; 1993.
45. Houldin AD, Salstein SW, Ganley KM. *Nursing Diagnoses for Wellness: Supporting Strengths.* New York, NY: JB Lippincott Co; 1987.
46. Eisler RM. Promoting health through interpersonal skills. In: Matarazzo JD, Weiss SM, Herd JA, et al, eds. *Behavioral Health: A Handbook of Health Enhancement and Disease Prevention.* New York, NY: John Wiley & Sons; 1984:351–362.
47. Mitchell RE, Billings AG, Moos RH. Social support and well-being: implications for prevention programs. *J Prim Prev.* 1982;3(2):77–98.
48. Rook KS. Promoting social bonding: strategies for helping the lonely and isolated. *Am Psychol.* 1984;39:1389–1407.
49. Bloom JR. The relationship of social support and health. *Soc Sci Med.* 1990;30(5):635–637.
50. Dean K, Holst E, Kreiner S, et al. Measurement issues in research on social support and health. *J Epidemiol Community Health.* 1994;48:201–206.

V

PART FIVE

Approaches for Promoting a Healthier Society

13

Protecting and Promoting Health Through Social and Environmental Change

- Health as a Social Goal
- Health in a Third-Wave Society
- Expanding Choices and Behavioral Options Through Healthy Public Policy
- Promoting Health Through Environmental Control
    - A. Eliminating Health-damaging Features of the Environment
    - B. Augmenting Health-promoting Features of the Environment
- Voluntary Change versus Legislative Policy
- Economic Incentives in Society for Disease Prevention and Health Promotion
- Directions for Research
- Summary

The relationships among individuals, families, friends, neighborhoods, organizations and the larger political, social, and environmental structures are critical determinants of health.[1] Effective health-promotion efforts, therefore, must take into consideration the dynamic relationships between evolving individuals and families and changing social and environmental contexts.[2] Health and social policies that fail to directly address harmful living conditions such as poverty, abuse, violence, hunger, and unemployment, as well as environmental threats such as pollution in worksites and communities sustain rather than ameliorate conditions damaging to health. Individual and family efforts to adopt healthy behaviors are likely to be highly frustrated and ineffective as a result of environmental constraints and prevailing policies that impede healthy living. Any strategy for health promotion that focuses only on behavior change is doomed to failure without simultaneous efforts to alter the physical and social environment and collective behavior.

In the Health Promotion Model, interpersonal influences and situational factors are proposed as affecting decisions to engage in health-promoting behaviors. Creative initiatives to foster social and environmental conditions that actively promote health are addressed in this chapter and Chapter 14.

• HEALTH AS A SOCIAL GOAL

Health needs to be identified clearly as a social as well as an individual goal. The health of societies, of communities, of families, and of individuals are integrated and inseparable. Life opportunities, justice, available behavior options, and extent of control over one's destiny afforded by a society are powerful influences on health. The negative effects of a social system that is oppressive rather than liberating are highly visible in the living conditions of many disadvantaged groups throughout the world. It should be of utmost concern to democratic societies to build sound social structures that enhance the wellness of their populations. Foundations for enhancing wellness include, but are not limited to, the integrity and fairness of social settings with which children and adults interact; the extent to which the larger society and its structures are just, empowering, and engendering of hope; the support available within family and peer groups; the quality of children's developmental and educational experiences; and the extent to which experiences in society support the development of generic life competencies such as problem solving, communication skills, interpersonal support building, and conflict resolution skills. The enormous costs of failing to lay a firm foundation for health in the early years of life are apparent every day in spiraling health care costs, the prevalence of mental distress, patterns of delinquency, and the heavy caseloads of criminal justice and legal systems.[3]

Health as a social goal requires that we integrate theories that address social change (eg, critical social theory, ecologic framework, community organization, community empowerment) with theories that address individual behavior change (eg, social cognitive theory, cognitive evaluation theory, theory of reasoned action) and family change (eg, family stress theory, family development theory, family systems theory). The three theoretical perspectives are complementary. Butterfield[4] has commented that people's cultural heritage, social roles, and economic situation combine to influence patterns of health behaviors. Meleis[5] has challenged nurses to consider the social conditions that limit achievement of human health potential in many communities and societies. When nurses think only in terms of one-to-one relationships, they severely limit the range of intervention possibilities.[4] Rather than focusing downstream when the damage is already done, thinking "upstream" focuses the efforts of health professionals on modifying economic, political and environmental factors that have been shown to be the precursors of poor health throughout the world.[4]

The pursuit of health as a social goal requires competent communities that are committed to building healthy public policy, creating environments supportive of health, strengthening community action capabilities, and working to reorient health services to meet the needs of their citizens.[6] Particularly in primary health care, addressing social and environmental barriers to good health is key to realizing improvements in health status for individuals, families, and communities. Goeppinger[7] defines competent communities as those capable of (1) collaborating effectively in identifying the problems and needs of their community, (2) achieving a working consensus on goals and priorities, (3) agreeing on ways and means to implement the agreed-upon goals, and (4) collaborating effectively in the required actions. As a community gains competence in negotiating for resources to address a particular problem, the community enhances its capacity to cope with other problems as they arise. The emergence of community competence is dependent on three levels of change: positive changes in perceptions and behaviors of individuals, increases in the social support functions of social networks, and readjustment of health services and health policies of relevant institutions.[7(pp4–5)]

Eng et al[1(pp2–4)] describe an ecologic framework for health promotion in which the determinants of health are organized into the following five categories: (1) intrapersonal factors (knowledge, beliefs, attitudes), (2) interpersonal factors (social support, nature of client-provider interaction), (3) organizational factors (health services available, school and worksite conditions), (4) community factors (social norms), and (5) policy factors (rules and regulations, entitlement to services). Each category suggests a related set of interventions that can be approached from either a social control or social change perspective. These perspectives are contrasted in Figure 13–1. Social control views communities

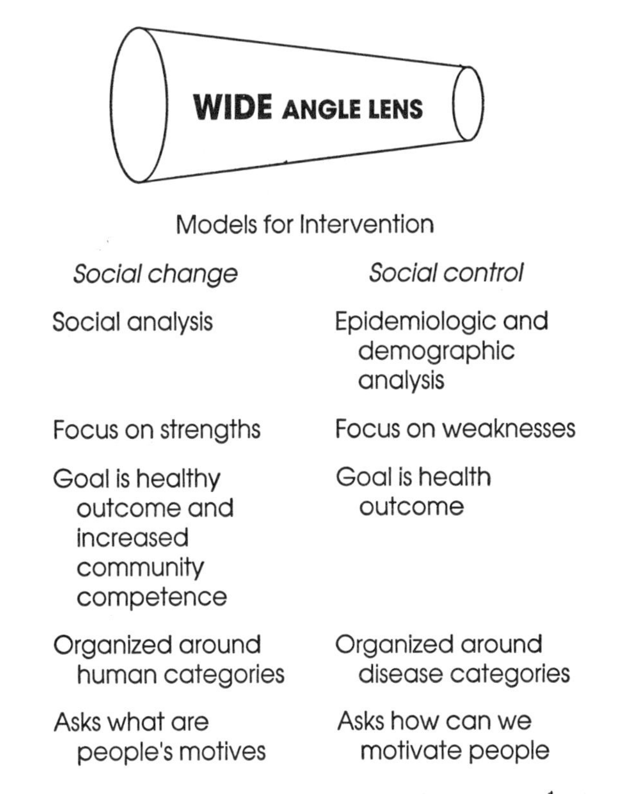

Figure 13–1. Comparison of social change and social control models. (From Eng et al,[1] with permission.)

as dependent and in need of an expert spokesperson with external rewards needed to "bring about" the desired behaviors. Social change focuses on a community's strengths and how these strengths can be used to best advantage in fostering continuing development of community competence. A social change perspective is consistent with an expansive view of health, which incorporates the ideas of growth, expression of human potential, and positive transformations.

Nurses, as part of their education and practice, need to spend more time immersed in the community and its varied settings as opposed to the narrow confines of hospitals and community clinics, for it is in the community in which people live out their daily lives that the ideas and power exist to fuel widespread health promotion efforts. Enduring, large-scale behavior change is best achieved by changing the standards of acceptable behavior in a community rather than by attempting to change the behavior of individuals against overwhelming social odds.

Health professionals should focus not on directing social change but on supporting social change in communities. The healthy development of societies calls for major input from citizens as well as from scientists and practitioners beyond the traditional health professions. There need to be formed new health alliances that include broad representation from target populations as well as professionals such as economists, urban planners, political scientists, and representatives from legal, welfare, and criminal justice systems.[3(p408)] Through strategically building coalitions, societies can make the pursuit of health as a social goal a reality.

• HEALTH IN A THIRD-WAVE SOCIETY

Despite the absence of comprehensive enabling legislation, health care reform in the United States is proceeding at a rapid rate propelled by social, environmental, and economic forces. Toffler and Toffler have identified the changes of major proportions that are now occurring globally as the information revolution or the **third wave**. They identify the other major changes or waves in history as the agricultural revolution (**first wave**) and the industrial revolution (**second wave**). They encourage all citizens to engage in analysis of the third wave so that key changes can be identified as they emerge and positively influenced by society.[8]

Characteristics of the third wave with critical importance to the promotion of health include: (1) demassification of society, (2) decentralization of decision making, (3) empowerment of the family and the home, and (4) minority-based or multicultural democracy.[8(pp82–88)] The increasing availability of information technology will move health care away from standardized health care protocols for the masses and toward highly customized health care plans and services for individual clients. Based on comprehensive, computerized health assessment, a number of information systems have already been developed to tailor health-protection–promotion interventions to the knowledge, beliefs, motivations, and prior health-behavior histories of diverse individuals and families.

In the third wave it is predicted that decision making will be decentralized rather than under the control of a select group of health professionals. Information is power, and the public will have self-assessment tools, diagnostic technology, decision-making protocols, and information input capabilities available to it as never before. The public will increasingly have available to it a broad range of information and related technologies to assist in making informed health care decisions. The balance of power in health care will change, enabling citizens to more directly impact the social and environmental conditions integral to their health and well-being.

Information systems will also enable large segments of any community to be in touch with each other about the social problems that they face and their potential solutions. Furthermore, a composite plan for addressing health-related social and environmental conditions can be jointly developed by citizens without their even leaving their homes. Information technology offers the possibility of direct contact with policy makers in relation to health issues, formation of national networks to enhance local coalitions, and development of multiple communication links between health facilities and grassroots community groups.[9]

The information era will also bring about changes that will empower families. Parents will often work at home as well as receive health information and health care at home through taking advantage of interactive computer technology.

The Tofflers project minority-based or multiculturally based democracy that can facilitate cooperative human existence. In a demassified society, it is not majorities but minorities that count. The rising activism of minorities reflects a need for social systems that are more varied, open, and responsive to their needs.[8(pp92–96)] In a multicultural democracy, cultural differences can enrich our portfolio of health-promotion interventions through the study and use of interventions that are now marginalized as outside of "mainstream" health care. Rather than looking for majority health care issues, health professionals will seek to understand the rapidly shifting health care needs of targeted segments of a multicultural society. Rapid response to health care needs of communities by health professionals who are culturally competent will be essential to meet consumer demands for "user-friendly" health care.

The information revolution will challenge health professionals to think creatively about the future of health care and new ways of educating health professionals to be more flexible and responsive to the needs of a multicultural society. Futurist perspectives should be critically analyzed by nurses so that the profession stays at the forefront in helping clients to enhance health amid conditions of rapid social and environmental change.

• EXPANDING CHOICES AND BEHAVIORAL OPTIONS THROUGH HEALTHY PUBLIC POLICY

The importance of shaping healthy policies in the public and private sectors as the primary vehicle for achieving major improvements in health status for populations has been widely advocated by Milio.[10–12] The following six propositions are proposed by Milio in her framework for prevention:

1. The health status of populations is the result of deprivation (eg, inadequate food and shelter) or excess (eg, obesity and alcoholism) of critical personal or societal health-sustaining resources.

2. Behavioral patterns of populations are a result of habitual selection from limited choices, and these habits of choice are related to (a) actual and perceived options available and (b) beliefs and expectations developed and refined over time by socialization, formal learning, and immediate experience.
3. Organizational behavior (decisions or policy choices made by governmental or nongovernmental, national or nonnational, nonprofit or for profit, formal or nonformal organizations) sets the range of options available to individuals for personal choice making.
4. The choice making of individuals at a given point in time concerning potentially health-promoting or health-damaging selections is affected by their efforts to maximize valued resources.
5. Social change may be thought of as changes in patterns of behavior resulting from shifts in the choice making of significant numbers of people within a population.
6. Health education, as the process of sharing health-supporting information, can have little impact on behavior or personal choice making of groups without the easy availability of new, or newly perceived, alternative health-promoting options.

Malnutrition is a good example of a health problem prevalent at all socioeconomic levels, but for different reasons. Malnutrition among the affluent results from excessive consumption of calorie-rich, nutrient-poor foods that have popular appeal or are convenient to eat or prepare. Individuals and families that can afford to eat frequently in restaurants where food costs are high often consume nutrient-poor meals that are cost-effective for restaurants to offer. Lower socioeconomic groups are often malnourished because of deprivation resulting from inability to purchase nutritious foods with limited resources. In addition, low-income families may not fully understand how to invest their food dollars for maximum nutritional quality. If individuals feel powerless in controlling their environment and lives, they may continue to limit personal choices even when a broader range of health-promoting options becomes available.[10(p436)]

Milio contends that health-damaging options are more accessible than health-promoting options among low-income groups. The cigarettes, sucrose, alcohol, and pollutants unregulated by healthy public policies are readily available to the poor, while at the same time they are deprived of the level of protection afforded by the quality of food, shelter, and environment that sustain the more affluent. Compounding the problem of choices for all socioeconomic groups, health-damaging options are not only more readily accessible but often are more attractively packaged and less costly than health-promoting options. Although individual and family behavior can change, often such changes must be made in the face of counterforces consisting of advertising, reference group norms, and the prevalent American lifestyle. Organizational control of advertising, production, and pricing policies sets the parameters of choice for many Americans. Advertising appeals to the emotions, priorities, preferences, and even self-concept of many Americans. Influential, attractive, and successful people are used to promote products that are actually health-damaging rather than health-promoting.[10(p436)]

Milio has proposed that choice-making behavior at any point in time reflects individual and organizational efforts to maximize valued resources. The value atmosphere or hierarchy characteristic of a particular society will determine those resources that are valued and consequently maximized. In Western culture, many individuals and groups make choices based on cost versus actual or perceived gain. As an example, for some individuals the cessation of smoking may be perceived as too great a sacrifice for the benefit of healthy lungs 15 to 25 years hence. For industry, the profit available from the manufacture of tobacco products appears to offset any concerns about the potentially lethal effects of smoking. Thus, profit from the manufacture and sales of products that put the health of individuals and society at risk is a powerful financial incentive for industries, organizations, and the government itself. Because health promotion represents a new direction in health policy, the profit-generating potential of health-protecting and health-promoting products and services is just beginning to be explored and tapped. Citizens and health care professionals should foster expansion of this market by **creating the demand** for such products and **inventing** new self-care products that protect and promote health.[10(p436)]

• PROMOTING HEALTH THROUGH ENVIRONMENTAL CONTROL

The quality of the physical environment in which people live is critical to the short-term and long-term health of populations. Not only should health-damaging features of the environment be eliminated, but health-enhancing features should be augmented and actively used to promote improved health and well-being.

Eliminating Health-Damaging Features of the Environment

The harmful effects of toxic substances in the environment are vividly illustrated by the fact that nearly 3 million poor inner-city children are "at risk" from elevated lead levels. Lead can be found in urban areas not only in paint but in dust and soil. Exposure to high levels of lead can be fatal, but even low exposures can be toxic to the central nervous system, resulting in delayed learning, impaired hearing, and growth deficits. Such disorders severely limit the potential of children to compete successfully in school and make affected children prone to early dropout and compromised adult lives. *Healthy People 2000* has set as one of its objectives to eliminate blood lead levels above 25 μg/dL in children under age 5 years.[13]

Leading indoor air hazards to which many thousands of people are exposed each year are **tobacco smoke** and **radon.** Environmental tobacco smoke is a cause of disease including lung cancer in nonsmokers. Children of parents who smoke are more likely to develop lower respiratory tract infections and middle ear infections than children of parents who do not smoke. A national health goal for 2000 is to reduce to 20% from 39% the number of children with smokers in their homes.[13(p150)]

The Environmental Protection Agency reports that although inexpensive kits are available for radon testing, only 5% of homes have actually been tested. As many as 8 million homes may have radon at a level requiring correction. Radon, when inhaled, releases ionizing radiation causing damage to lung tissue and lung cancer. The goal in *Healthy People 2000* is to raise the number of homes tested and found to be safe to 40%.[13(p320)]

Nursing as a health care profession must take responsibility for protecting and maintaining an environment that is health-strengthening rather than health-damaging. Five categories of environmental agents that can contribute to increased human health risks are presented in Table 13–1. The categories of health-damaging agents are: pathogenic agents, natural and synthetic chemicals, radiation, nutritional substances, and physical objects. Noise, which is not included in any category, is also a feature of the environment that can be potentially stressful and health damaging. Hearing loss ranks among the top 10 occupational hazards. Developing interventions to foster the use of hearing protection at worksites has been the target of on-going research efforts by Lusk and her colleagues at the University of Michigan.[14,15]

TABLE 13–1. FIVE CATEGORIES OF ENVIRONMENTAL AGENTS THAT CAN BE PROXIMATE CONTRIBUTORS TO INCREASED HUMAN HEALTH RISKS*

PATHOGENIC AGENTS	NATURAL AND SYNTHETIC CHEMICALS	RADIATION	NUTRITIONAL SUBSTANCES	PHYSICAL OBJECTS
Many microorganisms (bacteria, fungi, viruses, parasites)	Natural products (chemicals in foods, beverages, plants, animals, insects) Industrial products and by-products Consumer products Pesticides, agricultural chemicals Medicines, medical and diagnostic devices Chemicals used for clothing, shelter, other physical structures and objects Tobacco and its combustion products Substances used for fuels and their combustion products Substances of abuse By-products and wastes from above	All forms of ionizing and nonionizing radiation (including heat, sound)	Constituents of foods and beverages that are not necessary for nutrition	Weapons Machinery, equipment, tools Moving vehicles Components of physical structures Water Natural formation and products

From Rodricks JV,[18].

* Some subgroups contain many individual agents; naturally occurring chemicals in the diet probably make up the single largest subgroup of individual chemicals. Distinctions are made between pathogenic microorganisms that cause harm by invading the body and growing there and those that produce chemical toxins outside the body that cause harm when ingested; the latter are in the group of natural chemical products. Similarly, though the constituents of physical objects are all chemicals, the agents of harm are the objects themselves, and the harm they may create (usually some form of physical trauma) is not related to the hazards of their chemical components.

It has been estimated that there are as many as 2000 airborne chemicals to which persons in the workplace and the community could be exposed. Of these, occupational exposure limits have been set for approximately 700 chemicals, and only 30 chemicals have limits for ambient air.[16] A broad range of legislation is aimed at regulating natural pollutants as well as pollutants generated by human activities. However, a lack of knowledge regarding the exact links of many substances to disease causation, lag time before symptoms appear, and multiple exposures to many different substances complicates the assessment of human health impacts.[17] Despite limitations in methods and techniques, efforts must be made to both **assess** and **manage** risks imposed on the citizenry by the environments in which they carry out their daily lives.

The estimation of health effects resulting from chemical exposure is important to the development of appropriate standards for regulating the manufacture, use, and release of chemicals into the environment. By means of various procedures, the risk caused by inhalation of chemicals, dermal contact, and incidental ingestion can be extrapolated from animal and human data. Efforts have been made to further refine these procedures on the premise that health resources should be devoted to reducing risks in proportion to the toll they take on human health.[18]

Risk assessment is the means by which currently available information about environmental public health problems can be organized and understood. The National Research Council has described four major steps in this risk assessment process: (1) hazard identification, (2) dose-response assessment, (3) exposure assessment (estimation of human exposure over time), and (4) risk characterization (determination of risk for human populations under various exposure scenarios).[19] In **hazard identification,** the range of toxic effects for a substance are identified from the literature. The second step, **dose-response assessment,** is used to describe as accurately as possible the relationship between magnitude, duration, frequency, and timing of chemical exposure and the frequency of manifestation of the chemical's adverse effects. **Human exposure assessment** identifies the range of exposures experienced by the target population of concern. In the fourth step, **risk characterization,** the particular risks that are likely to be experienced by the population of interest under actual expected exposure conditions are described. This four-step assessment framework can be applied to many types of health threats that arise within the environment, including potential threats arising from the introduction of new technologies. Comprehensive risk assessment directs attention to those sources of risk that, if reduced, will yield the greatest public health benefits.[18]

It should be noted by health professionals that the tolerance for risks on the part of individuals and families is based on the characteristics of the risk itself. For example:

1. Voluntarily assumed risks are tolerated better than those imposed by others.
2. Risks over which scientists debate and are uncertain are more feared than those scientific consensus endorses as a risk.
3. Risks of natural origin are often considered to be less threatening than those created by humans.

Affective responses that differ according to the characteristics of the risk being considered can result in undue alarm or apathy. Individuals should be encouraged to consider objective information about the nature and extent of various environmental risks, rather than relying on feelings and emotions. Further, some societies base risk-reduction priorities on the relative ease with which risk reduction can be achieved. Ease of resolution sometimes has a poor correspondence to the public health importance of the risks being attacked. Environmental risk-reduction objectives should be based on the best available scientific knowledge regarding the relative risks of various pollutants to health rather than on what is emotionally appealing or politically attractive at a particular point in time.[18]

Many major environmental risks require intensive, multifaceted, and often long-term interventions to influence related attitudes and to reallocate resources for their control.[18] By focusing on environmental issues at worksites and in the community such as waste minimization, recycling, worker protection from toxic substances, and prevention of noise-induced hearing loss, nurses can play a proactive role in promoting health through environmental management.[20,21]

Augmenting Health-Promoting Features of the Environment

Kaplan and Kaplan[22] have gone beyond the maintenance of a safe environment to view the natural environment as a means of promoting health and well-being. They describe restorative environments in which the recovery of mental energies and personal effectiveness is enhanced. Restorative experiences in the environment create a sense of escape or "being away," immerse the individual "in a whole other world," offer fascinating multisensory stimuli, and foster a "sense of oneness" with the environment. Although the environment has long been considered to be the domain of the artist, the poet, the landscape architect, and the naturalist, increasingly it is considered to be much more than decorative. Understanding the uses of nature and its restorative properties may result in the development of innovative health-promotion modalities for use by care providers in optimizing health and well-being.

Increasing evidence supports the importance of natural environments in assisting individuals to deal with mental fatigue and, specifically, to regain directed attention capacities. Cimprich[23] has developed nursing interventions that use the environment to assist cancer patients to cope with attentional fatigue created by the demands of their illness. In a study of breast cancer patients, the intervention protocol consisted of explanation of the restorative experience, choosing of restorative activities that would be performed for 20 to 30 minutes at least three times a week, contracting in writing to carry out the activities, and keeping track of restorative experiences. Examples of restorative activities selected were sitting or walking in the backyard, a garden, or a park; tending green living things; sitting by a pond, lake, or stream; and observing wild life, birds and animals. A comparison of intervention versus nonintervention groups on attentional performance across various tasks (eg, Digit Span and Symbol Digit Modalities Test, Necker Cube Pattern Control, etc) revealed that the intervention group showed a significant and steady improvement in attentional performance over time, whereas the nonintervention group showed inconsistent performance.

Tennessen and Cimprich,[24] in a subsequent study, explored whether undergraduate students with more natural views from their university dormitory windows scored better than those with less natural views on tests of directed attention. Window views were categorized into four groups ranging from all natural to all built. When a battery of objective measures was used to measure directed attention, natural views were associated with better performance.

The research of Cimprich and her colleagues has important potential implications for creating health-strengthening environments for individuals of all ages in a wide array of contexts. Natural environments, as used in the above studies, undoubtedly provide the best restorative milieus. However, the effects of simulated restorative environments could also be explored, as natural environments may sometimes be unavailable or too dangerous to use for restorative purposes.

Discovery of strategies for fostering health and well-being through use of restorative environments in inner cities, at work sites, and in school settings is likely to be a significant breakthrough in prevention and health promotion. Several important questions arising include: What are the health promoting aspects of the environment? How do features of the environment actually affect mental or physical health? What is the range of psychologic and biologic processes that can be affected positively by restorative environments?

• VOLUNTARY CHANGE VERSUS LEGISLATIVE POLICY

In a democratic society, it is widely assumed that matters of risk critical to survival and security are predominantly subject to regulatory decisions, whereas risks not clearly vital to general health and welfare are issues for personal decision and action. In a democracy, even vital risks may be left to individual decision, providing that they do not infringe on the rights of others. The question can be posed as to what government's role is in legislating environmental and behavioral changes that promote good health and increase longevity. If the government uses the means at its disposal for regulating changes in behavior, it may be faced with problems of an ethical nature. On the other hand, educational approaches may fall short of achieving widespread change in self-damaging behaviors.

Government involvement in lifestyle reform is to some extent supported by the longstanding role of the federal government as a health care provider. In the face of costs of almost insatiable demands for health care, it could be cost-effective for the government to consider legislation that required individuals to assume more self-care responsibility. While such federal regulations might be cost-effective if health-promotion interventions are shown to reduce health care costs substantially, many individuals would resist legislation of preventive and health-promotion measures as unethical or undue intrusion upon individual freedom. Ethical issues, including individual autonomy, must be thoughtfully considered in matters of health.

Over a decade ago, Pellegrino[25] suggested certain guidelines in considering tradeoffs between individual freedom and social responsibility in relation to health. These guidelines are still timely today.

1. Certain lifestyles result in disease, disability, and death, with economic consequences damaging to the whole society. Thus, there is a social mandate to encourage healthier lifestyles in all citizens.
2. In a civilized and democratic society, individual freedom must be protected

and is to be limited only when it violates the freedom of others. In an interdependent society, free acts are subject to justifiable restriction.

3. Coercive measures should be considered only when their effectiveness is unequivocal for large numbers of people and when control extends over a limited sector of life.
4. Even if a societal control measure meets all of the above criteria, it must accommodate as closely as possible the democratic principle of self-determination. Voluntary measures must be clearly inadequate at the outset or must have failed before coercive measures are contemplated.

While government regulation is sometimes deemed necessary for the public good, self-direction is valued by Americans because most individuals believe that they themselves are the best judge of what is good for them, and the process of choosing is considered a good in itself, even when the outcomes are health-damaging. Some persons may voluntarily opt for a brief life span full of unhealthy practices. It can be argued that if the practices are not detrimental to others and are carried out in full awareness of the consequences, these people should be allowed to pursue the course they want. However, the role of the nurse is to make sure that individuals have as much information as possible on which to base informed decisions concerning lifestyle and health-related behavior.[25]

Deciding whether social changes to enhance health should be voluntary or mandatory presents society with a complex dilemma. Should coercion be used, and if so, how and to what extent? Is it coercive to increase cigarette taxes in order to help defray the cost of smoking-induced disease? Would such a move also imply that highly refined sugar products and high-cholesterol foods should also be taxed more heavily to pay for the cost of health problems induced by obesity and atherosclerosis? Should tax on large, high-speed automobiles be proportionately higher than taxes on smaller cars with limited speed and greater fuel economy? Should overweight individuals pay higher taxes than individuals of normal weight, with the excess taxes and interest to be paid back at the time individuals lose weight and arrive at the norm for their height–weight category? Which lifestyle, organizational, and social changes should be voluntary and which should be mandatory through enactment of legislation? Some blend of voluntary and mandatory action is needed. However, the ethical dimensions of such health-related decisions should be given careful consideration.[25]

• ECONOMIC INCENTIVES IN SOCIETY FOR DISEASE PREVENTION AND HEALTH PROMOTION

The dependence of the American people on diagnosis and treatment of disease for improving health and increasing longevity is economically and socially rooted in our culture. Americans have been willing to spend escalating proportions of both personal and public dollars on an increasing array of medical services, hoping for "magic bullets" to cure all ills. It is now apparent that few chronic diseases, once established, can be reversed, although many can be prevented through environmental and behavioral change. Furthermore, the cost of care for chronic illnesses in the United States is extremely high.

Thus, the time is right for restructuring health care policy and the health care system to achieve a balance among prevention, promotion, and treatment services. If disease-prevention and health-promotion services are to be widely available to consumers in the 21st century, the public must be convinced of the value of staying well, the effectiveness of environmental and behavioral change in promoting health and preventing disease, and the economic and human advantage of shifting a portion of health care dollars from the treatment of illness to keeping people healthy.

Public policy experts have already voiced concern that although prevention and health-promotion programs may be cost-effective, the primary goal of such programs should be enhanced health, not financial profit.[26] Because of a persistent history of double-digit inflation in health care costs, disease-prevention and health-promotion interventions will be critically scrutinized to determine their cost-effectiveness and cost-savings potential. They will be put under the "microscope" in the 21st century, as few other services have been, by skeptics who believe people and environments cannot be changed and by groups who reap major profits from illness care. Nurse scientists and nurses in practice who develop health-promotion interventions should be particularly sensitive to the need for cost evaluation as well as health-outcome evaluation.

Two frequently used cost-study methods are: cost-effectiveness analysis (CEA) and cost-benefit analysis (CBA). Each method answers a different question. CEA answers the question, What results were obtained for the money spent? In CEA, benefits or outcomes do not have to be expressed in dollars but may be expressed in days of illness prevented, number of quality-adjusted life years, or decrease in the incidence of domestic abuse and related arrests. Consider comparison of two community interventions for changing fat consumption in the population, one using only mailed self-change kits and the other using mailed kits plus telephone follow-up. The cost of each program per gram of decreased fat consumption in the two groups of participants could be calculated.[27]

In contrast, CBA answers the question, What financial returns are received from the money spent? In CBA, both costs and outcomes are measured in monetary terms. Then a ratio between monetary benefit and cost is constructed. For example, consider the impact of an aerobic exercise program on level of work absenteeism before and after entry into the program. If absenteeism decreases in the experimental group in comparison to a control group, the dollars saved can be contrasted to the cost of offering the program. A benefit-to-cost ratio of 1 : 1 indicates that the program broke even; a ratio of 2 : 1 indicates that the benefits exceeded the costs; and a ratio of 1 : 2 indicates that the program was more costly than economically beneficial.[27]

Positive effects from any health-promotion program requires a chain of events: a structured program, participation continuing over time, and health enhancement or reduction of risk as measured by specified outcome criteria. For many disease-prevention and health-promotion programs, costs are incurred now and benefits derived later. Although an extended time period between costs and benefits can be reconciled mathematically with cost-analysis procedures, it is important to consider how much consumers are willing to spend to improve their health status when they feel well or to protect themselves from a health problem with a 20-year latency. Emphasizing short-term as well as long-term benefits may enhance consumer acceptance of disease-prevention and health-promotion interventions that require marked environmental and behavioral change.[28]

Current insurance coverage offers little in the way of incentives to increase motivation for engaging in prevention and health-promotion activities. For individuals and families that have insurance coverage for hospital care, few have coverage for disease-prevention and health-promotion services because such services cannot be related to a specific diagnosis or medical complaint. Even more distressing is the higher incidence of preventive screening in low-risk groups than in high-risk groups, when the latter group could benefit more from such services but do not have insurance to access them. This is referred to as reverse targeting. During the 1990s an increasing number of Americans found themselves uninsured or underinsured for health care costs. Woolhandler and Himmelstein,[29] in a study of 10,653 women between the ages of 45 and 64, found that the **relative risk of inadequate screening** for uninsured, socioeconomically disadvantaged women was 1.60 for blood pressure check-ups, 1.55 for cervical smears, 1.52 for glaucoma testing, and 1.42 for clinical breast examination. Thus, the people who could benefit most from preventive screening lack access to these services, severely curtailing the potential societal benefits of screening. The disparities in disease and mortality rates among population groups will continue as long as this state of affairs persists.

Managed care organizations have the potential for incorporating prevention and health-promotion activities into the services provided. Rather than discouraging prevention and health promotion, as our present reimbursement system does, economic advantages for using such services should be brought directly to consumers. The following suggestions for financial incentives are offered:

1. Expand insurance coverage to include primary health care services for prevention and health promotion.
2. Offer partial insurance premium refunds for maintaining good health or improving health status.
3. Develop a sliding scale for insurance premiums based on documented attendance at health-education programs and use of early detection screening services.

Nurses, because of the high esteem in which they are held by the public, are in a key position to work with consumer groups to shape health and social policies to offer more incentives for prevention and health promotion. Further, because of their person-environment orientation, nurses can work in collaboration with other professionals and with target populations and communities to promote local, national, and global changes supportive of health and healthy lifestyles.

DIRECTIONS FOR RESEARCH

Environmental and social change approaches to protecting and promoting health offer new vistas for nursing research. Social change approaches to the realization of human health potential will receive more attention than ever before in the next century. The roles of public and organizational policy in managing risk and fostering health need rigorous evaluation. Suggested directions for nursing and interdisciplinary research efforts are as follows:

1. Test the effects of combined family and community health-promotion interventions on positively altering health-related social norms among children and adolescents.
2. Evaluate the effectiveness of interventions to decrease the exposure of children to passive smoke from parental smoking in their homes.
3. Develop and test models for proactive management of the environment to reduce health threats that are man-made or of natural origin.
4. Assess the synergistic effects of various environmental interventions and behavior-change programs on health behaviors and short-term and long-term health outcomes.
5. Test the effectiveness of various economic incentives in increasing health-promoting environmental and behavioral change.
6. Analyze the cost benefits of managed care plans that place extensive focus on health-promotion and disease-prevention services.

The study of interactive effects of human and environmental factors in health and disease is a fascinating area. The complexity of these issues will require interdisciplinary research collaboration to address the many gaps in knowledge that now exist.

• SUMMARY

The focus of this chapter has been on society as a collective and the impact of public policy and social and physical environments on the health status of individuals, families, and communities. Attempts to change health behaviors without changes in the environments in which people live will result in frustration and failure of health-promotion efforts. A balanced approach to disease prevention and health promotion within the United States requires attention to (1) the quality of the environment, (2) the health-promoting and health-damaging options available within the environment, particularly to those most vulnerable, and (3) the health-related behavior norms prevalent in various subgroups within society.

REFERENCES

1. Eng E, Salmon ME, Mullan F. Community empowerment: the critical base for primary care. *Fam Community Health.* 1992;15(1):1–12.
2. McCool WF, Susman EJ. The life span perspective: a developmental approach to community health nursing. *Public Health Nurs.* 1990;7(1):13–21.
3. Cowan EL. In pursuit of wellness. *American Psychologist.* 1991;46(4):404–408.
4. Butterfield PG. Thinking upstream: nurturing a conceptual understanding of the societal context of health behavior. *Adv Nurs Sci.* 1990;12(2):1–8.
5. Meleis AI. Being and becoming healthy: the core of nursing knowledge. *Nurs Sci Q.* 1990;3(3): 107–114.
6. Turner J. WHO charter for health promotion. *Lancet.* 1986;2:1407.
7. Goeppinger J, Lassiter P, Wilcox B. Community health is community competence. *Nurs Outlook.* 1982;30:464–467.

8. Toffler A, Toffler H. *Creating a new civilization: the politics of the third wave.* Atlanta, GA: Turner Publishing; 1995.
9. Milio N. Information technology and community health: invitation to innovation. *J Prof Nurs.* 1991;7(3):146.
10. Milio N. A framework for prevention: changing health-damaging to health-generating patterns. *Am J Public Health.* 1976;66:435–439.
11. Milio N. *Promoting Health Through Public Policy.* Philadelphia, Pa: FA Davis Co; 1981.
12. Milio N. *Primary Care and the Public's Health.* Lexington, Mass: Lexington Books; 1983.
13. *Healthy People 2000: National Health Promotion and Disease Prevention Objectives.* Washington, DC: US Public Health Service; 1991:317. US Dept of Health and Human Services publication PHS 91-50212.
14. Lusk SL, Kelemen MJ. Predicting use of hearing protection: a preliminary study. *Public Health Nurs.* 1993;10(3):189–196.
15. Lusk SL, Ronis D, Kerr MJ, et al. Test of the health promotion model as a causal model of workers' use of hearing protection. *Nurs Res.* 1994;43(3):151–157.
16. Paustenbach DJ. Health risk assessment and the practice of industrial hygiene. *Am Ind Hyg Assoc J.* 1990;51(7):339–351.
17. Harvey PD. Educated guesses: health risk assessment in environmental impact statements. *Am J Law Med.* 1990;16(3):399–427.
18. Rodricks JV. Risk assessment, the environment, and public health. *Environ Health Perspect.* 1994;102(3):258–264.
19. Kimmel CA. Quantitative approaches to human risk assessment for noncancer health effects. *Neurotoxicology.* 1990;11:189–198.
20. Garman C. The nurse and the environment: how one thinks globally and acts locally. *Holistic Nurse Pract.* 1995;9(2):58–65.
21. Clark MJ. *Nursing in the Community.* Norwalk, Conn: Appleton & Lange; 1992:120.
22. Kaplan R, Kaplan S. *The Experience of Nature: A Psychological Perspective.* Cambridge, England: Cambridge University Press; 1989:177–200.
23. Cimprich B. Development of an intervention to restore attention in cancer patients. *Cancer Nurs.* 1993;16(2):83–92.
24. Tennessen CM, Cimprich B. Views to nature: effects on attention. *J Environ Psychol.* In press.
25. Pellegrino ED. Health promotion as public policy: the need for moral groundings. *Prev Med.* 1981;10:371–378.
26. Warner KE. Selling health promotion to corporate America: uses and abuses of the economic argument. *Health Educ Q.* 1987;14(1):39–55.
27. LaRosa JH, Kiefhaber A. Cost analysis and workplace health promotion programs. *Occup Health Nurs.* 1985;33:234–236,262.
28. Leviton LC. Can organizations benefit from health promotion? *Health Serv Res.* 1989;24(2):159–189.
29. Woolhandler S, Himmelstein DU. Reverse targeting of preventive care due to lack of health insurance. *JAMA.* 1988;259:2872–2874.

14

Partnerships for Health Promotion

- The Nature of Health Partnerships
- Why Partnerships?
- The Role of Partnerships in Education, Research, and Practice
- A Community–University Health Partnership Model
- The Role of Schools of Nursing in Developing University–Community Partnerships
- Directions for Research
- Summary

The opportunity to create a new health care system, integrated within and tailored to communities and built on the strengths of an informed and involved citizenry is before us. The current health system is not working well, is too costly for what it yields, and is no longer accepted on "blind faith" as infallible by the American people. We need a coherent approach to restructuring health care amid the high-speed change that will characterize society and politics in the 21st century.[1] We need the spirit of change as opposed to vested-interest efforts to maintain the status quo. Toffler aptly describes the "rear guard . . . who wish to preserve or restore an unworkable past, and those who are ready to make a transition to . . . a 'Third Wave' information-age society."[1(p11)] Milio[2] calls for transition to a renewed health care system that includes developing provider–community alliances and coalitions of consumer groups, who both represent diverse publics and transmit information through multiple channels back to them. She characterizes future health care changes as **outward**—outside large institutions into communities. Milio speaks to a new world that is one of "interdependence among nations, communities, and groups; between environments and individuals; between policies and patterns of action. It is a time when what is bad for some will eventually spill over onto many; when, as we nurture others and our environment, we ourselves are nurtured. It is a time for collaboration, a time for partnership in order to realize to a greater extent our humanness and our health potential in a changing world."[3]

Health partnerships represent "third-wave" thinking in health care. They offer new approaches for linking health providers and communities to create health care systems that are information-intensive and responsive to local needs. Mass-production health care, based on how many patients can be seen in a day, no longer appeals to the public, if it ever did. Green and Raeburn[4] comment that "Industrialized societies have placed their management of health . . . into the hands of 'experts' who in turn are typically associated with large, centralized bureaucracies. Thus a relatively impersonal service takes over some of the most intimate and important human concerns—birth, death, sickness, health, education, care of the elderly and disabled, to mention just a few." The time has come to "repersonalize" health care.

The increasing diversity of cultures in America is creating demands for culturally competent health care that is tailored not only to racial and ethnic groups but to subcultures and individuals within those groups. Cultural fit can only be achieved through community partnerships that recognize the value of community representatives and health care providers coming together to create new health care systems that are user-friendly, accessible, and culture-sensitive. Partnerships optimize the combined resources of all partners so that mutually valued goals are achieved. Braithwaite and colleagues[5] advocate for health partnerships as a way of using community organization to achieve health empowerment and subsequently decrease excessive deaths and illness and improve health in communities of color. Significant advances in health for various racially and ethnically diverse populations will result not only from individual change but from social-structural change that removes constraints to good health and augments opportunities to pursue optimum health and well-being. There must be enacted comprehensive health policies that build a health-sustaining infrastructure within communities.[7]

• THE NATURE OF HEALTH PARTNERSHIPS

Partnership structures may vary by community type and size, past organizing experiences, program goals, racial and cultural preferences, and the nature of the lead organizations. Organizational members may be school districts, corporations or businesses, voluntary organizations, health care provider groups or agencies, churches, self-help groups, community service organizations, and colleges or universities. Particularly exciting is the trend toward formation of partnerships between health professions schools in universities and school districts, worksites, and communities to provide health services as part of the educational experiences of health professions students. This **serve-and-learn** approach is gaining momentum nationally as efforts are made to reawaken the ethic of "community service" among Americans of all ages. Serve-and-learn health partnerships seek to foster the provision of health services that augment the health-enhancing features of social and physical environments as well as improve the health of the people served. Community–university health-promotion partnerships are discussed later in this chapter.

Bracht and Gleason[7] have described five types of health partnership arrangements:

1. Coalition. Existing organizations combine talents and resources to collaborate in addressing community issues or problems. Coalitions tend to be fluid, with organizations free to enter or leave. Considerable effort must be directed toward interorganizational communication.
2. Leadership board or council. Existing leaders and community activists work together toward a common goal. Board leaders are generally from a number of community sectors. Additional volunteers are often recruited to serve on action-oriented task forces.
3. "Lead" or official agency. A single existing community agency or organization is identified as the leader for community action because of expertise or reputation in the target area, political prowess, or potential for generating resources.
4. Citizen panels. Appointed or elected panels work with bureaucratic organizations to monitor activities and advocate for citizens. They may shape policy, monitor program implementation, or evaluate program performance.
5. Networks and consortia. These often develop spontaneously, bringing people together who have a common commitment. They can act as a catalyst for community action. They tend to be short-term for addressing a specific problem.

To establish successful health partnerships, a relationship must be established with communities that clearly communicates respect for their right to identify problems and potential solutions to those problems. When a community is defining its own problems and controlling its own programs, normative changes in beliefs and behaviors are more likely to occur and persist than when attempts are made to impose new norms from outside the community.[8]

At the beginning of a community partnership, it is important to determine the community's norms for participation. Is community problem solving, at present, primarily an individual or collective effort? How in touch are citizens with each other? What are the units of interaction (eg, neighborhoods, townships, housing complexes)? Do crime or other factors deter citizens from interacting on an on-going basis? Some communities may already have structures set up for purposes of community planning that address health concerns. Current patterns of citizen involvement, working relationships among community organizations already in existence, and organizations known for activating community involvement (eg, churches, recreation centers, service clubs) should be analyzed to determine how partnerships for health promotion might be shaped in any given community. For some communities, flexible coalitions might be the appropriate organizing framework to address community health needs, whereas for others, a leadership board or council may be needed to combine the power of key community activists.

An important goal of community partnerships focused on health promotion is empowerment of the community. Community empowerment is defined as a social-action process in which individuals and groups act to gain mastery over their lives through changing their social and political environment.[9] Together the members of a partnership should create conditions that empower their joint efforts. Community partnerships for health promotion have the potential for bringing about institutional and policy changes that affect many people. It is widely recognized today that the prerequisites for health are no longer only disease-prevention services and appropriate health behaviors but include food, shelter, education, income, peace, social justice, equity, and a stable ecosystem.[10] It is to the broader goals of both social-structural and individual change that many community partnerships are committed.

Community activists and professional advocates often come together in partnerships with differing views and approaches to change and different perceptions concerning their power or powerlessness. A period of discussion and even conflict may occur before all partners feel comfortable in the relationship. Conditions for effective partnerships have been proposed by LaBonte as follows[11]:

1. All partners have established their power and legitimacy.
2. All partners have well-defined mission statements; they have a clear sense of their purpose and organizational goals.
3. All partners respect each other's organizational autonomy by finding a visionary goal that is larger than any one of their independent goals.
4. Community group partners are well rooted in the locality and have a constituency to which they are accountable.
5. Institutional partners have a commitment to partnership approaches in working with community groups.
6. Clear objectives and expectations of the partnership are developed.
7. Written agreements clarifying objectives and responsibilities are made; periodic evaluation allows adjustment to agreements.
8. All partners strive for and nurture the human qualities of open-mindedness, patience, and respect.
9. The political dynamics of a community are attended to, such as its collective cohesiveness, organizing capacities, and community competencies.

The will to work together to accomplish highly cherished social and health goals will sustain a community partnership over time despite points of disagreement and difficulties.

• WHY PARTNERSHIPS?

Why are health promotion partnerships of increasing importance as we approach the 21st century? Partnerships are not only important but critical because the nature of health problems faced by populations has changed dramatically throughout this century. At least 70% of major health problems today are caused by the environment or personal and family lifestyles. A comparison of diseases often **cited** as the major causes of death and the actual causes of death appears in Table 14–1. Both environment and behavior heavily impact availability of addictive substances and firearms as well as norms for sexual behavior, diet, and activity.

The potential for fostering healthier lives for citizens of all ages lies in the power of partnerships that are multisectoral and reach well beyond the bounds of traditional medicine. However, if partnership approaches to national and global health problems are to be successful, national investment strategies must change. In 1994, **99%** of health expendi-

TABLE 14–1. CAUSES OF DEATH: 1990

10 LEADING CAUSES OF DEATH*		ACTUAL CAUSES OF DEATH†	
Heart disease	720,058	Tobacco	400,000
Cancer	505,322	Diet and inactivity patterns	300,000
Cerebrovascular disease	144,088	Alcohol	100,000
Unintentional injuries	91,983	Certain infections	90,000
Chronic lung disease	86,679	Toxic agents	60,000
Pneumonia and influenza	79,513	Firearms	35,000
Diabetes	47,664	Sexual behavior	30,000
Suicide	30,906	Motor vehicles	25,000
Chronic liver disease	25,815	Drug use	20,000
HIV infection	25,188		
TOTAL	**1,757,216**	**TOTAL**	**1,060,000**

* From National Center for Health Statistics, "Advance report of final mortality statistics, 1990," *Monthly Vital Statistics Report,* 41(7).

† From McGinnis JM, Foege WH. Actual causes of death in the United States. *JAMA.* 1993;270:2207–2212.

tures went for "one-on-one" medical treatment with only **1%** spent on population-wide public health initiatives. This should be contrasted with the fact that **70%** of early deaths could be prevented by public health and prevention initiatives, whereas only **10%** of early deaths could be prevented by medical treatment.[12] Figure 14–1 depicts the deplorable lack of investment in health promotion and prevention. How could our health investment strategy be so irrational?

The irrationality of our investment in health stems from an industrially oriented way

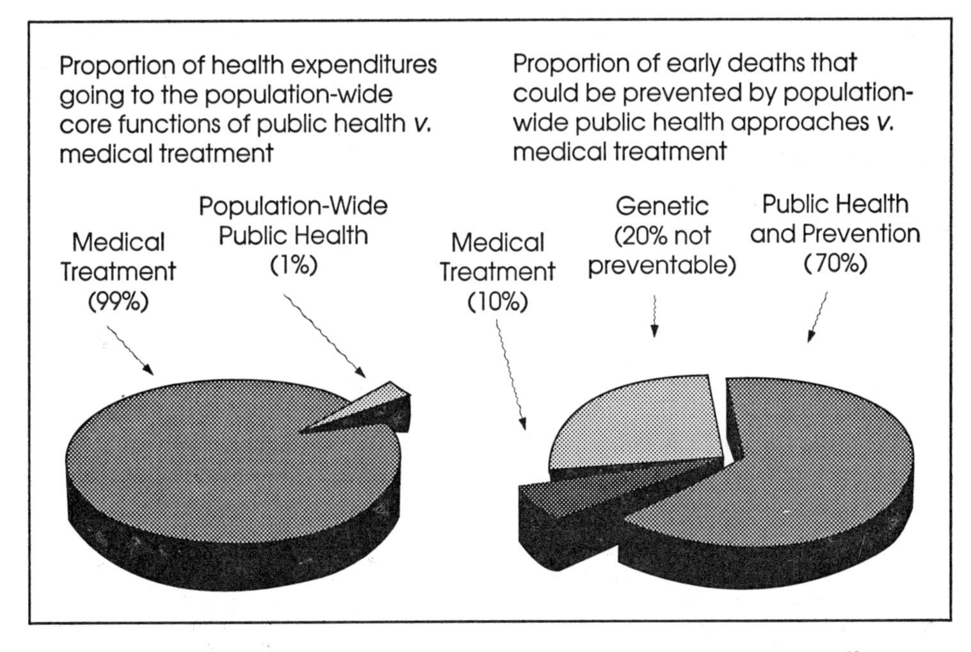

Figure 14–1. Is this a rational investment strategy? (From Health Care Reform and Public Health,[12] and Public Health Foundation, *Measuring State Expenditures for Core Public Health Functions,* Washington, DC: PHF; 1994.)

of life that has characterized American society. First, the health industry is a powerful political force that impacts how federal and state monies allocated for health are spent. Second, citizens have for many decades had blind faith in modern medicine as a panacea for all ills. Thus, if some money spent on traditional medical treatment is good, even more has to be better. Third, citizens are fascinated by high technology, and medical treatment is increasingly high-tech. Fourth, although almost all persons state that they place a high value on health, few individuals, families, and communities commit the time needed to pursue health before they face immediate health threats. Society needs to reexamine its approaches to fostering health and how health care dollars are spent. Data are beginning to accrue to indicate the cost-effectiveness of partnership arrangements to improve the health of communities. For instance, the Johns Hopkins University Center for Health Promotion reports that a community partnership that included the training of community health workers for health-promotion counseling, monitoring, linkage, and referral services reduced the morbidity and mortality in an African-American community as a result of improved control of hypertension. The program has begun to decrease the health status gap between African-Americans and Euro-Americans and has provided proof of its sustainability over time.[13] With increasingly diverse populations, decisions concerning health expenditures may best be made at the grassroots level. Communities have considerable expertise in identifying their problems and the most feasible solutions.

Community health partnerships can bring greater "rationality" to health care expenditures by insisting that prevention and health-promotion programs and services be adequately funded by national, state, and private insurers. Politically active health partnerships can reshape the health care system so that resources are allocated as depicted in Figure 14–2, with major emphasis on population-based health services, primary health care, and clinical preventive services. Over time, this "upfront" support of public health and primary care efforts should decrease or delay the need for secondary and tertiary care services until later in life as people lead healthier more disability-free lives.

Partnerships also are needed to appropriately plan, implement, and evaluate varying community-based health-promotion interventions. For example, if crime is a problem in a community, a wide array of youth activity programs can be offered to both foster greater cardiovascular fitness through physical activity as well as prevent crime. Partnerships can facilitate the safe transport of youth to programs and assist with the assessment of community change to determine if the desired program outcomes were attained. Community partnerships can set priorities for use of health resources in ways that are likely to work in their community, whereas an imported solution may be unacceptable because it is neither culturally or socioeconomically appropriate for a given community.

Community partnerships constitute an effective approach for addressing the needs of vulnerable populations. The vulnerable in our society are increasingly apparent as we go about our daily lives: The homeless at intersections with signs asking for work, children with AIDS who sit in our schools, pregnant adolescents who drop out of school, and the uninsured who labor beside us at work. Community partnerships seek to establish networks of cooperation and support rather than bureaucratic structures of indifference to respond to the vulnerable. The waste of human talents among the vulnerable who cannot live up to their potential because of inadequate education, joblessness, poverty, substandard housing, and often poor health is staggering.[14] For example, a study of the outpatient

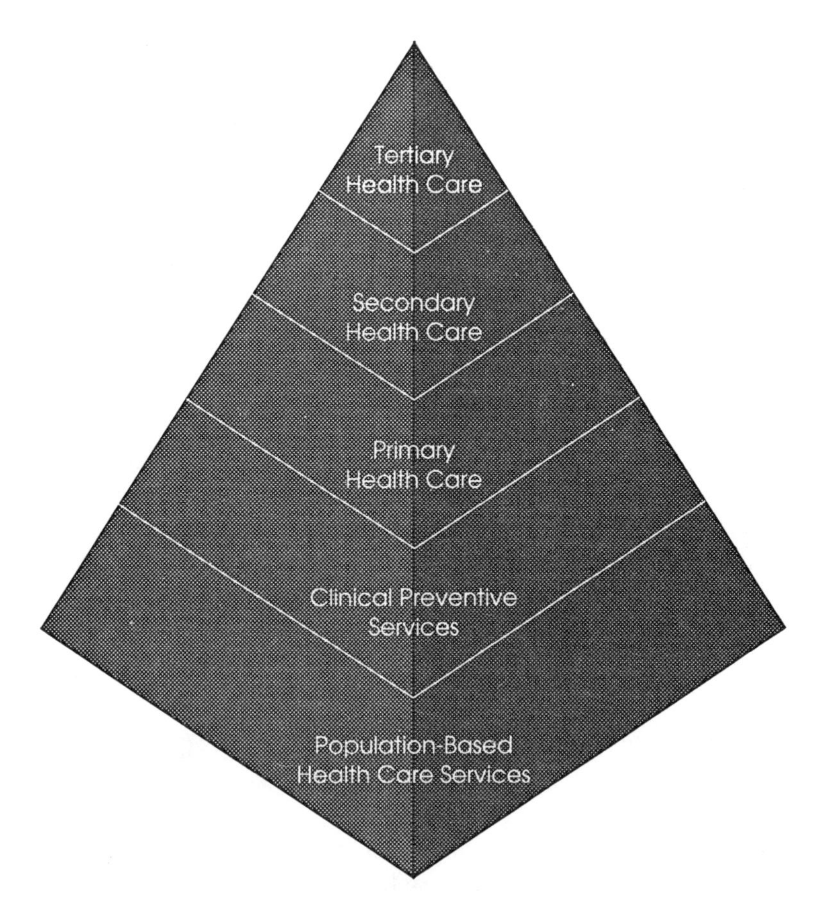

Figure 14–2. Health services pyramid. (From US Public Health Service. *A Time for Partnership: Report of State Consultations on the Role of Public Health, Prevention Report.* Washington, DC: US Public Health Service; *December 1994/January 1995.)*

medical records of 265 homeless children 5 years of age and younger in New York City compared with children of similar socioeconomic status but not homeless revealed major differences. Homeless children were more likely to have delayed immunizations, elevated blood lead levels, higher rates of hospital admission, and higher rates of reported child abuse and neglect—all conditions that affect their current and future prospects for health and well-being.[15] We as a nation are poorer because the potential contributions of our vulnerable citizens are compromised. Through the power of community partnering, the socioeconomic and health roots of vulnerability can be better addressed and community efforts can be directed at the prevention of vulnerability and its associated problems.

Health partnerships can be a source of empowerment to communities. The active involvement of disenfranchised persons in governance and national, state, and local decision-making processes that impact quality-of-life issues is empowering. Advocating for community reliance and self-reliance involves more than lip service. It involves inclusion of underserved populations in problem identification, planning, and implementation and evaluation of program and policy initiatives. Action research is an inclusive approach to community assessment and evaluation because it employs focus groups, key informant interviews, participant observation, analysis of existing records, community mapping, oral histories, and event analysis. Action research involves community members and provides important information for community organization.

A community development and organization approach to health-promotion partnering is based on the concepts of self-determination, shared decision making, bottom-up planning, community problem solving, and cultural relevance. The philosophy underlying this approach is that health promotion is likely to be more successful when the community at risk identifies its own health concerns, develops its own intervention programs, forms a decision board to make policy decisions, and identifies resources for program implementation.[5]

Communities that are empowered through organization and active participation develop leadership skills and the ability to attack an array of conditions that compromise their health and well-being. Empowerment as a process occurs over a period of time. The long-term goal of empowering health partnerships is to favorably impact on health services available in the community and improve the health status of the population. The impact of targeted individual behavior-change efforts is limited without efforts to bring about systematic change at a number of social levels through health partnerships.[5]

• THE ROLE OF PARTNERSHIPS IN EDUCATION, RESEARCH, AND PRACTICE

New models for health professions education, health care research, and community-based health care practice are needed. Education within community partnerships offers students opportunities to experience community-based leadership and ownership of programs, collaboration with indigenous community health workers, joint planning of strategies to address various problems in a culturally sensitive and competent manner, interdisciplinary practice and training opportunities, and prospective planning for evaluation of the effectiveness of health stategies. Furthermore, community partnerships create the opportunity for health professions faculty and their students to contribute to structuring seamless care systems that link primary care with ambulatory and in-patient facilities.[16]

Multidisciplinary education, community partnering, and collaborative work experience with community residents such as community health workers are critical to prepare health professions students for the diversity of health care roles that they will assume in the years to come. With the movement toward community-based care and away from traditional institutional care, except for the critically ill, knowledge of how to function in a community setting will be essential to meet the health needs of individuals and families. Communities need integrated networks of providers and community health workers to provide services that are currently unavailable. Bartering student and faculty services for access to educational experiences can be a win-win situation for both schools of nursing and communities. For example, students in the early stages of baccalaureate nursing education can experience various aspects of the role of community health worker by distributing health education materials in a community, participating in blood pressure screening programs, helping organize health fairs, collecting data from communities using preconstructed questionnaires, and surveying vending machines and fast food stores in a community to determine the availability of health-promoting options. More advanced baccalaureate students can both serve and learn by providing nutrition classes at schools and worksites, conducting stress management classes, assisting community residents in identifying environmental risks to health, and providing self-care education to groups of individuals who have similar health-risk profiles.

Graduate community health nursing students can assist community partnerships in assessing the needs of subgroups within the population and planning appropriate community interventions. Graduate-level nurse practitioner students can provide health assessment and anticipatory guidance to youth and their families, enhance the competence of families to deal with chronically ill children, and provide health supervision to children and adolescents. Graduate students and faculty provide a superb team for training community health workers in underserved communities. In order to build a successful cohort of community health workers, schools of nursing must: (1) establish rapport with the community; (2) collaborate with the community in the assessment of health needs; (3) hire workers who are sufficiently language- and culture-fluent to gain the trust and participation of community residents; (4) share program ownership and decision making with community health care workers, empowering them to evaluate and refine program goals and redesign strategies for greater effectiveness; (5) allow program flexibility so workers can adapt it to changing needs; and (6) closely link workers with community health and social service agencies so that professional backup is available as needed.[17]

Nursing students should increasingly be placed in educational settings where they can become culturally competent to provide care to populations that they have had little life experience with. Health professions education must provide learning experiences with various ethnic and racial groups within their indigenous neighborhoods or communities. Unfortunately, classical approaches to teaching often disempower residents of communities and students alike by assuming that they can only acquire knowledge but not produce it. It is time to focus on multicultural pedagogy that recognizes the rich knowledge that resides in community intelligence. The valuing of the knowledge held by community members must be transmitted to students.[6]

Through community–university partnerships that focus on education, communities benefit from the services of nursing students appropriately supervised by university faculty and, in turn, contribute to the competencies of nursing students, who are more likely to practice within diverse communities following educational experiences there.

Community–university health partnerships are valuable allies in research efforts. Increasingly, communities are seeking to share in shaping the studies that community residents participate in. Community leaders and citizens want the time that they devote to research participation to address questions of importance in fostering positive social and behavioral change within their community. Assessment is a natural activity of community partnerships to enable them to understand the nature of the problems that they face and are trying to resolve. Assessment to obtain baseline data is also critical before implementing health-promotion programs directed at large-scale social or environmental change. If baseline data are not collected, the partnership will be unable to assess the impact of health programs on community norms and values and on the health-related behaviors of community citizens. Partnering with universities throughout all stages of planning and conducting research creates a sense of community ownership of the study. This fosters more enthusiastic participation, greater attentiveness to subject recruitment, more thoughtful interpretation of findings in relation to a particular locality, and greater commitment to application of the findings to community programming.

Finally, community partnerships can improve the nature and quality of health services delivered in their community. This is sometimes achieved locally through restructuring services but often through involvement in statewide and national health-planning and policy-making activities to influence health care and wider social policies. A social system that maintains widespread inequities in distribution of resources and opportunities and deficit images for other than the majority group cannot be effective in revitalizing disenfranchised communities. An approach to health care that considers the social roots of problems as well as constructive social means for addressing them will avoid a blame-the-victim mentality.[6]

Each community, by the makeup of its population, requires a different mix of services to meet its needs. By using community health partnerships to monitor emerging health problems and the nature of services being delivered, the impact of services on the overall health of the community can be optimized. Partnerships can develop task groups to interact with health care providers to improve the acceptibility and accessibility of health care. Furthermore, they can catalyze meaningful interaction of the health care sector of the community with the education, employment, housing, food production and sales, transportation, communication, and recreation sectors to broaden the scope of factors addressed that impact on health. Community partnerships can play a strategic role in creating the total community capacity to respond to health needs. In addition, they can set the expectation that the health care system will function as a copartner with other systems in the community to shape public policy and conditions for healthy living.

A COMMUNITY–UNIVERSITY HEALTH PARTNERSHIP MODEL

The model described here for a community–university health partnership recounts the establishment and on-going development of a partnership between the public school district in Pontiac, Michigan, and the University of Michigan School of Nursing. The Pontiac–University of Michigan Alliance, hereafter referred to as PUMA, is directed toward increasing the accessibility and appropriateness of primary health care services and comprehensive health education to junior high school children and their families. School and university personnel are committed to working together long-term to affect the health of the community through planned partnership activities that use the resources of both partners to the best advantage.

In 1991, the idea for this community–university partnership emerged from relationships developed with a number of school districts during the course of planning and implementing research activities under the auspices of the Child and Adolescent Health Behavior Research Center (CAHBRC) within the School of Nursing. The CAHBRC was funded by the National Institute of Nursing Research, National Institutes of Health. Between 1991 and 1995, seven research studies that focused on the health beliefs and behaviors of preadolescents and adolescents were initiated and completed. Study topics included cognitions of self as regulators of adolescent exercise and alcohol use, influences of self-efficacy and exercise on the sexual behaviors of African-American females, antecedents of alcohol use and misuse, antecedents of sexual activity, effects of school transitions on exercise and physical activity, correlates of risk behavior and health outcomes in youth with diabetes mellitus, and stress as a biobehavioral correlate of sexual activity in black middle school children. Research projects conducted within the center are designed by scientists from nursing, medicine, public health, psychology, and kinesiology. The studies provide information useful in understanding the determinants of various health-related behaviors of youth and provide data upon which future studies of health-promoting interventions in schools, families, and communities can be based.

As part of the CAHBRC, a community liaison committee was established to serve as an on-going channel for sharing information and addressing future plans for partnership activities among the participating school districts. The codirector of the research center chaired the committee, which met twice a year throughout the duration of the center grant. The committee consisted of representatives from school districts participating in the research projects; recreation centers serving the target youth; community health departments providing services to preadolescents, adolescents, and their families; and the state public health department division responsible for developing health services for adolescents throughout the state. Out of the community liaison committee emerged a steering committee for the PUMA initiative consisting of representatives from the school district, the county health department, and the School of Nursing. The steering committee is jointly chaired by a member of the faculty of the School of Nursing and the director of the Pontiac School District Comprehensive Health Education Program. The director of student services for the school district and a number of University of Michigan faculty provide consultation. Junior high school students were identified as a target population for enhanced primary care services and expanded comprehensive health education.

The city in which PUMA is located has 71,166 residents, with 51% white, 42% black, and the rest of other ethnic origins, primarily Hispanic. The school district serves almost 13,000 students with over 2500 in the four junior high schools. Unemployment and poverty are problems faced by a number of junior high school children's families. Of all households with children, 53% are headed by single parents. With a shortage of health professionals in the city, there is a definite need for expanded health care and health education for junior high students in the school district. Thus, the school district and the School of Nursing saw multiple challenges that could be addressed through working together in a community–university health partnership. They identified the following health issues among the junior high population: (1) limited access to primary care, (2) increasing health-related absenteeism, (3) need for better coordination of health education and health services, and (4) no systematic way to identify health needs or students at high risk as a basis for prevention efforts or tailored interventions, according to B. Guthrie, PhD, RN.[18]

The community–university partnership has been structured as a community-driven endeavor with the opportunity for involvement of multiple health professionals. The University of Michigan faculty member who codirects the project devotes 30% of her time to PUMA partnership activities, with a comparable amount of time committed by school district personnel. The partnership has adopted a community service-learning focus to engage faculty, school personnel, and graduate students in meeting junior high school students' needs. The emphasis of the partnership is on health promotion and prevention to assist preadolescents and their families in fuller realization of their health potential. Specifically, the goals of the partnership are to: (1) provide a comprehensive health-education program focused on health promotion to junior high school students, (2) expand primary care services, (3) decrease preventable problems and related absenteeism, (4) enhance the school district's database reporting system to track health needs and intervention effectiveness, and (5) institutionalize collaborative community service-learning for master's degree students in health professions education at the university, according to B. Guthrie, PhD, RN.[18]

Service-learning activities to date have used the professional expertise of graduate-level nursing students for a variety of health-related activities identified as primary areas of need by the school district. For example, graduate nursing students have refined and offered comprehensive health-education activities for eighth-grade students, focused on the topic of developing healthy sexuality as an integral part of healthy self-image and self-esteem. Nurse practitioner students have conducted physical examinations for students in collaboration with the Adolescent Health Center located at one of the community high schools.

The need for coordination of student health services with health education is vital so that health messages are reinforced and the environment is "loaded" with cues that encourage healthy behaviors. Further, the School of Nursing is partnering with the city recreation department to integrate health promotion into evening and weekend recreation center activities. The development of a culture of peer support for healthy living is a primary goal as service-learning partnership activities evolve.

PUMA is an indication of the commitment of the Pontiac Schools and the University of Michigan School of Nursing to work together to improve the health of Pontiac youth. Future PUMA efforts will be directed toward:

1. Collaborating with school personnel to further refine and evaluate existing comprehensive health education programs and develop new educational interventions that are theoretically, culturally and developmentally appropriate to the populations served.
2. Hiring of parent community workers to assist with preadolescent and family health-education and health-care initiatives.
3. Enhancing the school district's existing database to track students' health needs and the effectiveness of interventions.
4. Providing preparation for University of Michigan nursing and social work faculty to enhance expertise in working with communities in implementing service-learning activities.
5. Developing collaborative service-learning courses and projects across the University of Michigan Schools of Nursing and Social Work to assist students in gaining skill to work with communities in a collaborative and culturally competent manner.
6. Planning research projects in collaboration with school district personnel to test interventions for their effectiveness in increasing the frequency of

health-enhancing behaviors and decreasing the frequency of health-damaging behaviors.
7. Appointing community-based professionals to adjunct faculty appointments at the University of Michigan.
8. Conducting an annual community service-learning seminar.
9. Placing graduates in employment sites that provide health care to underserved preadolescents and adolescents and their families.

The PUMA partnership, which began as an idea in the CAHBRC community liaison committee, has now become a reality. The challenges that lie ahead include garnering additional funds from varied sources to sustain the partnership and associated primary care and health education activities, recruiting nursing and social work students into multiprofessional service-learning curricular offerings, increasing junior high school students' and their families' involvement in partnership activities, and conducting studies of interventions that are state-of-the-science to determine their effectiveness in changing health-related social norms and behaviors among the junior high school population. The continuing partnership offers the promise that the health and life potential of preadolescents and adolescents can be enhanced through the joint efforts of the Pontiac School District and the University of Michigan Health Professions Schools.

THE ROLE OF SCHOOLS OF NURSING IN DEVELOPING COMMUNITY–UNIVERSITY PARTNERSHIPS

The need has never been greater for schools of nursing to take an active role in developing enduring health-promotion partnerships. Community leaders, health professionals, and community residents can work together to gain new knowledge through collaborative research and education programs in order to improve the health of underserved populations. The orientation of nursing to the whole person and the critical nature of the person–environment interaction in shaping health provides the professional background needed to work collaboratively with others to accomplish health goals. With escalating reform in health care and the economic pressures to provide cost-effective, quality care with a mix of professionals different from that in the past, nurses are in an excellent position to make a difference in the health care systems developed for the next century.

Nurses should be at the forefront in developing user-friendly, community-based health care. By strategically forming community partnerships, we can be. Partnerships can enrich the profession by providing diverse environments in which to educate students and by offering opportunities for students to work with communities in designing and conducting community-based studies of health-promotion interventions. Incentives that have been identified to foster greater emphasis on partnering with communities for health improvement include:[13]

1. Provision of reimbursement for disease-prevention and health-promotion services provided collaboratively by health professionals and community health workers
2. Provision of federal grant funding to schools of medicine, public health, and nursing that are engaged in true partnerships with underserved communities

3. Provision of incentives in the form of grants, matching funds, and low-interest loans to communities that are engaged in partnerships with academic health centers
4. Provision of federal incentives in the form of tax benefits to businesses and financial institutions that provide direct support and low-interest loans to such community–academic health partnerships

DIRECTIONS FOR RESEARCH

Investigative efforts of community health partnerships often focus on preintervention research to:

1. Describe the health strengths of the community
2. Describe the health-risk profile of the community
3. Interview key informants to determine community health priorities
4. Describe patterns of citizen involvement in the community
5. Develop valid and reliable measures of outcomes the partnership wishes to achieve, including community level assessments of quality-of-life indices

Although some anecdotal evidence suggests that community partnerships make a difference in health practices and the health of the community, few systematic studies have been conducted to determine the effectiveness and sustainability of community partnerships, particularly in communities with underserved populations.[5] Partnership intervention studies that build on information obtained from preintervention investigations are critically needed. The intervention process should be carefully documented to facilitate identification of its most effective components and to allow replication. Numerous measures should be used to assess the behavioral, social, and environmental outcomes of partnership activities.

In research conducted by community–university partnerships, all partners should have a sense of ownership. However, the participating parties may have different primary interests in the project. University partners are often most interested in the evaluation of an intervention and the wide dissemination of the results through publications. Community partners will likely be more interested in how the intervention affects health outcomes in their particular community. Both needs can be met as long as the intervention is "fitted" to the community, meticulously carried out, and outcomes carefully measured.

SUMMARY

Community partnerships for health promotion must build on the strengths rather than the deficits of a community's culture.[19] Partnerships can be empowering to the agencies that undertake them and to the entire community. The health problems of today can best be addressed by many sectors coming together to impact on the social and environmental conditions that compromise health. Partnerships offer a means of communication and collaboration and, thus, power to achieve solutions that organizations on their own do not have.

Particularly exciting is the opportunity for schools of nursing to join with other health professions schools in building partnerships with communities to facilitate service-learning arrangements. These arrangements benefit communities through the services provided and enrich the educational experiences of students so that they are better prepared to provide community-based care to diverse populations.

REFERENCES

1. Toffler A, Toffler H. *Creating a New Civilization: The Politics of the Third Wave.* Atlanta, Ga: Turner Publishing; 1995.
2. Milio N. Stirring the social pot: community effects of program and policy research. *J Nurs Adm.* 1992;22(2):24–29.
3. Milio N. Developing nursing leadership in health policy. *J Prof Nurs.* 1989;5(6):315–321.
4. Green LW, Raeburn J. Contemporary developments in health promotion: definitions and challenges. In: Bracht N, ed. *Health Promotion at the Community Level.* Newbury Park, Calif: Sage Publications Inc; 1990:29–44.
5. Braithwaite RL, Bianchi C, Taylor SE. Ethnographic approach to community organization and health empowerment. *Health Educ Q.* 1994;21(3):407–416.
6. Neighbors HW, Braithwaite RL, Thompson E. Health promotion and African-Americans: from personal empowerment to community action. *Am J Health Prom.* 1995;9(4):281–287.
7. Bracht N, Gleason J. Strategies and structures for citizen participation. In: Bracht N, ed. *Health Promotion at the Community Level.* Newbury Park, Calif: Sage Publications Inc; 1990:109–124.
8. Eisen A. Survey of neighborhood-based, comprehensive community empowerment initiatives. *Health Educ Q.* 1994;21(2):235–252.
9. Wallerstein N, Bernstein E. Introduction to community empowerment, participatory education, and health. *Health Educ Q.* 1994;21(2):141–148.
10. Labonte R. Health promotion and empowerment: reflections on professional practice. *Health Educ Q.* 1994;21(2):253–268.
11. Labonte R. Health promotion and empowerment: practice frameworks. In *Issues in Health Promotion,* Toronto, Ont: Center for Health Promotion, University of Toronto and ParticipACTION; 1993.
12. Health Care Reform and Public Health: A paper on Population-Based Core Functions. The Core Function Project, US Public Health Service; 1993.
13. Levine DM, Becker DM, Bone LR, et al. Community-academic health center partnerships for underserved minority populations. *JAMA.* 1994;272:309–311.
14. Aday LA. *At Risk in America: The Health and Health Care Needs of Vulnerable Populations in the United States.* San Francisco, Calif: Jossey-Bass Inc Publishers; 1993.
15. Alperstein G, Rappaport C, Flanigan JM. Health problems of homeless children in New York City. *Am J Public Health.* 1988;78:1232–1233.
16. Levine DM, Becker DM, Bone LR. Narrowing the gap in health status of minority populations: a community–academic medical center partnership. *Am J Prev Med.* 1992;8(5):319–323.
17. Sherer JL. Neighbor to neighbor: community health workers educate their own. *Hosp Health Net.* October 20, 1994;68(20):52–56.
18. Guthrie B. PUMA: Building community partnerships for healthy adolescents. *Office of Vice Provost for Health Affairs.* University of Michigan, Funded Grant; 1995.
19. Montes JH, Eng E, Braithwaite RL. A commentary on minority health as a paradigm shift in the United States. *Am J Health Prom.* 1995;9(4):247–250.

Index

A

D

E

F

G

H

I

L

M

N

O

P

R

S

T

U

V

W

Y